KT-574-708

Fix Your Life

1,500 holistic fixes for everyday problems

NIKKI BRADFORD

HODDER
MOBIUS

We have made all possible efforts to ensure that the information we offer readers in *Fix Your Life* is accurate. However, because every single person who reads this is an individual, with an individual's medical, emotional and spiritual history, needs and life circumstances, we also recommend that professional advice is sought for specific customised information regarding health and well-being. Facts, figures, prices and contact details are all correct at the time of going to press. Neither the author nor the publisher accepts any legal responsibility for any personal damage or loss arising from the use or misuse of the material in this book. *Fix Your Life* is intended as a positive adjunct to, rather than a substitute for, good professional treatment – medical or otherwise.

Copyright © 2008 by Nikki Bradford

First published in Great Britain in 2007 by Hodder & Stoughton

This paperback edition first published in 2008

The right of Nikki Bradford to be identified as the Author of the Work has been asserted by her in accordance with the Copyright, Designs and Patents Act 1988.

A Mobius Book

1

All rights reserved. No part of this publication may be reproduced, stored in a retrieval system, or transmitted, in any form or by any means without the prior written permission of the publisher, nor be otherwise circulated in any form of binding or cover other than that in which it is published and without a similar condition being imposed on the subsequent purchaser.

A CIP catalogue record for this title is available from the British Library

ISBN 978 0 340 84043 6

Typeset in Formata Light by Hewer Text UK Ltd, Edinburgh

Printed and bound by Clays Ltd, St Ives plc

Hodder Headline's policy is to use papers that are natural, renewable and recyclable products and made from wood grown in sustainable forests. The logging and manufacturing processes are expected to conform to the environmental regulations of the country of origin.

Hodder & Stoughton Ltd
A division of Hodder Headline
338 Euston Road
London NW1 3BH

Contents

General

Women

Men

Young Children 0–11

Home improvements: home feng shui top 10 (452) Household pests: Flies (467) Moths (467) Mice (467) Cockroaches (468) Woodworm (469) Loo rings (446) Loo position (460) Laundry (486) Moving home (470) (471) Paints: eco-friendly (473) Plant re-potting trauma (474) & Ponds (478) Power lines & pylons (479) Room-clearing (473, 435) Seedlings: Super-size them using healing (474) Music to enlarge plants (477) Sofas (466) Stains (483) TVs (484) Tiles (471)

Work & Office

Burnout (488) Bullying (495) Brain-booster breakfasts (513) Calming your colleagues (496) Tiring co-workers? (496) Concentration (502) Computers (507) Commuting (532) Desk-Improvers (506) Day from hell: clear it *now* (504) Energy: more *now* (500, 503) Emails (509) Eyes: dry (510) or Strained (511) Ethical Jobs (521) How to focus faster (500) Goal achievement (515) Headaches: see Lighting (518) Desktop plants (506) The tug (355) and Tiger Balm (57) Keyboard hands (508) Insomnia: work-related (529) Interviews (517) Lunch (515) Lighting (518) Mid-afternoon slump (502) Making more money (520) Networking (521) New job (526) Productivity (501) Laugh your way to promotion (527) Performance anticipation stress (530) Speed-napping (503) Super-snacks (514) Sick Office Syndrome (528) Stress-busters (530) Stuck (531) Travel for business (534) Working late (503)

Finding Everything

How to find the products, professional associations, complementary therapists and training organisations mentioned in this book: they are all listed alphabetically with websites, telephone numbers and contact addresses in the Directory on page 551.

Shopping

If it's a **product** you need, perhaps a specific aromatherapy oil or a nutritional supplement, herb, homeopathic tablet, essence remedy or maybe a holistic device such as a particular backrest, please look under the name of the manufacturer or distributor given in the relevant Fix. So, for Lambert's Multiguard mineral and vitamin supplement, look under 'L' in the 'Shopping' section, which starts on page 551.

Therapies and Therapists

If you need a **professional therapist**, whether it's a homeopathic vet, an experienced healer, a hypnotherapist who is also medically qualified, a chiropractor or an applied kinesiologist practitioner, see under 'Therapies and Therapists', which starts on page 576.

Training Courses

For where to find the **training courses** mentioned in this book, from transcendental meditation to animal whispering, see 'Training Courses', which starts on page 585.

Useful Helplines, Websites and Contacts

If you want to find out more about a specific condition or subject, from fertility to volunteering, or would like to get in touch with a **support body** or **helpline**, please see 'Useful Helplines, Websites and Contacts', which starts on page 590 where all the ones I mention are listed alphabetically.

Introduction

There are books about emotional intelligence, books about neuro-linguistic programming, books about every conceivable complementary therapy from acupressure to herbs. There are books about communicating with angels, animal whispering, geomancy, crystal power, biodynamic gardening, spiritual healing, body language, facial exercises, meditation, mindpower and feng shui too . . .

But there is nothing that unites all these immensely useful subjects into one coherent, practical, problem-solving whole, bursting with strategies and tips that you can *take away and use yourself*. Now. Immediately.

Wholly Healthy

Nothing until now, that is. *Fix Your Life* contains all of the above, having sought out some of the very best, fastest and most effective self-help techniques from almost every area of complementary medicine, combining them with emotional and mind strategies and spiritual techniques for the most holistic book ever to hit the shelves. We call this the **'Whole Self Health'** approach, as it involves keeping the whole of you healthy and using every part of yourself to do so. That whole is made up of your:

MIND,
BODY
and
SPIRIT

There is no separating the three. They are all extensions of each other, all linked, all merging into one another.

Spiritual is the new Complementary

Today, spiritual therapies and the idea of spiritual well-being are where complementary medicine was 16 years ago, when people still called it 'alternative health' and most doctors raised their eyebrows whenever acupuncture was mentioned, even as their patients went for it in their thousands on the quiet. Tomorrow, spiritual therapies will be an intrinsic, indispensable and powerful part of healthcare, both offered by professionals and used DIY at home.

No Separation

If a problem kicks in at one level – say, the emotional – it affects the next (your physical self) pretty smartly, and then goes on to the next (your spiritual self). For instance, if a child is being hurt *emotionally* – perhaps they are being bullied at school – on the *physical* level, this often goes on to produce, say, abdominal cramps that have no clinical cause your doctor can find, and on a *spiritual* level, the child becomes increasingly weakened or 'open', which attracts even more bullying.

You can:

- offer hot-water bottles and paracetamol when the tummy pains strike, and give vitamin B-complex to replace the reserves that the stress of being bullied has depleted, leaving the child exhausted *(physical-level help)*
- give confidence-boosting essence like the effective Confid, or Lion Cub, to help them access their own courage reserves *(emotional-level help)*
- get the support of their teachers *(emotional-level help).*

But the child can also be backed up (on the spiritual level) by, say:

- a healing session or two to boost energy levels
- you regularly asking for powerful angelic help to:
  a) support your child in developing strong protective boundaries around themselves
  and
  b) actively encourage harmony and friendship between your son or daughter and the other children at school.

Once in place, each of these strategies will work together, each one reinforcing the others to help the child recover fully, from both the stomach cramps and the underlying causes (bullying, lack of support) which caused the pains in the first place. This is Whole Self Health in action.

Mind, Body, Spirit Reality

Most people are right behind the mind-body idea, but the spirit bit . . . who's proved that's even definitely there? Perhaps that's something for every person to make their minds up about themselves, whenever they feel ready to do so. Yet everything I have seen and experienced over the last 20 years supports the idea that there is far, far more to life than what most of us can see with our eyes or touch with our hands. And it has become blindingly clear to me that someone's spirit (inner self, soul, what 'makes them, them') is real all right – as real as the chair you're probably sitting on as you read this. Which came as something of a surprise to someone who was a facts-only investigative medical journalist and obedient member of the Royal Society of Medicine.

Over the last six years especially, more and more people of all ages and walks of life are re-evaluating their beliefs, often as the result of what Australians call the 'being hit by a Mack truck' effect: a major life event such as an illness, burnout, divorce, family crisis, redundancy or general epiphany that pulled them up short and led them to take another look at some of the beliefs they'd always held.

Triple-Action Power

Complementary medicine is now moving towards the triple-action mind, body, spirit approach of Whole-Self Health.

It is even increasingly seen in orthodox medical facilities (billed as 'fully integrated healthcare') such as hospital cancer units, pain clinics and hospices, where standard surgical and medical care are offered alongside a range of complementary therapies from massage to aromatherapy, and where there is often also a spiritual healer or reiki practitioner on the staff as well.

But Whole-Self Health is also perfect to use yourself for everyday things at home, both the Big Stuff (perhaps something like painful arthritis, ADHD, nervous breakdown, or infertility) and the Smaller but Still Important Stuff (frown lines, thinning hair, spots and hangovers) because . . .

> . . . whatever the problem,
> there *is* a holistic fix that can help.

That's why this book is subtitled *1,500 Holistic Fixes*, as, counting them all up, there are many more than the 500 broad sections. I could cheerfully have written thousands more and still not finished.

It is said that no matter how difficult things may be, we will always find the very thing that will help us when we need it most . . .

May you find some of the information you need, for whichever challenge or health problem you are facing, every time you look between these pages.

General

In this chapter you'll find everything from which aromatherapy oil to sniff to suppress cigarette cravings to the spiritual technique for ensuring the entire day goes your way (yes). Whether you might be interested in how a kindly phone call can measurably reduce someone's pain levels, find out which herb really works for arthritis, discover the instant no-pills approach to boosting your sex life or find the one brilliant backrest that actually makes a bad seat good, just flick through to the section you want and nab all the information you need.

Accidents and Shock

1. Upsets
If you, or anyone around you, is really upset after a row, shock or near-miss, there is something gentle but remarkably effective you can take that can help immediately. Bach Rescue Remedy may be the well-known and much-loved traditional 'upsets' treatment, but two newer products not only work gently as Bach's does, but also seem to be stronger, as well as working immediately: **Emergency Essence** from Australian Bush Flower Essences, available direct (30 ml, £7.95) or from Healthlines, and **Soul Support** by Alaskan Essences, available in the UK from Healthlines (60 ml, £8.95). You can buy Soul Support direct in the US and Canada.

They are a must-have for every home, school or office first-aid kit. Like Rescue Remedy, both treatments are taken as drops under the tongue or in water. However, for elderly people, very young children and babies, the gentler-acting Rescue Remedy is still often the best choice. It too is available from Healthlines (10 ml, £3.99) or via Healing Waters in the US..

For all contact details, see under 'Shopping' in the Directory.

2. Shocked? Spacey? Try the Three-Breath Quick Fix

Need to come back down to earth? This is the five-second quick-fix version of the basic spiritual ritual for grounding and protection, for use in emergencies – when you don't have much time and need to keep going.

Perhaps you've just been told a piece of news that has knocked the ground from under your feet. Or you were crossing the road hurriedly, late for an appointment, and a speeding car missed you by millimetres. Maybe someone came up a second or two ago, said something unexpected or unpleasant and moved swiftly on. Whatever it was, you can re-establish your equilibrium immediately:

1. Take a deep breath in.
2. As you let it out, *blast* it down through your body deep into the earth to re-ground yourself.
3. Take another strong breath in. As you breathe this one out, imagine an arrow of light whipping round you once in a clockwise direction, beginning at your feet, swinging up round one side of you, over your head and down the other side to join where it began at your feet. It forms a shining, unbreakable circle.
4. Take your third breath in. As you let it out, see your circle filling out into a big sphere of gold light. Seal it at the top with a golden disc.
5. If you've got time, repeat this three times. If not, just the once should steady you until you can have a break and take stock.

Anal Fissures

These small splits in the skin, sometimes also involving upper soft-tissue layers, may be caused by anything from a large, hard stool to anal sex. They can make emptying your bowels pretty uncomfortable, and if they reopen as the skin stretches to allow faecal matter past, they may get reinfected and therefore be quite hard to get rid of. If they've become infected, see your GP right away. If they're not infected, try the following self-help fix.

3. Self-Help Measures

1. Keep your stool as soft as possible. Besides drinking as much water as you can and eating plenty of fruit, vegetables and other good sources of fibre, sprinkle **millet seeds** (yes, the stuff budgies like) over your cereal, salad or vegetables. Once in your digestive system – which extends from mouth to anus – they act like tiny ball bearings and help you pass faeces through the lower section much more comfortably. Try a brand like **Linusit Gold** from a local health food shop – e.g. Holland & Barrett (250 g, £3.95). For contact details, see under 'Shopping' in the Directory.
2. Wash the anal area with cool water and gently pat dry with soft loo paper (avoid wiping briskly in the usual way) every time you pass a motion, even a small one.
3. Apply a little very mild antiseptic cream, like Savlon, to the area each time you use the toilet. If the fissures extend up the rectal passage, use a clean finger to try to slide a small amount inside. Then wash your hands (and under your nails) well with hot, soapy water.

Anaesthetic Recovery

Some people report that a general anaesthetic makes them feel worse than the actual operation. After-effects are usually gone within 24-72 hours, but depending on the anaesthetic mix and your particular reaction to it, side effects such as tiredness, feeling spacey and loss of mental sharpness may persist for weeks. However, the following can be immensely helpful:

Drinking Up
• Drink plenty of pure plain water. Start once you wake with small sips as soon as you feel like it. It may take a while to build this up as you can wake up feeling nauseous at first.

Essences that 'Bring You Back'
• Try taking a mixture of two excellent essences: **Sundew** (for vagueness, disconnection, not feeling 'all there', not feeling like you're in your body) and **Fringed Violet** (for shock or trauma). The latter's often given after surgery as it also helps to repair any splits or breaks in the protective aura around the body, which can be damaged by the physical impact of an accident or by invasive surgical procedures.

Put seven drops of Sundew and seven of Fringed Violet in a 30 ml dropper bottle. Top up with two-thirds pure spring water and a third brandy, as a preservative, and shake gently. Take seven drops three or four times on day one, then seven drops just twice a day, morning and evening, thereafter until you are feeling better.

Both Sundew and Fringed Violet can be mailed direct from Australian Bush Flower Essences or go to their website for your nearest local retailer or mail-order distributor. They can also be bought via Healthlines in the UK (15 ml, £8.95 each) or Earth Spirits Herbal Apothecary in the USA. For contact details, see under 'Shopping' in the Directory.

Anger and Aggression

5. Keeping Anger in Check

The gentle but deep-acting **Anger and Frustration Essence** by Bailey Flower Essences can be very helpful for people of any age, from toddlers to teens and adults, who find that they:

- fly into a rage easily
- have trouble controlling the course of their anger when it's in full flood
- often become very angry very quickly through sheer frustration.

Therapists and health workers all over the world, including psychiatrists, child psychologists, healers and homeopaths, are now using this gentle form of natural 'energy' medication, and the feedback is that it:

- balances
- stops you rising to the bait so easily
- takes the sting out of situations
- offers you more control over your 'fire energy' (something everyone needs in order to prevent being walked all over, so it's not something to suppress or extinguish but to direct and control)
- helps people grasp situations more accurately and respond more appropriately.

Take two drops of Anger and Frustration Essence under the tongue three times a day, or when in need. It can be purchased in the UK direct from Bailey Flower Essences (10 ml, £5.15) or via Earth Spirits in the USA. For contact details, see under 'Shopping' in the Directory.

6. The Three-Step Nutritional Rescue Plan

It is now well accepted that what someone eats can have a powerful effect on their mood and consequently on their actions. If you would like to help calm aggressive or consistently confrontational behaviour in yourself, a child, teenager or another adult, it is well worth doing the **Three-Step Nutritional Rescue Plan** before you try anything else.

1. Take essential-fatty-acid (EFA) capsules. For the types you need here, which are **omega-3** and **omega-6**, try Udo's Choice Ultimate Oil Blend Omega-3, -6 and -9, available from Body Kind (500 ml, £15.45).
2. Use a good-quality one-a-day **general mineral and vitamin supplement**, such as Lamberts MultiGuard from Planta (90 capsules, £16.16) or Solgar's V-Formula (£17.50 for 60 capsules)
3. Remove as many additives, refined foods and refined sugars from your diet as you possibly can.

For all contact details, see under 'Shopping' in the Directory.

Keep this up for three months and then review the situation. Research suggests that you are likely to see a *substantial improvement of between a half and a third*. If the person needs additional support (such as behavioural therapy, complementary treatments or counselling) it is also likely that they will now find it easier to work with their therapist(s), and are more receptive to any help that is offered.

See also Teenagers: Aggression and Disruptive Behaviour on page 313.

7. After Antibiotics
A course of antibiotics not only deals with infection by killing the bacteria responsible, it can also wipe out all the 'friendly' (i.e. useful) bacteria in your gut, causing problems ranging from troublesome skin to bloating, tiredness, depression and poor food absorption. The answer is to take a probiotic (ready-made mixture of millions of live 'good' bacteria) for four to eight weeks afterwards to get your levels back up to scratch. You've probably heard that one before, many times.

The only problem is, which one? There are literally hundreds of different combinations on the market, all claiming and counter-claiming, and some aren't very good. Luckily, the advice from top nutritionists is to 'keep it simple'. Meaning that in independent tests, the *Lactobacillus acidophilus* strain came out top, and there's a British company called BioCare that has been supplying this for years in powdered form so it can be added to food, cereals and smoothies, for both adults and children. They also do capsules, like Bio Acidophilus Forte (60 caps, £45.95), or the gentler Bio Acidophilus (60 caps, £17.95). For contact details, see under 'Shopping' in the Directory.

See also Young Children: After Antibiotics on page 242.

Anxiety

8. Calming Mild Anxiety

Sprinkle five drops of good-quality organic **lavender aromatherapy oil** on your neckline. Try Neal's Yard Organic Lavender Oil (10 ml, £8.95) or Baldwin's (10 ml, £4.95).

If you're feeling anxious but need to go out and about, you can carry your calming therapy with you all day, breathing it in as you go. Research in 2000 by the University of Exeter confirmed that no less than six randomised controlled trials found lavender oil calmed hospital patients' anxious feelings.[1]

As a backup, also slip a little bottle of Bach Rescue Remedy, Emergency Essence or Soul Support into your pocket. With the Bach, take four drops under the tongue every 30 minutes until you're feeling better; with the Emergency Essence, take seven drops under the tongue as often as needed; for Soul Support, take four to six drops under the tongue, or in small glass of water and sip frequently. If you can't drink, it can be rubbed on the lips, temples or pulse points. Repeat after 30 minutes if required.

You can buy Bach Rescue Remedy from Healthlines (10 ml, £3.99). Emergency Essence can also be bought via Healthlines or direct from Australian Bush Flower Essences (30 ml, £8.95). Soul Support is available via Healthlines in the UK (60 ml, £8.95) or direct from Alaskan Essences in the US and Canada.

For all contact details, see under 'Shopping' in the Directory.

9. The No-Worries Drink

Hot, milky drinks are traditionally calming because of the tryptophan (an amino acid) they contain; add some **cardamom seeds** for one of the best quick mood-soothers around. Cardamom has been used for 2,000 years in Indian Ayurvedic medicine to promote equanimity, deep restful sleep, a relaxed, focused mind and also to soothe the hot rush of an anxiety attack. Crush the seeds and sprinkle over warm milk, adding a little Horlicks or Ovaltine if you like it.

See also Women: Anxiety on page 116, Young Children: Anxiety on page 242 and Teenagers: Anxiety on page 242/327.

Arthritis

Arthritis is a general term that simply means inflammation of the joints. It is one of 200 different types of rheumatic disease, which includes gout, rheumatism (general aches and pains in the joints and bones), lupus and ankylosing spondylitis. The condition can have many different triggers, aggravating factors and causes. It also tends to be quite an individual thing, so as with other multi-causal disorders like asthma or PMS, different approaches will help different people and a combination of two or three (sometimes more) often works best.

Medical Treatments

There are several natural ways to relieve pain and reduce joint inflammation. These have been of increased interest since a study of 9,218 patients by the University of Nottingham suggested that taking the 'safe' and much-used ibuprofen-based family of painkillers appears to raise the risk of heart attack by between half (for a drug called Diclofenac) and a quarter (for ibuprofen, the best-known over-the-counter brand being Nurofen).[2] Pharmaceutical giant Merck whipped its top-selling ibuprofen-based pill, Vioxx, off the market immediately, and the 9 million people who have arthritis in the UK alone were left wondering what their options were and whether anything effective can be free of unpleasant and harmful side effects.

Natural medicines and strategies have fewer, and usually far more minor, side effects than man-made drugs, though the latter tend to be more powerful, so the best course of action will depend on how much discomfort someone is in and whether they are on a maintenance programme or responding to a really painful flare-up.

Orthodox medicine *and* complementary techniques like nutrition or herbs tend to be used together to good effect. However, many people, wary of the damage to the stomach lining and potential stomach ulcers ordinary painkillers Non Steroidal Anti-Inflamatory Drugs – (NSAIDs) can cause when used all the time, are opting for natural therapies and medicines that do not have the same unwanted side effects. Basically, if you don't want holes appearing in your stomach lining and guts, consider holistic approaches instead. For those who wish to go down the holistic route, some of the most helpful natural approaches are given below.

Complementary Treatments

10. Eating Right

For both osteoarthritis and rheumatoid arthritis for instance, 'red-light' foods to avoid or cut right back on include fried foods, dairy products, tomatoes, alcohol, caffeine (in tea, coffee, colas, Red Bull and other 'energy' drinks), potatoes, aubergines, all peppers, refined white sugar and red meat.

Many people find switching to organic food helps too. Those with rheumatoid arthritis may respond well to an eating regime that also cuts out animal fats, as certain types can trigger an autoimmune reaction and inflammation.

Finding a good nutritionist

If you would like to try the eating-plan route either on its own or with other complementary therapies or natural supplements, it is well worth seeing a professional nutritionist or naturopath. Word of mouth is a useful way to find a good one, or try graduates from the Institute of Optimum Nutrition or the British Naturopathic Association. If they are also an experienced Applied Kinesiology practitioner who can check you for food intolerances and allergies reasonably accurately, this would be extremely useful. For contact details, see under 'Therapies and Therapists' in the Directory.

11. Nutritional Supplements

- **Glucosamine** (a substance occurring naturally in the body and used to make cartilage) and **chondroitin** (another naturally occurring substance that helps protect joints from wear and tear): there's now a large body of evidence showing glucosamine helps for both osteo- and rheumatoid arthritis.[3] Look for a brand that combines glucosamine with chondroitin and, if possible, collagen, such as

Collagen Plus, a powdered product you can make into an orange-flavoured drink taken at breakfast. Try mail-order products from Arthro Vite (£26.99 for a month's worth), or Glucosamine and Chondroitin 1,500/1,200 from Victoria Health (120 tablets, £7.25).

Drink like a Fish

Water can also be considered a supplement – if you drink lots of it, that is. Research by Dr F Batamanghelidj (*Your Body's Many Cries for Water*) suggests that people with joint pains can reduce them by drinking 1 litre of pure non-carbonated water (he strongly recommends *not* Volvic though) per 50 lbs or 24 kg body weight, plus an additional 2 litres per day. And while most people simply wouldn't be able to do that, it can help to take even an extra 8-10 glasses of pure water daily – plus an extra one after each tea/coffee/glass of wine or other alcohol consumed – which is far more do-able for most of us.

- **Oils containing omega-3 fatty acids** (e.g. cod-liver oil): a recent major review of randomised controlled trials showed that fish oil, and also eating lots of oily fish, provides plenty of inflammation-calming omega-3 fatty acids such as eicosapentaenoic acid (EPA) and docosahexaenoic acid (DHA).[4] They have the added plus of being very good for the condition of your skin, hair and nails. The dosage is approximately 1–1.5g daily. Cod-liver oil capsules are inexpensive and available from any health store or good chemist.

- **Hyaluronic Acid:** its high viscosity ups the amount of water in joint fluid, resulting in better lubrication and shock absorption for those joints. It also does a nice job of plumping up the skin and reducing visible signs of ageing but that's another story (see Anti-Aging, in Women section, pp 108–115). Supplements are available as Hyaluronic Acid Undenatured from Time Life Vitamins (30 capsules £29.95) – you need to take two daily – via Victoria Health.

Other options

If you're taking fish oils in any quantity, watch out for 'fishy burps'. Should this happen, or if you are a vegetarian, you may prefer the plant-derived **borage (starflower) oil**, also an excellent source of omega-3 fatty acids.[5] The dosage is 1–1.5 g daily. It is available from any health food shop or good chemist.

Note: do not take with prescription medicine for schizophrenia, blood-thinning or liver disorders.

All-in-one supplement

A good all-rounder, which also has the distinction of being the only joint remedy to have been researched by Harvard University and endorsed by Boston Medical School, is **Advanced Joint Support Formula**, which contains many of the most helpful anti-arthritis nutrients in one convenient package (the cost of which, if bought separately, can really add up). It is manufactured by LifeTime and available from Victoria Health (90 tablets, £29.95).

This particular formula contains bromelain (an effective tissue-healer), MSM (a form of organic sulphur, which also helps heal tissue and can make hair thicker and glossier), glucosamine, chondroitin, type-II collagen (found in 80 per cent of the body's collagen framework) and hyaluronic acid, a well-documented tissue-regenerator.

For all contact details, see under 'Shopping' in the Directory.

12. Herbs and Spices

White willow bark extract

Aspirin is a synthetic copycat of the anti-inflammatory painkilling substances salicylates, which are found naturally in the bark of the **white willow** tree. However, the latter is far gentler on the stomach. Try BioCare White Willow Complex from the Nutri Centre (90 capsules, £15.15).

Note: white willow bark extract's active ingredient is also a blood-thinning agent, so check with your GP before taking it if you have any health issues relating to this. Avoid it if you already have an ulcer or gastric problems. It is not suitable in high doses in the long term, as it may eventually cause similar problems to aspirin-based painkillers and anti-inflammatories. Do not take with non-steroidal anti-inflammatory drugs (NSAIDs) or ibuprofen products. However, white willow is gentle and effective when used in the short term or in lower doses (60–120 mg daily). It takes a little longer to kick in than aspirin, but its beneficial effects last longer.

Nexrutine

If you are taking conventional anti-inflammatory drugs for arthritis and they are giving you stomach problems, consider using **nexrutine** to safeguard your gut lining. It was developed from the rue plant to prevent the common side effects of conventional anti-arthritis drugs – gastric irritation and erosion of the stomach lining – and has recently become available in supplement form. It's also a useful anti-inflammatory in its own right.

In clinical trials, nine out of every ten volunteers who took it for two weeks reported they had no gastric problems any more when taking their usual NSAIDs.

Try Nexrutine Cox-2 Inhibitor by LifeTime from Victoria Health (90 capsules, £19.95).

Black cumin

Also known as **black-seed oil**, black caraway or Persian shonaiz, this was once a highly valued and much-used anti-inflammatory healing oil. Mentioned in the Bible, written about by first-century Greek physician Dioscorides and popular in Islamic countries, this lovely oil is now making something of a well-deserved comeback. Compounds contained in the oil and seeds of this spice (especially thymoquinine, or TQ) have been shown to be powerful anti-inflammatories for conditions like arthritis.[6]

The suggested dosage is one teaspoon a day of black-seed oil, taken with food. It is available in the UK from Black Seed Europe in Eastbourne (100 ml, £7.95; 100 ml plus 200 x 450 mg capsules, £23); in the US, from Herbal Remedies (90 x 500 mg capsules, $12.98).

Ginger

Ginger can be very helpful for both travel and morning sickness, but it is also an anti-inflammatory, and research suggests it has similar properties to ordinary NSAID painkillers, including interfering with the usual pathway leading to chronic inflammation.[7]

One particular trial in 2000, which compared it with both a placebo and ibuprofen, found it did indeed reduce pain levels. Another double-blind placebo-controlled scientific study of 250 people who had osteoarthritis in the knee found that sufferers could stand with far less pain and cut back considerably on their usual drugs after taking ginger extract for six weeks.[8] The usual dose for inflammation is 250 mg three times daily. Try Nature's Best Ginger (90 capsules, £7.95); in the US, try Nutrivea USA (100 x 500 mg capsules, $29.45).

Turmeric

This is a member of the ginger family and adds a distinctive rich yellow colour to food. Its active ingredient, curcumin (an antibacterial agent), is an anti-inflammatory and works by depleting nerve endings of a chemical called substance P, a neurotransmitter that carries pain signals round the body. Add turmeric to cooking whenever you can – great in curries, egg dishes, some fish recipes – or take 400–600 mg daily in capsule form. Try Organic Turmeric Joint Formula from Pukka Herbs (90 capsules, £14.45).

Note: turmeric is usually a good gentle anti-inflammatory but can occasionally exacerbate arthritic symptoms, so keep a close eye on it and discontinue if necessary.

Devil's claw

Long used in Africa for relieving joint pain, clinical-trial results are mixed but coming down on the positive side: the majority suggest patients who use devil's claw can cut back on their NSAIDs. The typical dose is around 100 mg twice daily. It is available in the UK in good health shops and via Think Natural (60 x 450 mg capsules, £5.49). Try also Lichtwer Healthcare Devil's Claw. In the US, try the National Supplement Center (100 x 525 mg capsules, $10.39). Its active ingredient is the anti-inflammatory glycoside, called harpagoside, so look out for the stated percentage of this in standardised products.

Note: it may interfere with blood-pressure and anti-acid medication, so it's best to avoid it if you are taking either of those two.

Boswellia serrata

This is also known as salai guggal or Indian frankincense, not to be confused with *Boswellia carterii* (Bible frankincense, which has different properties). *Boswellia serrata* can be an effective anti-inflammatory and does not seem to cause gut irritation. It works by inhibiting enzymes that trigger the inflammation characterises arthritic conditions. Trials suggest it is as helpful as the conventional drug for rheumatoid arthritis, sulfasalazine.

The dosage is around 400 mg, three times daily. There's a useful *Boswellia serrata* and devil's claw combination capsule from Higher Nature (60 capsules, £8.90).

Yucca

Yucca extract has been clinically researched for rheumatism.[9] Yuccas are related to the desert's Joshua tree, and the Native American Indians have long made poultices from yucca to soothe many types of inflammation, including rheumatism. The usual dosage for capsules or tablets is around 1–1.5 g daily. In the UK, try Zipvit (90 x 450 mg capsules, £4.95); in the US and Canada, try Nature's Way Yucca from All Star Health (100 x 425 mg capsules, $9.99; special offer, $5.99).

For all contact details, see under 'Shopping' in the Directory.

13. Warming Anti-Arthritis Aroma Mix

Combine two drops of **ginger essential oil** (for its warming effect) with two of **juniper** (to encourage toxin elimination) and two of **rosemary**, which stimulates good circulation, thus enabling prompt removal of waste products in the blood, as waste products can further irritate inflamed joints, advises medical aromatherapist and ex-pathologist Dr Vivian Lunny, formerly of the Harefield Heart Hospital in the UK. Rub the mix gently on the areas that are sore.

Try Neal's Yard Juniper Essential Oil (10 ml, £11.95), Rosemary Essential Oil (10 ml, £5.50) and Ginger Essential Oil (10 ml, £7.95). Or, for a more budget approach, their Juniper and Ginger Warming Oil (50 ml, £5.55). Neal's Yard also has a US website that does prompt mail order. For contact details, see under 'Shopping' in the Directory.

14. Homeopathy

For best results with chronic arthritis, it pays to see a homeopath in person, who will probably give you a good constitutional treatment – i.e. individually prescribed to fit your specific symptoms and personality type.[10] However, for isolated flare-ups, top UK homeopath and author Dr Andrew Lockie suggests that the following can be very useful:

- **Byronia 30c** – if your particular pain is severe, movement and heat make it worse but cool compresses help
- **Aconite 30c** – for nasty flare-ups triggered by cold weather
- *Calcarea phosphorica* **6c** – can be helpful if you have osteoarthritis, your joints feel 'chilly' and numb, and the stiffness or pain is worse when the weather changes.
- *Rhus tox* **6c** – could be the one for you if heat helps but cold and damp make things worse; also if the pain is the sort that wears off when you move about but is worse in the early mornings.

Take three times daily for seven days.

Homeopathic remedies are available from Helios or Ainsworths (approximately £3.50 each). For contact details, see under 'Shopping' in the Directory.

15. Anti-Arthritis Jewellery
Rings on her fingers
Wearing a **gold ring** on every finger (as some wealthy Indian and Pakistani women traditionally do) could prevent, or at least delay, the onset of arthritis of the hands. Research from the Birmingham City Hospital suggests that the gold passes through the skin 'downstream' to the nearest knuckle joint in large enough quantities to protect it.[11] If the problem's beginning in just one or two digits, wear a gold ring on those.

Note: gold-salt injections are also used by hospital arthritis specialists and prove helpful for around 60 per cent of people, though a third of users have unpleasant side effects.

Copper bracelets
Using **copper bands** to soothe arthritis, often pooh-poohed as gimmicky, is in fact backed up by clinical trials.[12] It helps because the copper acts as an anti-inflammatory agent by kick-starting an anti-oxidant enzyme called superoxide dismutase (SOD), which protects the joints from inflammation. You can also buy SOD in capsule form (60 for £23.00 via Victoria Health).

Therapeutic magnetic jewellery

You can buy bracelets, necklaces, anklets, even pet collars for arthritic animals with tiny magnets embedded in them. The **jewellery** is slim, unobtrusive, as it's essentially therapeutic not decorative, and metal-plated (usually with gold, copper, silvery rhodium or titanium).

Does it help?

Trials suggest that you usually get real benefits after an average of two to three weeks but some people feel the difference within a few hours.[13] Work by the independent British electromagnetic (EM) research lab Coghill Laboratories in 2002 suggests that for arthritic pain a company called Magna's bracelets *cut discomfort by a third in the hands, wrists and arms*, and by around a sixth in other more 'distant' parts of the body. Costs vary from £30 to £50 ($58 to $96) for a bracelet from different manufacturers, which compares well with the average cost of a year's supply of ordinary anti-inflammatories at approximately £250 ($380).

How does it work?

Magnets are thought to help alleviate arthritis pain and other types of discomfort by creating a magnetic field around the problem area, which improves the blood flow to it, thus increasing oxygenation, reducing inflammation and encouraging localised cell rejuvenation and renewal. It is also suggested that the negative pole of the magnet interferes with the bioelectricity of nerve cells, compromising their ability to transmit pain signals to the brain, where they can be registered. For more information, see Notes on page 548.

How do you get the best results?

Magnetised jewellery works best when you can wear it *near the pain site* – i.e. a bracelet for arthritis of the hands or wrists – so if you have arthritis of the knee, look for a good-quality magnetised ankle bracelet. However, in 2005, when Exeter's Peninsula Medical School arranged for five GP practices in Devon to carry out a three-month stringent clinical trial of magnetised wrist bracelets involving 194 men and women aged 45–80 with hip and knee arthritis, the patients all reported some pain reduction, so it seems even 'distant' magnetic jewellery can be pretty useful. What's more, some of the patients in the trial had unknowingly been trying out dummy magnetised jewellery and they didn't report as much improvement, suggesting it's not just the placebo effect at work.

Get a money-back guarantee

. . . in case the jewellery doesn't help you. The following three all offer a money-back guarantee, as do several others: Magna Jewellery (gold-plated unisex magnetic bracelet, £29.99), Bioflow products from Magnetize Your Life and, in the US, AAAMagnetic (titanium magnetic bracelet, $95). For contact details, see under 'Shopping' in the Directory.

Note: magnetised jewellery is claimed to be side-effect-free, but this isn't strictly true. Some of those who wear a magnetised necklace, especially if they are particularly sensitive or have had a physical trauma to the head area (e.g. a blow, concussion, brain haemorrhage or a clot) in the short- to medium-term past, report the necklaces make them feel woozy, unbalanced, disorientated and that this became apparent rapidly, often within half an hour. If this is the case for you but you'd still like to try magnetic jewellery, try wearing a bracelet – or if the pain is around the back and hips, try a magnetised back support instead. Magna Therapy does a very good one (£32.99). For more information about magnetised back supports, see Fix 23: Back Pain When Sitting.

16. Colour Therapy

There is no specific scientific research to be found on this, but, anecdotally, the use of colour is said to be comforting and healing for many pain-related conditions, and it is certainly relaxing, non-invasive, side-effect-free and a pleasure to use.

Colour therapy is often given by professional therapists in the form of bathing the affected area in coloured light or using coloured oils. However, they also suggest the following DIY anti-arthritis strategies for people to use at home.

If you find warmth helps soothe your discomfort from osteoarthritis, try wearing **orange** over the affected areas. If it's your knees, go for orange tights; for feet or ankles, orange socks; for the hips, orange tights again or alternatively dye a strappy T-shirt dress, silk petticoat or half-slip. Silk is an especially good material to use as it takes dye very well. It is also warming when it's cold even when it's very thin, yet cool in hot weather. Cotton's fine too, nylon a third choice. Interestingly, many of the spices (e.g. turmeric and ginger) and metals (e.g. gold and copper) that are anti-inflammatory and used to help arthritis have warm orangey-gold colouring.

For people with rheumatoid arthritis whose joints are inflamed and therefore too warm already, try cooling **turquoise** instead.

For further information about colour therapy and its potential effects on health, contact the International Association of Colour. For contact details, see under 'Therapies and Therapists' in the Directory.

17. Turquoise Elixir

Gem therapists recommend trying **turquoise elixir** as a complement to other treatments. Turquoise gemstones – soothing, cooling, clarifying – have long been used for bone disorders, joint problems, rheumatism and arthritis (among other things).

Healer and gem therapist Jacquie Wilton, who is also the National Federation of Spiritual Healers' senior trainer for the South of England and runs year-long courses for professional gem healers in the UK, says the elixir is straightforward to make at home and suggests this method:

1. First, take a polished turquoise gem (2–5 cm long is fine: you don't need a big, expensive piece), cleanse and programme it – i.e. dedicate it for the job in hand if this has not already been done. This is quick and easy to do. See Appendix 1: Cleansing and Programming Crystals and Gems on page 536.
2. Charge up the gem with positive energy by placing it in the sunlight among green leafy plants for an hour or two.
3. Pour a litre of cooled fresh spring water into a glass, china or earthenware jug. Place the turquoise in the bottom, cover the jar and leave somewhere cool for eight hours.
4. You now have your gem elixir. Remove the stone, dry it and put it away.
5. Drink the elixir at intervals throughout the day and make more as necessary. Take initially for seven to ten days and continue if needed.

18. Blood Pressure
As an adjunct to controlling low blood pressure medically, with herbs and diet, wear **red**. Theo Gimbel, the UK's foremost researcher and practitioner of colour therapy, advises that red light or clothing can be used to raise and balance blood pressure – it's also used therapeutically to counter feelings of apathy and lack of interest in life.

Asthma

19. The Buteyko Method

People with asthma are usually given things to inhale or swallow to treat their symptoms. However, they may also benefit greatly from learning a system of exercises designed to slow the breathing rate called the **Buteyko method**, which seems to reduce (sometimes drastically) the amount of medication needed.

Developed in the 1940s, it is based on the idea that many of us breathe faster than we ought to, thus lowering the levels of CO_2 in the bloodstream and reducing the delivery of oxygen to the tissues – meaning we try to breathe even faster (hyperventilate) to compensate.

A small but encouraging study of 39 severe asthmatics at the Mater Hospital in Brisbane, run by some of Australia's leading asthma specialists, found that after three months the group who had been practising Buteyko were using 90 per cent less of their usual beta-agonist drugs and only half their former level of inhaled steroids, whereas the group who weren't doing Buteyko either increased their drug usage or stayed the same. For more information about research, see Notes on page 548.

Classes on Buteyko are also available worldwide. To find your nearest practitioner, visit the Buteyko Institute of Breathing and Health (BIBH) website, www.buteyko.info.co.uk. For more contact details, see under 'Training Courses' in the Directory.

Alternatively, LifeSource offers a good self-help package on CD-Rom called *The Breathology Programme* (£29.95), which is also suitable for children. For contact details, see under 'Shopping' in the Directory.

For how to practise the method, see Fix 235: Buteyko Breathing.

20. Nutritional Anti-Asthma Strategies

Try taking daily supplements of **vitamin C**, because there is some evidence that vitamin C can substantially reduce the number of asthma attacks.

One double-blind crossover clinical trial in Nigeria in 1980 found that if asthmatic adults took 1 g daily they had 75 per cent fewer attacks. It is thought that 50–100 mg daily is safe for one- to three-year-olds. Another advantage of vitamin C is that it may reduce the likelihood of, and certainly shortens, colds, which can plague asthmatic children all winter and exacerbate the condition.

For the best way to take vitamin C (as at high doses, you will pee much of it all out), see 'Hitting the High Note: Top C Tips' on page 36.

Essential fatty acids have also been found to have an effect on asthma. It is recommended that asthmatics have fewer foods containing omega-6, like margarines and 'ordinary' vegetable cooking oils (e.g. sunflower, safflower corn oil and fast or processed foods) and have more foods high in omega-3 such as oily fish, like mackerel, or take fish-oil capsules.

The rationale behind this is that the body converts omega-6 oils to substances that encourage inflammation and inflammatory reactions in the tissues, such as those that occur in the respiratory system and are associated with asthma.[14]

Other nutritional tips:

- **Cut salt intake as far as possible.** Research suggests it makes the airways more twitchy.[15]
- **Try magnesium supplements.** There is some evidence to show they help to prevent the breathing tubes going into spasm. Take 150–250 mg a day for a 40 kg child, proportionately more for a teen or an adult.
- **Check out food sensitivities (intolerances and allergies).** The most common offenders are wheat, dairy, eggs, chocolate, corn, citrus fruit and fish. One study showed 90 per cent of children with asthma or a runny nose due to allergy improved on a food-elimination plan.[16]

21. Coffee for Asthma

Asthmatics who wake up with breathing difficulties in the morning often find a **coffee** or two with breakfast does the trick. Drinking two strong cups (235 ml in total) can have you breathing more easily within an hour, and the benefits last six hours, say Canadian researchers who worked with both children and adults, because the caffeine dilates the bronchiole tubes.[17]

For more information and suggestions, especially those suitable for children, see Young Children: Asthma on page 244.

Athlete's Foot (Tinea Pedis)

Garlic & Tea tree Doubly Whammy

Besides showering daily and drying carefully between your toes – a supply of throwaway paper towels for your feet may be a good idea until you are better – try the killer combination of **garlic** and **tea-tree oil**. It is a mighty natural antifungal. Pierce a garlic capsule and squeeze its contents into your palm, add one to two drops of tea tree, mix and rub it into the affected areas morning and evening. Continue for 7–14 days.

One study found 27 out of 34 people were completely clear after seven days using just the garlic treatment,[18] and an Australian trial published in 2002 found using tea tree on the relevant areas for a month produced significant improvement for 70 per cent of those with athlete's foot.[19]

Both substances are effective fungicides and are sold in most health shops and almost every chemist's – e.g. Holland & Barrett (garlic, 100 x 1 g capsules, £2.49; tea tree, 10 ml, £3.99). For contact details, see under 'Shopping' in the Directory. See also the note on tea-tree oil on page 549.

The 3-step programme

As a back-up measure to the above, to ensure that athlete's foot stays well and truly gone for good:

1. If you wear trainers, wash them in as hot a wash as possible without denaturing them.

2. Throw away any old shoe liners you wear and buy new ones.
3. Walk around at home in cool, clean cotton socks (not bare feet – that'll spread it around). Ditto under your desk at the office or if driving to work alone.

See also Women: Feet on page 39–216 and Men: Feet on page 216.

Backache

22. Back to Bed
Had backache for ages but no one can tell you why? Recent evidence in *The Lancet* suggests that merely changing to a medium-to-firm mattress improves matters by up to 83 per cent within three months for people with chronic 'non-specific' lower-back trouble.[20]

23. Back Pain When Sitting
One of the best back supports I have ever come across for people who suffer from lower back pain (and I've tried a few, as I have a seven-year-old lumbar injury to manage and have access to some of the best chiropractors and osteopaths in the country) is the **Backfriend** from MEDesign (approximately £54).

Light, portable and minimalist, you can take it anywhere. Companies worldwide from Hewlett-Packard to Marks and Spencer have bulk-purchased these for staff, because, as *What Car?* magazine put it, 'This one makes a bad seat, good.'

Designed so it takes much of the weight off the base of the spine, it enables me to sit comfortably for four to five hours at a stretch, whereas before I'd have been lucky to manage one. And if it doesn't help you personally, you can return it within 14 days and get your money back.

Also check out the **Magna Therapy Back Support** for use when you're sitting, working or driving. This is a soft, comfy, padded lower-back support with judiciously placed magnets inside. The magnets are thought to work by stimulating blood flow to the area, which encourages new cell growth and repair there, and possibly also by interrupting the efficient conductivity of electrical pain signals to the brain through the nerves it is placed over. Published clinical research studies show that magnetic fields can reduce pain and inflammation of many kinds – e.g. post-polio, chronic pelvic, arthritis of the hip, knee and wrist, and back pain – and that magnets can help promote healing if there has been a mechanical trauma (i.e. surgery or injury).[21]

It helps by supporting the back too, since it's about 22 cm across at its widest point across the back, narrowing to nearer 12 cm for the wrap-over part. The Magna Therapy Back Support secures with Velcro, can be worn under clothes as long as they're not too skintight, or over the top for a sporty belt look. It's good to keep in an office drawer if you have intermittent back pain too.

If the support doesn't work for you, just send it back within 60 days for a full refund. You can buy it direct (£32.99).

For all contact details, see under 'Shopping' in the Directory.

> **Tip**
> For back pain with inflammation, a terrific instant fix from LifeTime is Stopain analgesic spray. It contains glucosamme, MSM and Boswellia and it does what it says on the bottle. Available from Victoria Health (£9.95, 118ml).

Bad Breath (Halitosis)

Besides having a dental check-up in case the problem's related to tooth decay, gum disease or a tonsil infection *and* seeing your GP in case there is an underlying gastrointestinal cause that can be easily sorted (e.g. a mild but ongoing digestive problem), there are a number of holistic fixes you can try.

24. Food Sensitivities

Check for food sensitivities and keep your diet as natural as you possibly can. An increasing number of cases of halitosis are thought to be linked with gut toxicity brought about by a diet high in refined foods and additives. In one study of hyperactive little boys (all pre-schoolers) published in *Pediatrics*, researchers found that when they took the problem foods out of the children's diets, their tendency towards halitosis also improved.[22]

See also Women: Bloating on page 128 and Young Children: Food Intolerances on page 281.

25. 'Good' Bacteria

Take **probiotics** (freeze-dried 'good' bacteria) for four to eight weeks. For maintenance, you could also eat a pot of natural live yoghurt every day, but the capsules (like Biocare's for instance, see Shopping) have many, many times more of those positive bacteria in them and will do a better fix-up job by far.

For instance, in March 2005, one Japanese study found volunteers who were given strict oral-hygiene instructions, then taken off yoghurt and cheese for two weeks and asked to eat 90 g natural yoghurt every day for another two weeks had an 80 per cent lower level of hydrogen sulphide (a smelly, volatile chemical that is a major cause of bad breath) when they ate the yoghurt.

See also Fix 7: After Antibiotics and Young Children: After Antibiotics on page 242.

26. For a More Kissable Mouth . . .

. . . scrape your tongue twice a week, as it removes the film of bacteria that is busy breaking down the remains of old food (a process that can create bad-smelling biochemical by-products).

Going out? Fast temporary fixes

If you need fresher breath *fast*, chew some **fennel seeds** or a few sprigs of fresh **parsley**. Fennel seeds are sold in health shops, or if you have no time for shopping, you can get them via fast mail order from Island Spice (320 g, 79p) and keep them handy. Also a great digestif containing fennel, ginger root and meadowsweet is **Digest-Aid Tonic** from the Natural Healing Centre (100 ml, £14.50).

For an instant antibacterial mouthwash, add one drop of **myrrh essential oil** to a cup of cool spring water or cooled boiled water, gargle and rinse. You can buy it from Baldwin's (5 ml, £4.79).

For all contact details, see under 'Shopping' in the Directory.

Women and bad breath

As already explained, the most common causes of bad breath are an infection of the gums, food intolerances and allergies, but for women in particular there's also being premenstrual and crash-dieting, both of which may affect saliva flow, and saliva usually washes away the odour-producing bacteria from the mouth.

Being premenstrual causes a rise in progesterone, which can make your gums swell, trapping tiny amounts of decaying food and bacteria in the crevices where tooth meets gum, resulting in a bad taste in the mouth and maybe a bad odour too. So if your symptoms are worse seven to ten days before your period, anything that balances out your progesterone levels with oestrogen will help. To tackle the cause, see Fix 187: Premenstrual Syndrome (PMS) for some effective options.

Broken Bones

Mending Breaks Fast

When you've broken a bone, speed up healing with an excellent homeopathic combination suggested by Helios, the pharmacy that supplies the famous Tunbridge Wells Homeopathic Hospital (one of six NHS-funded homeopathic hospitals in the UK), rather than arnica, the standard single remedy usually suggested. The special break-bonding formula is a potency-6 mix of **Symphytum** (homeopathic comfrey, also known as knitbone), *Rhus tox* and **Ruta**.

Any homeopathic pharmacy, such as Baldwin's or Helios, can make this combination up for you and send it by post (approximately £6). For contact details, see under 'Shopping' in the Directory.

Bruises

27. Arnica – the Expert Approach

Homeopathic **arnica** can work well, but people get variable results because they don't always take it at the right potency (usually chemists and health shops only sell 6c) or in the most effective way. For best results, if you have a bad bash and are expecting some impressive bruising:

1. Take one **200c arnica** tablet three times daily *and* gently rub a really good-quality arnica cream from a proper homeopathic pharmacy, like Helios (30 g, £4.99), rather than one from the local chemist (it works *way* better), into the affected area two to three times daily. After a bath or shower is a good time as the skin absorbs cream extra well if it's warm and damp. Helios does fast mail order, and having arnica tablets and a good cream to keep in the medicine box alongside the Germolene and ibuprofen can be invaluable anyway, especially if you have a family. For contact details, see under 'Shopping' in the Directory.
2. From the next day for up to five days, take a 30c arnica tablet three times daily and apply the cream topically three times daily. Then continue on with 6c tablets until your bruising starts coming out and the area begins to feel more comfortable.

See also Men: Black Eye on page 208, Fix 313: Bashes and Bruises, and Bromelain on pp 208–9.

Burns

28. Cool, Calm and Heal

1. **Cool it.** Do this immediately. You can use either cold running water or an ice pack (a few ice cubes in a plastic bag wrapped in a cloth or, better, a gel pack like Theraflex, page 84). Apply for 20 minutes, wait for ten minutes, then apply again. If it's a chemical burn caused by, for example, oven- or drain-cleaners, flush the area with cool water for 15–30 minutes and check whether there are any first-aid instructions on the label. If still very sore and not improving after 24 hours, go to A&E.
2. **Calm it.** Reduce the pain with a natural painkiller like white willow bark extract (Germany's Commission E, which is similar to the US's Food and Drug Administration, endorses this for pain relief), aspirin or paracetamol.

3. **Heal it.** Fast. Natural options include:

- **Honey** – especially, if you can get some, **manuka** honey with an AMF of ten or above. When Indian researchers treated burns either with the standard sort of dressing or one soaked in honey, the honey group healed in nine days instead of 18.[23] You can buy it direct from Manuka Honey. See also Fix 105: Bee Better and Fix 62: Wound, Ulcer and Sore Healing.
- **Aloe vera** – often used for burns and a 1995 study by Thai researchers illustrates why: when they treated one group of people with second-degree burns using dressings smeared in petroleum jelly and the other with aloe vera, the latter got better in 11 days, the petroleum-jelly group in 18.
- **Fireweed** from Alaskan Essences – this is used in the clinical Burns Unit at Sao Paulo's University Hospital in Brazil. For home use, on the day of the burn as an emergency measure, Alaskan Essences recommends taking one drop under the tongue or in water three times a day. Then add just two drops of essence from the tincture bottle to a 30 ml dropper bottle, filling it up with three-quarters pure water and a quarter brandy as a preservative. Take four drops of this three to four times a day; it also helps to pour a little on to the dressing over the burn. You can purchase it in the UK via Healthlines (dosage bottle, 30 ml, £5.50); in the US and Canada, contact Alaskan Essences direct.
- **Lavender aromatherapy oil** – apply two to three drops to the affected area. Lavender is a great burns healer. In fact, it was an accident in a French laboratory in 1910 that showed how powerful essential oils could be, when chemist René-Maurice Gattefossé burnt his hand and plunged it into the nearest liquid he could find to cool it – which happened to be a container of lavender oil. His burn healed so fast and with so little scarring that he was motivated to study the therapeutic action of plant oils and the art of modern medical aromatherapy was born. Doctors in France now use essential oils alongside conventional drugs. Organic essential oils are preferable if you can afford and find them. In the UK, try Neal's Yard Organic Lavender (10 ml, £8.95); Neal's Yard also have a site for US customers (0.34 fl

oz, $32). See also the organic lavender from Starchild, and also via the terrific Florihana (in Provence).

For all contact details, see under 'Shopping' in the Directory. Note: do not use any of these on broken skin without medical advice.

Circulation

29. Chilblains

These itchy, reddish-purple patches usually occur on the toes but may also affect the fingers and are caused by circulation problems: usually excessive narrowing of the blood vessels due to the cold. Sometimes if the feet get severely cold for a while (e.g. when skiing) they can have a predisposition to chilblains in the future.

Vitamin E can help. It probably does so by reducing the stickiness of the blood platelets, effectively thinning it so it flows better. **Ginkgo biloba** would be a sensible herbal supplement to take too. Used clinically to boost circulation (often in connection with memory enhancement in the elderly), in one German study researchers working with diabetic patients who had reduced circulation to their extremities found it increased blood flow there by around 40 per cent.[24] Try the ginkgo supplement Vein Tain from Nature's Best (60 capsules, £11.95). For contact details, see under 'Shopping' in the Directory.

Freelance feet

For the growing percentage of the workforce who are freelancers operating from a little wooden office (garden shed) at home – witness the rash of designer garden-office pods at London's 2005 Chelsea Flower Show – chilblains can be a bit of an occupational hazard.

If the floor is not extremely well insulated (sometimes even if it is) and your shed is built, as most are, on a concrete platform, the winter cold can come up in waves through the floor despite adequate heating in the room. From personal experience (having been a happy shed-worker for the past 17 years), it helps considerably to put my feet on a fat phone directory so they are not in direct contact with the ground during the coldest times, and wear ski or thermal socks (especially **red** fluffy comfort or ski socks, as this colour is thought to boost blood flow.

30. The Chilly-Feet Cherisher

To boost feet's circulation, massage them in the evening after a cold day with a palmful of carrier oil and two drops of warming, comforting **ginger aromatherapy oil**, like the ginger essential oil from Neal's Yard (10 ml, £7.95). For contact details, see under 'Shopping' in the Directory.

31. Phone Calls as Medicine

Know someone who has been ill for a long time? You can help them feel physically better without even going to see them.

Regular 'Hello, how are you?' phone calls can be as effective as medication from the doctor. In one study, when a group of elderly Americans with osteoarthritis were rung up for a chat *just once a month* for a year, their pain levels dropped, their stiffness eased, they were able to move about more easily, and also, unsurprisingly, they felt happier and more optimistic.[25]

Many other studies show that regular friendly calls help elderly people as much health-wise as visits to the clinic – so ring someone who is unwell now (no matter how old or young they are) for it really could make all the difference.

Clarity – 'What shall I Do?'

32. When You Can't See the Wood for the Trees, Try the Sky Stone

Though our intuition is one of the most powerful assets we have – the bit of us that is always right, the bit that cannot be fooled, the bit that just *knows* – it's not always possible to hear it above the static of everyday life. It can also be muddied by the thoughts that we already have about a problem.

The following is an excellent technique for accessing that intuition clearly and accurately. You'll need:

• **Angelsword** by Australian Bush Flower Essences. It is available direct worldwide. In the UK, via Healthlines, IFER and Flower Sense (15 ml, £9.95) or Earth Spirits in the US.

- a small **candle**: a tea light in a glass will do
- a **blue lapis lazuli stone**: one of the small, shiny, 'tumbled' stones from gift or gem shops costing about £2 or £3 will do fine. You can buy them mail order from Pretty Rock and the Litlington Crystal Store. For all contact details, see under 'Shopping' in the Directory. Lapis is the stone of objectivity and clarity. It encourages self-awareness and is also a traditional truth-revealer, helping you to confront the reality of a situation, no matter what it is. However, as with every gemstone you use therapeutically, it is vital to cleanse and programme it before you use it. This is quick and easy to do. See Appendix 1: Cleansing and Programming Crystals and Gems on page 536.

The Truth-Seeing Technique

1. Run a bath as hot as you like it and add seven to ten drops of Angelsword, also known as 'Angel's Word'. This essence helps someone distinguish between what's really true, and best for you personally, and what other people have been trying to convince you is good for you. *Note:* very sensitive people may find that even five to seven drops are enough.

2. Light your candle. As you do so, dedicate it in your mind to the angels of truth. Ask for their protection, then ask them to help you find the best solution to your problem *for the highest possible good.* For more about this, see 'Highest possible good' on page 69.

3. Get into your bath, lie back, soak and enjoy for a few minutes. You will be absorbing the Angelsword in the water through the pores of your skin and inhaling it as steam. Let your mind go quiet: try and dismiss or let go of any ideas or preconceptions you may have.

4. Centre yourself with an easy breathing technique: breathe in for six, hold it for six, breathe out for six. Do this ten times. Feel all your tension melt into the warm water, and any negativity (anxiety, frustration and confusion) melt with it.

5. Now, close your eyes and place the lapis in the centre of your forehead over your third eye, the seat of your intuition.

6. Ask to be told, or shown, that which you need to know to solve your difficulty.

7. Wait for a while, enjoying the peace and warmth you've created.

Don't try to work anything out or think it through. Just be and see what comes. You may receive a gentle impression as an answer, or even see something in your mind's eye. If nothing presents itself right away, that's fine. Some people receive no hints at the time but may dream of the answer that night, or simply wake up the next morning somehow knowing what to do.

8. Remove the stone.

9. Ask that your third eye be closed now and protected. Imagine a disk of golden light hovering a few inches above your forehead, protecting the third-eye area. This is important: if it is left open and unprotected, you can end up feeling drained and spacey. Thank the angels of truth for their help.

10. Take three deep breaths, feeling the bath against your body, and bring back your awareness of where you are.

11. Now open your eyes. Stretch a little and yawn if you feel like it. That's it.

12. As you get out of the bath, stamp your feet a bit on the floor to ground yourself and rub your body briskly with a towel. Let the candle burn down by itself rather than blowing it out. If you still feel at all vacant when you leave the bathroom, stamp about some more, then have a drink or a small snack.

33. Coeliac Disease

People with coeliac disease cannot tolerate gluten, which is a protein found in barley, rye, oats and wheat. Symptoms include diarrhoea, bloating, flatulence, feeling tired, mood swings and, in the long term, possibly osteoporosis and anaemia. Traditional advice is that those with coeliac disease must avoid any gluten-containing foods like the plague.

However, more recent research suggests most coeliacs can in fact tolerate **oats** just fine, meaning extra healthy, quick and convenient sources of energy and fibre like oatcakes, oat muesli, flapjacks and porridge are open to them after all.[26]

So if you or your child have been diagnosed with coeliac disease, it is well worth being tested to see if your gut is oat-friendly. A good nutritionist could help you here. For contact details, see under 'Therapies and Therapists' in the Directory.

Colds and Flu

34. Avoiding them

Cut the sugar and stay bug-free this winter. Next time you hear there is a nasty virus going about that has claimed several of your neighbours or work colleagues, cut right back on sugary foods – American studies show sugar disrupts the body's infection-fighting system.[27] Go instead for more complex carbohydrates like baked spuds and pasta to keep your energy levels up. This is a good temporary strategy to follow at the first sign of any infection.

35. Cold-Shorteners
Three of the Best
1. Vitamin C

If you have a cold and want an inexpensive way to shorten it, take a total of 1–3 g **vitamin C** daily. There are now around 30 good long-term trials to show that while it isn't necessarily going to stop you coming down with something, vitamin C can shorten the life of upper--respiratory-tract infections, cutting the runny nose and sneezing miseries (which usually last around four days) by at least 24 hours.[28] It is best to get the time-release so none is wasted, you get an even amount in your system all day long, and it is easier to digest.

> ### Hitting the High Note: Top C Tips
>
> - **Tail off any supplementing you do gradually** or you will end up back at square one because your body will be suddenly short of vitamin C and very likely going down with the next cold that comes along. According to top British nutritionist and applied kinesiology practitioner John Taberman-Pichler, if you flood the body with vitamin C, it can really banish the bugs, but if you suddenly stop taking it (thinking, 'Hey, I'm better, aren't I?'), that stimulates the release of an enzyme called ascorbase, which breaks down vitamin C and removes the lot from your system. So take it slowly. If you're on 3 g a day, drop down to 2 g for the next four days, then down to 1 g a day for three to four days, then down to 500 mg daily, then stop.

- **Hit a cold with frequent 500 mg doses of vitamin C throughout the day,** since your body can't absorb more than that at a time. Rather than, say, a hefty 1.5 g in the morning, then another 1.5 g at night, split it into six small doses. Take, for instance, each time you have some food – e.g. breakfast, mid-morning snack, lunch, mid-afternoon snack, suppertime – and then the final one at bedtime. If you don't, you will be peeing out much of your vital C and it's pointless taking it.

Easy Does It

The far less fiddly way to do this is to try taking a single slow-release Vtimain C tablet in the morning and one at night. This enables you to take far higher doses and not lose any. Try Nature's Best Time Release C (1500 mg, 60 tablets, £7.50).

2. Herbs

Echinacea, available as a tincture and as capsules, can help too, taken immediately a cold strikes, for three to seven days – one study showed it reduced the duration of a particularly lengthy cold strain from nine days to six.[29] For best results, *begin taking the instant symptoms begin*, and to really hammer the virus, add in 1 g time-release vitamin C two to three times daily for two to three days. **Astralagus**, the traditional Chinese immune system and energy boosting favourite, is great too – and was recently validated by the University of Texas. Try Solgar's capsules (approximately £17.99 for 60).

Which? echinacea product?

Not all are equally effective. In 2005, *Proof* (the UK-based complementary health equivalent of *Which?*) tested several in a private biochemical laboratory for strength of active ingredients and quality, but only gave a five-star rating to Solgar's **Echinacea Root and Leaf Extract** (60 capsules, £13.65). In the US, you can also try Nature's Answer Fresh Echinacea (1 oz, $9.99).

3. Bee propolis

Bee propolis extract, though more costly, is such an efficient antiviral, antifungal and antibacterial agent that it can cut the time you have a cold in half so long as, like echinacea, you start taking it at the very first sign of a sniffle.[30]

In the UK, try Apitherapy Health, a small family-run Norfolk company set up by Clive and Susan Brockdorff, a beekeeper and a nutritionist respectively (60 ml, £10.75; 45 x 1 g capsules, £10.75); in the US, see Beehive Botanicals, for a 65 per cent propolis tincture ($13).

For all contact details, see under 'Shopping' in the Directory.

36. Constipation
How to Get Going Again

Sensible anti-constipation self-help measures include:

- **upping your fibre intake**
  Eat plenty of fruit and vegetables. Also consider oat-based cereals and whole rye breads instead of wheat-based bread as these seem to be easier on the stomach and less likely to produce bloating, constipation and discomfort. You could also use a bulking agent if needed, such as psyllium husks or linseed. Try **Linusit Gold** from any local health shop – e.g. Holland & Barrett (250g, £3.95). Take probiotic capsules for four to eight weeks in case an imbalance in gut bacteria is the problem – try BioCare's Bio Acidophilus (60 capsules, £17.95). For contact details, see under 'Shopping' in the Directory.

- **drinking plenty of pure water.**
  According to water and health pioneer Dr F Batamanghelidj we need a litre per 50lbs (24 kg) of body weight plus another litre *on top* a day . . . of pure non-carbonated water. (He gives a big No to Volvic though: read his book named on p 14 for why). Oh – and each cuppa or glass of booze you drink means an equal amount of pure water extra. This is not an easy regime to follow but even 8-10 glasses of pure water a day can help flush our systems through, help shift any toxins and waste products in both circulatory system and alimentary canal (especially those which might have built up during a period of constipation) and will also help soften stools.

- **getting enough exercise** – pleasingly, just 20 minutes of brisk walking twice a day is thought to do the trick. Walking (or running, dancing, swimming, tennis – you name it, if it's making you move it's doing the trick) eases constipation because the muscular contractions made by the intestines as we move about help massage the waste along the lower digestive tract.
- **Taking a teacup of prune juice** with a tablespoon of lemon juice or a single **senna** tablet (such as Senacot, available in local chemists) as an occasional overnight treatment.

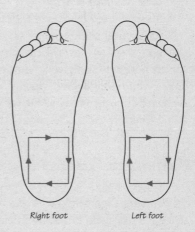

Right foot   *Left foot*

Move Along There! Press here

DIY anti-constipation reflexology on an ongoing basis can offer gentle stimulation and support for your gut and keep things moving. Work in the direction of the arrows (see illustration), pressing in small clockwise spirals along the 'box' outline, which mirrors the colon and contains the reflexology points that connect with it. Do so morning and evening for two to three minutes at a time.

See also Men: Flatulence on page 221, Young Children: Constipation on page 262 and Fix 205: Bunged Up.

Courage

37. Boost Your Bottle

When it's a one-off boost of sheer bottle that's needed, some go for a shot of brandy or vodka, but the new way (that will leave your head totally clear) is with **Andean Fire**. This is a remedy made from a rare and beautiful flame-coloured orchid, and its developers say it is *for those who need to make a leap*.

It is usually used by people (both adults and children) who are facing a major physical challenge like sky-diving, bungee-jumping, white-water rafting or abseiling down a cliff for the first time . . . but, on a more serious note, it is also given therapeutically to survivors of disasters and others who have suffered greatly. It is by Living Tree Orchid Essences and can be bought through IFER. For contact details, see under 'Shopping' in the Directory. (See also page 116 for confidence boosting tips.)

Cravings

38. Craving Cigarettes

Dying for a cigarette but trying to give them up? Carry a bottle of **black-pepper oil** around with you and sniff when the craving takes hold. In one study in 1994, 48 volunteer smokers had their cigarettes taken away overnight, then the next morning they were divided into three groups and given devices to puff on for three hours. One group had the black-pepper oil, one group had the scent of mint, and the other just had plain air. Those tooting the black-pepper oil found it significantly cut their desire for a fag.[32] If you can't find any locally, try Baldwin's (10 ml, £3.55). For contact details, see under 'Shopping' in the Directory.

See also 'Advice on stopping smoking' on page 218 and Men: Smoking on page 234.

39. Coffee Addiction

If you're finding you cannot do without your coffee-with-sugar intake every day yet you are also feeling a bit down or depressed, it is very possible that your cuppas are the culprit. The good news is that research shows if you can cut out coffee and sugar for *just one week*, it can lift depression fast.[33]

However, researchers also found that going back to coffee brought the symptoms straight back. These people were drinking 700 mg caffeine – about five cups – steadily throughout the working day. Perhaps if you feel depressed but need your caffeine hit, you could try just the one to kick-start your working day but stick to non-caffeinated drinks and fresh water after that. Or, if you want to go cold turkey, consider ordinary vitamin C to combat stress instead. Studies say this works – see Fix 483: Performance Anticipation Stress.

See also General: Depression on page 45.

Cystitis

Cystitis, or bladder infection, is the most common type of urinary-tract infection (UTI) and especially common in women: in fact, up to half of us will get it at some point in our lives – sometimes repeatedly. The treatment you would normally be offered by your GP is a course of antibiotics. However, it is thought that cystitis can also be related to an imbalance in 'friendly' microorganisms in the gut and genital area, which antibiotics themselves can cause, and if you already have an imbalance, they will certainly make it worse.

40. Drug-Free Approach

If you think that antibiotics may be making your cystitis worse in the long run, you are getting repeated attacks or you just prefer a drug-free approach, try **cranberry extract**. Plenty of research has been carried out in the past dozen years on the benefits of this and it has been found to contain substances called proanthocyanidins. These help stop the E. coli bacteria, which causes cystitis, from sticking to the bladder walls.[34]

The recommended dose is 200–400 mg dried extract daily. Dried extract is more effective than cranberry juice, which also usually contains sugar and artificial sweeteners.

Try Super-Strength Cranberry Extract from Higher Nature (30 x 500 mg capsules, £8.90). Also take a good probiotic (freeze-dried 'good' bacteria) capsule for eight weeks, like BioCare's Bio Acidophilus Forte

(60 caps, £45.95), or the gentler Bio Acidophilus (60 caps, £17.95). For contact details, see under 'Shopping' in the Directory.

See also the suggestions about cat's claw, echinacea and goldenseal in Fix 303: Natural Treatments.

Instant comfort for acute cystitis

Drink plenty of plain water (at least 2 litres a day) to dilute your urine so it stings less and creates extra volume to help flush out the infection.

Keep a jug of cool water by the loo and pour it over your vulva when peeing. This takes much of the sting away.

---

41. Top Loo Technique

Holding back very small amounts of urine in the bladder encourages cystitis in both sexes – if, for instance, you are doing exercises on the loo to increase pelvic-muscle strength and thus the intensity of orgasm when lovemaking – see Women: Pelvic-Floor Muscles on page 161 and Fix 224: Orgasm Power. (So be sure to empty totally afterwards!)

This is because those last few millilitres of wee provide the ideal breeding ground for any bladder bacteria to multiply faster than photons in a fast breeder reactor, says Julian Shar, consultant at the Institute of Urology in London. You'll get a similar effect if you hover over dodgy public toilets when passing water. Shar suggests that if the seat looks dirty, put some toilet paper on it and sit down.

42. Sit It Out

When the burning of cystitis is really bad and you need immediate relief, sit in a warm (not hot), shallow bath into which you have poured a litre of really strong **chamomile tea** – make with four tablespoons of chamomile steeped for 15–20 minutes. Either a herbal sachet brand will do or try Baldwin's for supplies of dried chamomile. For contact details, see under 'Shopping' in the Directory.

Lie in the bath, knees apart, for a good 20 minutes: perhaps take in a book or magazine to pass the time. Chamomile baths are also helpful for thrush discomfort.

Warning

If your cystitis attack has lasted *more than 48 hours without improvement*, if there is any blood in your urine or you are miserably uncomfortable, see your GP right away to avoid the risk of kidney damage.

For more advice and fixes, specifically those for children with cystitis, see Young Children: Urinary-Tract Infections (UTIs) on page 306.

43. Yeast Intolerant but Love Bread?
Toast it. It kills the yeast, says John Taberman-Pichler, a top nutritionist and applied kinesiologist who has a busy practice in Sussex.

Dandruff

44. Recurrent Dandruff
If you have dandruff that is 'kept down' by your usual anti-dandruff shampoo but tends to come back with a vengeance if you stop using it (and using the same shampoo for too long without a break can leave the hair looking dull anyway), it is likely that the root cause is a fungal infection of the scalp.

According to Dr Stephen Davies, one of the UK's top clinical nutritionists, founding chairman of the British Society for Nutritional Medicine and fellow of the American College of Nutrition, if you want to get rid of the dandruff for ever, go for a good general antifungal programme. Speak to a qualified nutritionist about the fine details of this, but general measures include:

• reducing refined carbohydrates
• cutting out yeast (e.g. in breads and Marmite)
• cutting out sugar and sweet things (e.g. cakes, biscuits, sweets, sweet fruit like bananas, apples and grapes)
• taking antifungal nutritional extracts such as grapefruit-seed extract – e.g. the splendid **Citricidal**: take 5–15 drops two to three times

daily in 145 ml water, starting with the low dose and working up over two weeks. In the UK, Citricidal is available from Higher Nature (45 ml, £6.90; 100 tablets, £10.50); in the US, it is called just grapefruit-seed extract and is available from NutriTeam (2 fl oz, $6.95). For contact details, see under 'Shopping' in the Directory.

- if you are not already doing so, using a selenium-containing shampoo like **Selsun** because selenium is, among other things, an antifungal. To turbocharge, add two drops of **tea-tree oil** (test first: see below) to the shampoo each time, or five drops of Citricidal. Massage in and leave in for two to five minutes before rinsing out well.

For best results, Dr Davies recommends that you would need to follow an antifungal routine for around three months, since the fungus will probably be lodged deep in the hair follicles.

To find a nutritionist near you, get in touch with the Institute of Optimum Nutrition, the British Naturopathic Association or one of the other organisations mentioned under 'Therapies and Therapists' in the Directory.

Anti-Dandruff Aromatherapy Rub
Mix together:

15 drops tea tree oil
15 drops rosemary
45 ml jojoba oil

Massage into clean hair, leave for an hour and rinse out well. It leaves your hair very shiny (thanks to the rosemary) and smelling good; the jojoba oil improves the flaky, dry condition of the scalp, and the tea tree is powerfully antifungal. In 2000 an investigation by Edzard Ernst, professor of complementary medicine at the University of Exeter[35] based on four strict randomised controlled trials showed tea tree zaps fungal infections, which often cause or contribute to dandruff. You can get tea tree, rosemary and jojoba from any good health shop, such as Baldwin's and Neal's Yard, which also has a US website. For contact details, see under 'Shopping'.

Note: tea tree is usually safe to use on the skin, but a few very sensitive people may find it does not suit them. To check, dab a little on the inside of your elbow 24 hours before doing the scalp treatment: if there is any redness or irritation, do not use it. See also the note concerning the use of tea-tree oil on page 549.

Depression

45. Antidepressants – Alternatives

One in every five people in the GP's surgery has depressive symptoms. Nearly half go unrecognised. If you are taking antidepressants such as Prozac but are concerned about their side effects, trying to come off them or finding they don't work for you, there is a substance found in fish oils called **eicosapentaenoic acid (EPA)** that appears to be as effective as conventional antidepressant drugs, yet can work faster.

EPA has no reported side effects – something that can't even be said about the other major natural treatment for depression, St John's wort.

Formerly used to help those with schizophrenia, and more recently bipolar disorder, most doctors may not yet be familiar with the use of EPA for depression, though recently there have been encouraging research studies on the subject.[36] To find out more, see the clear and comprehensive book *The Natural Way to Beat Depression* by Dr Basant Puri, a pioneering psychiatrist who successfully uses EPA to treat depression. He is consultant psychiatrist and senior lecturer at the MRI Unit at the Imperial College School of Medicine, London, and is also honorary consultant in imaging at Hammersmith Hospital's Department of Radiology.

The charity Food and Behaviour Research, which studies clinical links between human behaviour, mood and nutrition, also has a useful website with information on EPA usage and clinical trials, www.fabresearch.org.

Eight out of ten people with depression *will begin to feel better within a week* if diagnosed and treated correctly.[37]

EPA can also safely be taken with ongoing antidepressant medication, and research has found this speeds recovery. The suggested dose is 1 g daily for mild to moderate depression. Try **Eye Q** by Equazen, which is also used to treat dyslexia and dyspraxia. It is sold in Boots, Superdrug, Tesco and Morrisons and can also be bought from Equazen's website (60 x 500 mg capsules, £7.99). For contact details, see under 'Shopping' in the Directory.

Note: if you're taking anticoagulants for heart disease, check with your cardiologist before taking EPA.

Detox

46. By Hand in 30 Seconds

Instant tox test

With the first finger and thumb of one hand, 'milk' the webbing, applying reasonable pressure but not so hard it would usually hurt, between the fingers of your other hand. Hurts, huh? Then you need to detox – the following technique, done daily, will help.

This easy hand-reflexology technique can enhance any detox programme you're on and takes as little as 30 seconds, explains Angela Parker, an ex-NHS premature-baby nursing expert and now reflexologist and aromatherapist who has a busy private practice in Brighton.

1. With your left hand, use the tips of your index finger and thumb to gently but firmly grasp the webbing between the index and middle fingers of your right hand.
2. Work and roll this area *gently* for anything between 10 and 60 seconds, until you feel some discomfort. This may be a bit sharp if you have a lot of detoxing to do: if uncomfortable, proceed more softly.
3. Repeat for the other two fleshy webs between the fingers of your right hand.

4. Switch and do the same on your left hand.
5. When you've finished, rub your hands lightly together – first rub both palms together, then use your palms to rub the backs down past the wrist. Give your hands a gentle shake or two.
6. Repeat three times daily in quiet moments – and drink as much pure water as you can.

47. Herbs 'n' Husks – When You Just Don't Fancy Fasting

If you need to detoxify but the traditional combination of fasting (groan) and digestive-system cleansing (often by colonic irrigation) doesn't appeal one little bit, an easier and less invasive alternative may be the **Herbs 'n' Husks method**.

Psyllium husks are important for colonic cleansing – they work by absorbing moisture from the gut walls and swelling so your faeces is bulked up and can move through more comfortably and efficiently. These husks are thought to help clean the colon walls of old toxic waste matter, which can cling in nooks and crannies, and it also stimulates peristalsis (the rhythmic contractions of the gut that keep waste moving). You can get them in capsule form. Try @!@ (200 capsules, £11.96); in the US, call Solgar toll free. See 'Shopping' for details.

Lepicol, a comb of husks, pre- and probiotics, is another possibility. You can purchase it direct from Leppin Health. Unfortunately, it tastes like sawdust.

There is also **triphala**, a cleansing Ayurvedic herbal medicine. It contains *Terminalia chebula*, *Terminalia belerica* and *Emblica officinalis*, which encourage those smooth, healthy gut contractions. Try the tincture from Pukka Herbs, which you could use as well under the guidance of an Ayurvedic practitioner.

Note: take it gently. Stop if the combination of both proves a bit robust and you get tummy pains – just go for whichever one seems to suit you best.

For all contact details, see under 'Shopping' in the Directory.

See also Men: Detoxification on page 209.

Difficult Day Coming Up?

48 How to make sure it all goes your way . . .

Use the **Silver-Violet Flame** technique – imagine it *blasting along the entire timeline of your forthcoming day.*

Typical results include a seat suddenly being available to you on a packed commuter train where you usually have to fight for standing room, a potentially awkward meeting where everyone remarkably sees your point of view . . . even shopping for that elusive perfect pair of bottom-flattering jeans and finding them in the first shop you visit. This fix ensures your day *works.*

1. Close your eyes. In your head or out loud, ask for help as follows:

> **Dear Silver-Violet Flame of Transmutation and Grace, given to us by mighty Archangel Zadkiel to increase the level of positivity on this beautiful planet, in the name of Light, I ask for your help.**
>
> **Please create a positive pathway before me for this whole day.**
>
> **Blaze through my morning, my afternoon, my evening and my night, transmuting *everything and anything* that is of a negative vibration, within or upon the way I go, to 100 per cent positive vibration and burn away all dross and blockages from the path I tread.**
>
> **Please – do this NOW.**

2. As you say this, see in your mind's eye a great shining wave of silver-violet fire rearing up and sweeping along ahead of you, starting at whatever time it is *right now* and creating a shimmering pathway all the way through to your bedtime. Imagine it burning up all negativity and rubbish along the route and leaving it perfect.

3. Afterwards, say thank you three times.

Special days

If you have a day coming up that is potentially especially complicated or in which there are many things that could go wrong – such as a long journey abroad with very young children in tow or moving into a new home – repeat the above three times.

The esoteric Law of Three is that if you ask for something to be done 'in the name of Light' three times – providing it harms no one, is for the highest good and doesn't impinge on anyone else's free will – it will be.

Disability

Disability could be loosely defined as any chronic condition (physical or mental) that prevents you from doing what you wish to do or from living your life to the full.

49. Partners for Life
There are many different strategies, approaches, therapies and organisations that can help with almost every aspect of disability to some degree. Yet, having seen them at work and talked with those who have them, **Canine Partners (CPs)** seems to be one of the most loving, positive and supportive holistic measures around.

Canine Partners are highly trained, loving assistance dogs, and they can help people with many different types and degrees of physical disability. Able to respond to over a hundred different commands, these dogs can help a disabled person with a multitude of tasks that enable them to live an independent life – from unloading the washing machine or picking selected items off the supermarket shelf to operating a lift. Just as importantly, these remarkable dogs also offer unconditional love, a sense of security, backup and are great conversation-starters when they and their owner are out and about.

For contact details, see under 'Useful Helplines, Websites and Contacts' in the Directory.

50. Wild Potato Bush
Well worth taking for someone who is feeling frustrated or corralled by their disability is the gentle **Wild Potato Bush**, which can bring a sense of greater freedom and calm, no matter what your physical circumstances. It is indicated for those who feel weighed down, 'physically encumbered' or frustrated by the limitations of their body.

In Australia, essence therapists often give Wild Potato Bush to those who are paraplegic, quadriplegic, very overweight or who have an illness that restricts them physically. It is available direct from Australian Bush Flower Essences (15 ml, £8.99) or via Healthlines (£8.95) in the UK or Earth Spirits in the US. For contact details, see under 'Shopping' in the Directory.

52. Exercise for Memory

Can't remember things as well as you used to? Put on your trainers and take a walk every day . . . Anyone over the age of 40 worried about memory loss (from the age of 25 we're losing 1 per cent of our brain cells and, just as importantly, nerve cells each year) can slow any mental decline not with expensive supplements but plain old ordinary exercise. Even a brisk walk for 20 minutes a day will do and helps offset the fact that by the time we're 70 over a third of the brain cells we had in our youth will have gone.[38]

53. Fight Falling Arches

Shoeless toe-scrunches (as if you're trying to pick up a pencil) strengthen the muscles supporting your arches. You can do this under the desk at work, while you're on the phone, while cooking or washing up at home or watching TV. Aim for 100 casual scrunches a day.

54. Ear and Eye Infections
Beating Both . . .

An excellent all-rounder to keep in your bathroom cabinet is the home-opathic remedy *Mimosa pudica* 6c. Trials show it's useful for treating not only colds and flu, but also sinusitis, runny nose, acute ear infections, eye infections like conjunctivitis and general allergy-style sensitivities such as hay fever.[31]

To purchase this remedy, try a specialist homeopathic pharmacy such as Ainsworths, Baldwin's or Helios (£3.50–£4.50). For contact details, see under 'Shopping' in the Directory.

Fibromyalgia

Fibromyalgia can be absolutely miserable. As one long-term sufferer said, 'There's nothing visible for people to see, but all you can do when it gets bad is sit in an armchair and *hurt*.'

It is not easy to treat successfully either, though as with other chronic pain conditions like arthritis, different things help different people and the range includes a variety of medical and natural strategies, from anti-inflammatories to herbs.

Medical Treatments

Medical treatments include painkillers, anti-inflammatories, low-dose anti-depressants and trigger-point injections of the powerful painkiller lignocaine.

Complementary Treatments

Gentle soft-tissue massage, herbs, acupressure, nutritional supplements and chiropractic can often help. There is also a particular homeopathic preparation that is well worth trying. It's gentle, non-invasive and when it works, it does so very fast – it certainly sorted out my vicious bout of fibromyalgia last year within a week, when it had dragged on for six months. The pain has not so far returned.

55. Homeopathic Help

Take **Ledum 30c** twice daily for two days: if there's improvement, continue for seven days. It is likely to help if the pain:

- is in the soles of the feet and the hands
- affects the wrists, ankles and other joints, making them painful and feel hot
- is in the trigger or acupressure points down the meridians running along the outer sides of your arms and legs.

Ledum can be bought via Helios or Ainsworths (£4.75). For contact details, see under 'Shopping' in the Directory.

Note: if the homeopathic route seems to work for you, it is also a very good idea, when you feel up to it, to go and see a good homeopath for a full consultation and a customised remedy. A professional consultation with a homeopath costs £25–£70. If you wish to find a professional who is a medical doctor trained in homeopathy, get in touch with the British Homeopathic Association, and to find one who is a lay (non-medical) practitioner, contact the Society of Homeopaths. For all contact details, see under 'Therapies and Therapists' in the Directory.

See also General: Pain (Chronic) on page 67.

---

56 . . . Hay Fever Cuppa

When the pollen count's up, it's worth knowing that for someone with hay fever, the equivalent of two strong cups of **coffee** (this seems to be the optimum dose to calm symptoms without sending someone into orbit) can reduce an average of 27 hearty sneezing fits a day to a couple of small ones plus a mildly itchy nose, according to work by Dr Philip Shapiro of the Albany Medical Center, New York.

See also Fix 267: Hay Fever.

Flirting: Upgrade Your Pulling Power Instantly . . .

57. Just give them The Look

The Look is one of the most important sexual body-language techniques on the planet. Why? Psychological research suggests that even in an ordinary face-to-face conversation your words account for just 7 per cent of the impact you make (the figure's even lower in a chat-up context) but the tone of voice you use scores 38 per cent, and your body language (including facial expressions) accounts for more than 55 per cent of the impression you make on others (to find out more about that, see Bob Etherington's *Presentation Skills for Quivering Wrecks,* Cyan).

The Look is also the first thing to do when you are trying to catch the attention of someone you are attracted to – Step 1 in the art of effective flirting. Do it right and it will seriously enhance your pulling power. Do it wrong and you may turn off that cute woman or man over there in a New York second, by coming across like a guy who needs to go shave his back or a footballer's wife on the drink.

It is one of the great inequalities of life that some people can just do the Look instinctively, while others can't. But fortunately, according to body-language guru Judi James, though 'body language is one of the most powerful influences on the meet-date-mate process', you don't have to be born talented in this direction: you can learn it.

Learn how to do the Look step by step, practise in secret, then when you're good and ready, unleash it on the next gathering you go to, to gratifying effect.

Ms James, an author, ex-catwalk model and former model-agency owner, has taught thousands of people the secrets of body language and is much in demand with both blue-chip corporates (seminars on effective non-verbal signalling for work situations) and the TV networks. She has her own show on Channel 5.

Here is her gold-standard advice for intriguing the one you want across a crowded room. James calls this 'not exactly industrial-strength flirting, but the first step in the dance'. And it works.

OK, you've seen someone who interests you and have been watching them covertly for a while. It's time for the Look. So:

1. **Make your first eye contact.** *Women:* 'Glance for one second, then look away – *but only for a bit*. The trick is to then look back again, this time with a more meaningful glance and a slight smile.' *Men:* a longer, slightly bolder stare, as though you are smitten. James's tip: 'For God's sake, *do* practise it first. I thought I was quite good at it at one time, until I checked in the mirror and discovered I was mimicking the expression Alan Rickman wears in his role of Professor Snape in the Harry Potter movies.'
2. **Keep quiet and stand tall.** Don't mention you've made eye contact with Cute Person if you are with a group of friends, or they'll all turn round to look as well. Instead, 'Stretch your spine as if trying to touch the ceiling with the top of your head. Take and release a deep breath.'

Women: arch your back very slightly and tilt your head back subtly, displaying your throat. 'The small throat gesture works, I promise,' says James. 'Men think it looks polite but raunchy.' *Men:* pull your stomach in, but without sticking out your chest (because that looks Neanderthal).

3. **Talk to your friends, but glance back occasionally.** Carry on talking to your friends (and appear interested) so you don't look like a misfit, showing animation without overdoing it. Then: 'Glance back again. Smile if they're looking. Make it a secret-looking smile, with no teeth showing but lots of eye-softening.'

4. If you want to try and move things along now, try keeping this up for 5–15 minutes, then detach yourself from your group and wander over to the bar or drinks table. Loiter for a couple of minutes, then you'll either look round and see Fit Person loitering there too or, if they're still returning your looks but haven't budged, just do it. Take a drink over to them with a questioning smile. If you can't see what they've already got, wine of any colour is usually acceptable to all.

Absoultely essential reading: see James's book *Sex Signals: Decode Them and Send Them*.

Face-saving retreat tactic

If they're not receptive, merely shrug elegantly, smile tolerantly, return to your group and immediately offer the glass to a friend.

For more detailed advice specifically for each sex, see *Parties* pp 179, and on page 179 , in Women's section, see : *Pulling Men and Chatting Them Up* pp 70–74, and *'Facial Expressions That Score* pp 181–2. In the Men 's section, see also *Attracting Women: the Top 10 Posing Tips* page 235; and *The Drop Dead and Worship Me Saunter* pp 237.

Hangovers

58. Hangover From Hell

If you wake craving a fry-up after a hefty night's drinking, it may not be the healthiest breakfast in the world (saturated fat and then some), but your animal instincts are good. According to hangover expert Dr Andrew Irving, that high-protein plateful gently corrects your blood sugar level, which has dropped dramatically and is now making you feel, well, pretty bad.

How to feel better fast

You need to get your blood sugar up quickly, because all that alcohol has upended your body's ability to control the amount in your system, and too little sugar in the bloodstream affects the brain, making you feel sick and wobbly.

Remember the staggers, shakes and intellectual impairment that come with a major dose of drunkenness (when you were younger, naturally)? They were brought on by low blood sugar (hypoglycaemia), which is produced when large amounts of insulin are released by the pancreas to help break down the sugar-rich alcohol. So far, so good. Except that when you *stop* drinking, the insulin output falls but you are still left with too much in your system, causing even less sugar to circulate round the body and feed vital parts of it like your brain.

There are two main causes of hangover headache and disorientation: dehydration (alcohol is a great diuretic) and hypoglycaemia. The following will address both:

Dr Irving's easy hangover-cure breakfast

It helps if someone would be kind enough to make this for you. Often cooking with a hangover is more than flesh and blood can stand, at least until you have finished Step 2.

1. Two glasses of sweet tea or fruit juice, sipped down as gingerly as you like when you wake, *not* coffee – it'll dehydrate you even more.
2. A little porridge and sugar. Better still, chop half a banana over it. This gets blood sugar levels inching back up *steadily*: the oats are complex carbohydrates, which release their energy sugars slowly into the body, and bananas are slow-release too.
3. Grilled bacon and sausage, a poached egg, plus a piece of wholemeal toast. This is high in protein, which again helps restore blood sugar levels. Much nicer than the Middle Ages recipe for hangovers, which followed exactly the same protein principles but involved a chopped eel mixed with bitter almonds and diced owl's eyes.

59. Hangover Homeopathy

Homeopathy can work well fast – *Nux vomica* 6c taken at 15-minute intervals is the standard remedy. If a headache is the main symptom, however, choosing the right remedy for the specific sort of pain brings the best results:

• For a *throbbing head* that is worse in hot sun, and if your face feels a bit flushed and your pupils are more dilated than usual, take **Belladonna 30c** at 30-minute intervals. Take up to three doses.
• If it feels like a *nail's being driven into the side of your head*, try **Ignatia 6c.**
• When your headache is *sharp and stabbing*, and is worse when you move, take **Byronia 30c.**
• For *tightness, head-band-fashion*, round your skull that arrived suddenly, try **Aconite 30c.**

Homeopathic remedies in potency 6c are usually available from your local health shop or independent chemist. If the odd hangover is not exactly unknown in your household, it can be useful to have some of the remedies sitting in the bathroom cabinet for when you need them, so for potencies 30c and below, try a good specialist homeopathic pharmacy like Ainsworths or Helios, which also deliver mail order (usually within 24 hrs) in the UK, but also promptly to Europe and the US. Remedies cost from £3.50. For contact details, see under 'Shopping' in the Directory.

60. The Ultimate Morning-After Pick-Me-Up

The naturopath's favourite: tomato juice with plenty of crushed ice helps replace lost water and salts, plus a piece of wholemeal toast and Marmite, Vegemite or Bovril to settle the stomach and replace the B vitamins depleted by alcohol.

Headache

61. (One *Not* Caused by Alcohol)

For quick results, try **Tiger Balm**, the strong-smelling traditional Chinese balm containing camphor, peppermint, cloves, menthol and many other 'secret' ingredients. It's as good at getting rid of headaches as the common over-the-counter painkiller acetaminophen and works faster, according to one piece of Australian research in 1996.[39]

Tiger Balm's widely available in health shops, but if you can't find any locally in the UK, try Extra-Strong Red Tiger Balm from Express Chemist (19 g, £4.39); in the US, try the Tiger Balm patches from By the Planet (4 in. x 2.75 in., $5.30). For contact details, see under 'Shopping' in the Directory.

Healing and Recovery

62. Slow Recovery

If you want to speed up someone's injury healing – of any sort – lay on the love and harmony. Recent American research by Ronald Glaser (professor of virology at Ohio State University) and his psychologist wife, Jan Kiecolt Glaser, offers the solid biological proof that *happy people get better faster*.

They saw 42 married couples for two visits and, using a small suction device, made little blisters on their arms, monitoring how those healed up over 24 hours.

In the first visit, the couples were encouraged to talk about their marriage, supported positively and encouragingly by Jan. In the second, they were merely asked to relive a time when they'd had a blazing row – and remember how bad they'd felt. The little wounds from the second visits took twice as long to get better. Sadly, in couples who said they were usually pretty argumentative and hostile with each other, the wounds took 40 per cent longer still.[40]

63. Wound, Ulcer and Sore Healing

Slow wound healing is one of the biggest post-surgical problems for patients, and open 'minor' wounds such as leg ulcers in particular (for instance in bed-bound elderly people) can also be notoriously hard to resolve.

One of the best ways to heal a persistent sore is to apply honey to the area, and there are many reports in medical literature indicating honey to be an effective and healing dressing for wounds, sores, burns and skin ulcers.[41]

Hooray for honey

Honey's terrific. It
- fights infection effectively
- brings down inflammation
- reduces swelling, pain and any bad odour
- encourages the shedding of dead tissues, so surgery to remove it isn't needed after all
- speeds healing
- heals with minimal scarring
- reduces the need for skin grafting.

However, not all honeys fight infection equally well (in fact, they can vary hundredfold), due mostly to the differing amounts of hydrogen peroxide they contain. The best sort to use medically is the **manuka** variety, found by the Central Public Health Laboratory of London to be effective even against resistant strains of bacteria like the infamous MRSA. Check it has an AMF rating of ten or above. It's available in good health shops by the names MediBee or Comvita. Failing that, it can be ordered over the Net through Manuka Honey. In the US, you can get it via GloryBee. For contact details, see under 'Shopping' in the Directory.

If you're using it as a wound dressing or for something like a pressure sore or varicose leg ulcer:

- Ensure even coverage of the wound area, including any cavities, by warming the honey first so it goes runny. Cover with a second dressing to prevent leaks or, better still, use a waterproof occlusive dressing – no leakage or stickiness.

- If the area is very sore, spread the runny honey on the dressing pad, not the wound.
- Change honey dressings daily.
- Use 20 ml honey on a 10 cm x 10 cm dressing.

Family first-aid

Manuka honey is also invaluable for family first-aid, and for anyone with children, it ranks alongside arnica and Emergency Essence in the frequent-use stakes.

According to the Honey Research Unit at the University of Waikato in Hamilton, New Zealand, this variety – made by nectar from the manuka bush (*Leptospermum scoparium*) – is highly effective for the smaller stuff too and acts as an anti-infective healing agent for cuts and grazes (see Fix 256: Grazes). Dab a bit on topically, either directly on to cleaned skin or on the gauze or plaster, and put it over the sore area. It can be used for throat infections (see Fix 105: Bee Better), mouth ulcers, minor burns (see General: Burns on page 30), diarrhoea, gastroenteritis, even diluted into an oral wash and used for eye infections. I now keep a little pot in the fridge to use whenever needed – it lasts for years.

64. Bee'ing Herpes-Free

Even persistent herpes sores clear up smartly if they're treated with **propolis**, the substance bees make to put on the walls of their hives (especially in the chambers where their larvae hatch) in order to keep the infection rate down. A big multi-centre trial in 2000 found this resin-like natural material is so effective against viruses, including herpes, that it works better than the usual drug of choice, Acyclovir.[42]

In the UK, propolis is available in good health shops or via Apitherapy (60ml tincture, £10.75); in the US, it can be purchased from GloryBee. For contact details, see under 'Shopping' in the Directory.

IBS

65. Have Words With Your Gut

IBS sufferers who had tried everything else may well find that either **light self-hypnosis**, during which you 'talk' directly to your own gut, or **deep relaxation with an affirmation** (e.g. 'I will be totally free of tummy pain tomorrow') do the trick.

Clinical research at Manchester's Withington Hospital found this simple DIY therapy got a success rate of more than 80 per cent with people who were at their wits' end because no other treatment or strategy they'd ever tried had worked.

This adds up because the mind has a particularly powerful connection with the digestive system, which itself is bristling with so many nerve cells that if you rolled up all the neurones in your gut together, they'd make a ball the size of your brain. No wonder it responds so sensitively to stress or so well to mind-control and relaxation techniques – an estimated half of all hospital in-patient gastro cases have an unknown but 'probably' psychological cause.

To find a professional therapist who can teach you how to put yourself into light hypnosis and send your abdomen the instructions it needs, see under 'Therapies and Therapists' in the Directory. **Autogenic Training** is another highly effective way to do this, as several research studies into idiopathic gastric problems (stomach complaints for which no one can find the cause) show. For information and classes in autogenic training, contact the British Association for Autogenic Training and Therapy (BAFATT), or if you live in south-west England, contact the Centre for Autogenic Training (CAT). For contact details, see under 'Training Courses' in the Directory

Immunity

66. The Happiness Boost

If you want to stay healthy and keep your immune system strong, *deliberately relive your favourite happy memories*. Regularly. Also deal with, and move on from, the bad memories – if you dwell on them, they'll make you ill. (See Forgiveness Process page 326.)

A study in 2004 by the Association of Research Into the Science of Enjoyment (ARISE) at the University of Reading found that when volunteers were made to relive traumatic or guilt-ridden experiences, their antibody production slumped, yet reliving happy times doubled their output of these disease-battling cells.

Set aside a few minutes a day (tucked up in bed at night or relaxing in a warm bath) to replay the happy times in your head and just see how many fewer infections you catch this winter.

67. Indigestion: music to avoid

Should you suffer from indigestion, don't listen to rock music when you're eating: it raises levels of stress and excitation hormones like adrenaline and cortisol, can produce anxiety symptoms like muscular tension in the gut and may also interfere with your stomach's production of digestive enzymes.[43]

Insect Bites

68. Colour as a Mosquito Repellent

If you want mosquitoes to steer clear of you this summer, wear light colours for an evening drink outside, as well as repellent. They don't care for **yellow**, **orange** or **white**, says Neil Holliday, head of the Department of Entomology at the University of Manitoba, but will zone in on people wearing **navy**, **burgundy** or **brown**.

69. Wipe Away winged biters

Question: what smells good (contains essential oils whose mix is based on research by the Benakeio Foundation in Athens, Greece), sends biting insects packing and also soothes post-leg-wax soreness? Answer: the Greek anti-insect wipes from Apivita and Propoline: five for £5 (or 100ml lotion for £5.70) via Victoria Health. This one's multi-purpose and really good to put on itchy bites too, providing the skin's not broken or oozing.

70. The All-Round Remedy

Ledum 30c is the best all-round insect-bite remedy to keep in your bathroom cabinet. It is available in the UK from homeopathic pharmacies like Ainsworths (£4.75).

Use unless the area is really red, swollen and hot, as with some European mosquito bites, in which case try **Apis 30c** instead.

There is also a great topical natural spray called **SOS Rescue** that soothes cuts, grazes and insect bites, and is gentle enough to use on babies – many anti-bite preparations aren't. Recommended by the alternative *Which?*-style magazine *Proof*, this is a must for every bathroom cabinet and can be bought from Barefoot Botanicals (75 ml, £9.95).

If you don't have these to hand and you need something immediately (rather than pre-ordering for, say, a holiday medical kit), ferret in the kitchen cupboard for some **baking soda**. Dissolve it in iced water until it tastes quite strong and apply to the sting to reduce itching.

For all contact details, see under 'Shopping' in the Directory.

Jet Lag

71. Smart Stuff That Helps

- **Reset your watch** to the time of your destination the minute you board. Begin getting used to the fact that this is the time you are living to from now on.
- **Take an essence.** Australian Bush Flower **Travel Essence** or **Travel Ease** from Alaskan Essences are both very helpful and suitable for all ages. Place drops under the tongue throughout the journey.
- **Avoid alcohol.** It ups the risk of dehydration, which makes jet lag worse.
- **Drink water.** If you're long haul, take a 1.5 litre bottle of spring water for each person and sip throughout.
- **Eat right.** You should have a high-protein breakfast (e.g. bacon and eggs or a boiled egg) and a high-carb supper (e.g. pasta or bread). Protein promotes wakefulness; carbs encourage sleepiness.

Travel Essence can be bought via Healthlines (bottle, 30 ml, £7.95; spray, 50 ml, £8.95), as can Travel Ease (bottle, 30 ml, £10.95; spray, 60 ml, £11.95). For contact details, see under 'Shopping' in the Directory.

72. Melatonin Magic

You can buy a synthetic form of **melatonin**, the hormone that relieves jet lag by regulating the body clock. Its release is stimulated by dark and suppressed by light.

Melatonin has been subject to many clinical trials. [44] The majority of research suggests it is effective for jet lag in most people, but concern over both short-term side effects (abdominal cramps, fatigue, dizziness, headache and irritability) and the possibility of long-term ones have meant that you can't buy it over the counter in many European countries, Australia or Canada though you can in the US. In the UK, you can order melatonin from Biovea (60 x l mg tablets, £6.97). For contact details, see under 'Shopping' in the Directory.

Note: the correct timing of the dosage is crucial or you may make your jet lag worse.

73. Bright Light

You can correct your body clock by stimulating the release of natural melatonin and the mood-enhancing hormone serotonin using full spectrum or natural light.[45] If you are going east, you need to get plenty early in the day after arrival; if you're going west, it needs to be at the end of the day.

The light intensity you'd need to take effect is 3,000 lux, which is not always available outside, depending on cloud cover and weather, and may not be easy to get if you are expected to stay inside – e.g. if on a business trip.

If you have the money, frequent long-haul travellers could buy a small **lightbox** (£100–£280). Type 'broad-spectrum lightboxes' into the Internet and you will be deluged. One very good company in the UK, however, is Outside In.

If you've not tried light therapy for long term use before, it is suggested you start with a unit that beams out 10,000 lux and sit at arm's length away from it while eating breakfast or even first thing at work with the unit on your desk (it's the size of a slim briefcase) for approximately 40–45 minutes and see how you feel. You can lower the dose a bit if need be (to, for example 35 minutes). One of the best-value products sold by Outside In is called a Pharos (£220). In the US and Canada, see Alaskan Northern Lights.

You can also try a battery-powered **light visor**, which can be worn on the journey (approximately £160). Outside In can give a detailed practical explanation of how to use a light visor depending on the number of time zones you will be crossing.

For all contact details, see under 'Shopping' in the Directory.

For more information, see General: Seasonal Affective Disorder (SAD) on page 85, Fix 298: Light Therapy and Notes on page 548.

74. Homeopathy Route

A combination homeopathic pill called **No-Jet-Lag** has been developed in New Zealand. A small but strict double-blind placebo trial with skiers travelling from Auckland to Frankfurt through 12 time zones found it was effective for three-quarters of them.

The passengers taking it found it easier to sleep during the flight and regain normal sleep patterns afterwards. They also found that they had less leg and ankle swelling during the journey and didn't feel so tired after the flight. Further research carried out in 1994 with 288 cabin crew on punishing long-haul flights between New Zealand, Asia, North America and Europe, in conjunction with their professional union, found 'good to very good' all-round results for 75 per cent, and 87 per cent said it relieved their tiredness. [46]

You can buy No-Jet-Leg direct from the manufacturer or, in the UK, from NZ Health (32 tablets, 50 hours' flytime, £6.50). For contact details, see under 'Shopping' in the Directory.

Migraine

75. Herbal help

Feverfew used to be the herb of choice for migraine sufferers, but another one called **butterbur** (*Petasites hybridus*) is now becoming a favourite, partly because it seems to work faster.

Its active extract works by blocking the action of the body's natural production of prostaglandins and leukotreines, which cause inflammation.

Butterbur extract is now licensed in Germany as a pharmacy medicine after trials suggested a 60 per cent reduction in the frequency of migraine attacks.

A recent piece of strict double-blind placebo research carried out by nine different clinics and hospitals across America on 245 migraine sufferers found that two daily doses of either 50 mg or 75 mg active ingredient a day cut the number of attacks by half.[47] Other trials have found butterbur helps children with migraine too.

In the UK, butterbur extract is available from Victoria Health, who also distribute the anti-migraine nasal spray Sinol (£12.95) and the soothing Hot & Cold Magnetic Relief Mask (£14.95), which is useful as an adjunct to other anti-migraine measures and medications, natural or drug-based. For information on how magnets can relieve pain as effectively as strong painkillers, see page 20.

Petadolex, the standardised active ingredient of butterbur root developed in Germany and used in the trials, is available through Physician Formulas in the US and worldwide. For contact details, see under 'Shopping' in the Directory.

Migraine-Buster Tip

Keep a full hot-water bottle in the freezer, suggests the Migraine Action Association. When the early-warning signs begin, wrap it in a tea towel and lay your head against it for a few minutes. For some, this can stop an attack in its tracks.

See also Teenagers: Headaches on page 354, Houses and Gardens: Electromagnetic Fields on pp 479–83 and Work and Office: Desks and Workstations on pp 506–9.

Panic Attacks

Unless someone has experienced a full-blown panic attack themselves, they may not know how immensely distressing these attacks are. They are disabling surges of overwhelming fear and distress that arrive like a tidal wave, seemingly from nowhere. Your heart rate shoots up, breathing can be difficult, you may pour with sweat, shake, feel irrationally terrified, fear that you are actually going to die and think you are losing your grip on reality.

In any one year, one in three Americans has a panic attack, and so do an estimated half a million to a million people in the UK, making it the most common psychological problem on both sides of the Atlantic, way ahead of depression, which receives a lot more attention, recognition, public sympathy and support. For some contacts, see under 'Useful Helplines, Websites and Contacts' in the Directory.

Medical treatments
The usual treatment is with anti-anxiety drugs such as Xanax.

Complementary treatments and psychotherapy
The most commonly used non-drug treatments are hypnotherapy, psychotherapy ('talking' therapies), meditation and **timeline therapy (TL)**, an adjunct to neuro-linguistic programming, which can work, if it's going to, very swiftly. To find a TL therapist near you in the UK, get in touch with the Association of NLP Practitioners; in the US, try NLP-Practitioners.com. For contact details, see under 'Therapies and Therapists' in the Directory. Regular Tai chi and qi gong, which can also be very grounding, and calming as well as being good exercise and flexibility-promoters, are popular as longer term approaches to anxiety and panic control too.

Re-programming the Brain for Calm
However, there is another approach that's well worth looking at as it seems to be getting good results and claims a 96 per cent sustained success rate. It is a self-help system that combines some basic re-programming of the brain's response to stress and panic triggers with behavioural strategies.

Called the **Linden method**, it is based on targeting the amygdala area of the mid-brain, the neurological centre responsible for our emotional and panic responses. The programme offers the 'how-to' system itself in a series of simple teaching modules on CD-Rom or video to use at home, plus unlimited access to trained counsellors and, encouragingly, a 12-month money-back guarantee on its standard £117 package, which can be bought from the Linden Centre. For contact details, see under 'Training Courses' in the Directory.

Pain (Chronic)

76. White Willow Bark Extract

People with chronic pain like lower-back pain, arthritis and fibromyalgia who find the usual non-steroidal anti-inflammatory drugs (NSAIDs) such as aspirin upset their stomach lining could find both decent pain relief and an end to stomach problems if they switch to **white willow bark extract**.

White willow bark also contains buffering agents, absent in its artificial form, which help to protect the stomach: a major plus-point since in the UK alone the yearly bill for treating the gastric bleeding caused by anti-inflammatory drugs is currently around £380 million. Its major active ingredient is salicin, which has been (artificially) synthesised as aspirin. When buying white willow bark extract, check to see how much salicin each tablet contains – the recommended dose is 240 mg salicin daily (which could be split into three doses of 80 mg). The amount of salicin in different products varies, so make sure you are getting enough.

Several respectable double-blind placebo studies, including one of 210 arthritis patients in the *American Journal of Medicine* in 2000, confirm white willow bark's effectiveness.

See also General: Backache on page 26, General: Arthritis on page 12 and General: Fibromyalgia on page 51.

77. Nexrutine

If you would like to carry on taking NSAIDs rather than natural painkilling agents but are worried about the potential effect on your gut lining, consider using **Nexrutine** to help protect it. Nexrutine was developed from the rue plant to prevent the common side effects of conventional anti-arthritis drugs – gastric irritation and erosion of the stomach lining – and has recently become available in supplement form.

In clinical trials, nine out of every ten volunteers who took it for two weeks reported they had no gastric problems any more when taking their usual NSAIDs.

Try Nexrutine Cox-2 Inhibitor by LifeTime from Victoria Health (90 capsules, £19.95).

Parking

78. Parking Spaces and How to Get Them

Have you ever noticed that some people just seem to find parking spaces when they need them while others can't? Part of this may be because the former simply expect to do so: since energy follows thought, you prepare the ground for a thing to happen by believing firmly that it will.

However, if you feel it would take more than (possibly misplaced) confidence to get you a spot in the centre of town on a gridlocked Saturday when it's bristling with traffic wardens, ask for help from your guardian angel. You may be startled by how well this works: you'll usually find a space within a couple of minutes. Sometimes less.

How?

Personal guardian angels don't just deal with the big stuff (healing, protection, inspiration, guidance, comforting . . .) They can, and do, help with the small things that make life go more smoothly as well. You may think it's frivolous to ask something as remarkable and special as an angel to help you find a parking spot, but they will be happy to help you out as long as you:

- don't overdo it
- ensure it's your own angel you're asking
- ask with respect and love.

However, there is certainly an angelic hierarchy, so it probably wouldn't go down that well to ask, say, Zadkiel, the Archangel of (amongst other things) Abundance, to find you a meter with money still in it (beings like Zadkiel generally deal with larger issues). For more about this, see 'Which Archangel helps with what?' on page 540 Appendix 1.

For how to connect with your guardian angel in the first place, please see pages 546 to 547 in appendix 3. After you have done so fully the first couple of times, it will be much easier and quicker on other occasions

– such as when you are driving around town, where you don't have time for the peace, quiet and full 'tuning-in' ceremony.

At moments like that when you need help quickly, just ask your angel silently and politely in your head, with purpose and focus, to *'Please help me . . . (find a legal parking spot round here right now),'* or whatever it is that you need. And they will.

It's also important to say 'thank you' genuinely and wholeheartedly when that space, or other help you asked for, does appear. Everyone likes being thanked properly (apart from being good manners, it encourages others to help you again in the future) and angels are no exception.

Will this really work?
People tend to be thoroughly sceptical until they have tried it – then they find out it does work. However, there are a couple of provisos. One is that someone asks respectfully, believing and expecting help to come to them, rather than in the spirit of 'Duh! What a load of nonsense, but I suppose I might as well – the damn car park's full anyway.'

Also know that your guardian angel is more than happy to help you with anything at all, provided that it:

- harms no one
- isn't something that's needed more by anyone else at this time (e.g. in the case of a parking spot for a disabled person who cannot walk far)
- is for your highest possible good.

Highest possible good
What's that? Here's a small working example: you are driving round town, no parking slots to be had anywhere and you're getting late for an appointment. So you ask your angel to help find you a space quickly, *without* adding that you would like this to work out for your highest good. Sure enough, you see a vacant slot and in you go.

However, you don't notice that the spot you were in such a hurry to get was slap by a lethal T-junction, and when you return, you find that another vehicle has pulverised your car's nearside brake lights on their way round the corner. There is another space a bit further down the road – one where you wouldn't have got your lights smashed. Had you stipulated that it should be for your 'highest possible good', you would have been shown that instead.

Angel information

Background reading: if you are interested in finding out more about this area, there is a lovely, straightforward and extremely practical book by Diana Cooper called *A Little Light on Angels*, which makes a great starter title since it neither 'goes on,' nor gives too much personalised, anecdotal or whimsical information – which unfortunately, many other books on this subject can do.

Diana Cooper is a bestselling author and healer, and is also the UK's leading authority on angels and Atlantis. If you would like to read a bit further still, see also her other books, *Living With Angels* and *Angel Inspiration*.

Parties

79. How to Walk In and Be Accepted Immediately

Someone you've never seen before has opened the door, you walk in and are engulfed by a room full of people but you can't spot a single person you know. You are seriously considering sliding off home. But wait. Body-language expert Judi James's techniques will ensure you're welcomed and included right away.

Do some groundwork

- **Before you leave home**, check out the dress code. Wear clothes you can move in easily, that are comfortable but look good on you.
- Wear something minor as an ice-breaker that people can comment on or ask you where you got it, e.g. an eye-catching pair of earrings or a small designer pin stuck casually in the lapel of your jacket.
- Script yourself. Have a 15- to 30-second spiel ready on who you are and what you do.

- Prepare two or three cultural trivia nuggets and opinions, whether it's the newest superbug scare, last night's *Big Brother* or the return of the basque as outerwear.

Enter well: do the 3 Ps

- **Pause** before you go in. If you're already in, and panicking, make for the loo or coat room and shut the door to give yourself a moment.
- **Posture** – pull yourself up to your full height, push your shoulders back and down. It decreases anxiety and relaxes the hands.
- **Performance** – pretend you are an actor, a PR, press officer or anyone who is mixing socially because it is just an enjoyable part of your job – one that you are good at and do every day. Relax your facial muscles. Now smile.

Travel light

- Get rid of your coat, hide your bag (if you have one) and hand over your bottle so nothing's weighing you down.
- Get yourself a drink. Ensure you hold it with one hand near waist level rather than with both hands clutched round it at chest level: that looks anxious, hamster-like and as if you are putting up a barrier.
- Food – pick things that are easy and tidy to eat (pass on the chicken wings, flaky filo thing-ettes and noisy crisps) or leave it out altogether.

The approach

Go up to a group – any group you like the look of. Remember, if they don't work out there's lots of others. Look purposeful as you approach, keep your pace steady and don't rush.

Smile, and stand a metre away, turning your shoulder slightly towards whoever is speaking or appears to be dominant in the group. This indicates that you would like to 'insert yourself' into the company.

Wait just three seconds and certainly no longer than ten for them to let you in. They usually will.

However, if they've not done so by then, they're not going to, so to avoid being stranded there looking sad, behave (casually: no big grins or frantic waving) as if you've just seen someone you know and move *unhurriedly* away in that direction. Repeat as necessary, neither slowing nor stopping, until you have found a group you like that admits you.

You're in. Now what?

- Wait until whoever was speaking in the group has finished. Join in with a bit of nodding and eye contact.
- After a couple of minutes make a casual but positive remark about what they just said – e.g. 'You're quite right about . . .'
- Pick up on the next thing the dominant person in the group says and take it further: 'You mentioned you'd seen Razorlight play last week: doesn't one of them live in a former floating Chinese restaurant on the Thames?' Before you know it you are one of the group and chatting away nineteen to the dozen.

In general

- Mirror the group's behaviour: do as they do. This will help you achieve pack acceptance. If they're talking about new films, ask if anyone's seen a recent one you've seen and throw in a brief, informed comment on it. If they're telling jokes and laughing, listen appreciatively and laugh too, even if it's not really your sort of joke.
- Be slightly deferential to the person who appears to be group leader.
- Be a good listener. This means listening 'actively'. Also known as 'aerobic listening'. It makes other people feel appreciated and special, and they'll automatically like anyone who can do that for them.

People who can really listen are seen as terrific conversationalists, even when they've barely said a thing.

Active listening isn't just waiting until the other person's stopped talking. Good listeners will:

- look interested
- use eye contact
- turn towards the person you are listening to slightly, even when you are in a group
- mirror their body posture
- nod as you listen. Do this a little faster to show enthusiasm (careful, though: nod too fast and it means 'shut up' in body language) but slower for sympathy.
- make other visual responses where appropriate: smiling, raising an eyebrow, perhaps the occasional slight tilt of the head.

Use emphatic hand gestures as you speak: it makes more of an impact. People will take in at least 15 per cent more if a speaker is using their hands.[48]

Time to move on
Leaving a group
Leaving a group easily, with charm and without looking rude or hurting anyone's feelings can sometimes be as hard as joining a new group. But you don't want to get stuck. Here are some techniques that make breaking away simple and seamless:

- If you are in a group, turn yourself outwards a bit. The person next to you should mirror this, to help create a gap in the ranks. Do the same if you are in a pair, talking to one person – as you turn out a little, so should they.
- Say in a friendly way, 'It's been good to meet you, but I must just speak to X over there. See you later, I hope?' and leave gracefully.

Leaving one person
If you are with one person, a kind but effective withdrawal line would be, 'It's been really nice to meet you, but I think we're meant to mingle

a bit. Now, who else do you think looks good to talk to?' If they don't pick up on the hint (perhaps they really like you, or are shy), be nice. Help them out by taking them along. Try:

- 'I need to catch up with Y before he leaves – would you like to come over too?'
- 'Tell you what, shall we go talk to so-and-so?'
- 'By the way, have you met X? No? Must introduce you – I think you might like her.'
- 'Shall we go and say hello to Y over there?'

Should the person take up your offer to come with you rather than let you leave them behind, don't worry: it is far easier to gently detach from someone when you've both joined a new group.

Don't escape by saying say you must go and get a drink. They may interpret this as a sign they're meant to wait for you till you come back.

Getting stuck with someone

Try not to sit down to talk to someone (unless you know them well or want a long chat), especially if they are on the edge of the room. You are liable to get stuck there. If you do happen to get trapped:

1. Stand up slowly, but leave a hand touching your chair to suggest gradual separation, and carry on talking.
2. After a moment or two, remove your hand from the chair, turn slightly outwards away from the person.
3. Proceed with the options given above for 'Leaving one person'.

See also Work and Office: Networking on page 521.

Personal Space

80. Back *Off!*

This quick and easy visualisation technique can be invaluable when someone is in your face, pressurising you or trying to invade your personal space.

People report using it to good effect in a wide variety of situations: a barman serving a drunken customer who persists in talking *at* him; a young girl being chatted up by an older man of whom she is nervous; a mother driving her children to school while the car behind tries to make her go faster than is safe by sticking so close behind she can see the driver's face in her rear-view mirror.

The method is called the **Bulletproof Screen** and works immediately.

1. Take a deep breath.
2. As you let it out, send energy down through your feet and deep into the earth.
3. Now take another deep in-breath. Breathe out strongly and at the same time imagine you are pulling down (hard) in one swift, strong movement on the handle of a bulletproof Perspex screen, unrolling it between you and the offending party. Bang! It's in place.
4. Now the barrier is down, say firmly in your head, '*In the name of Light, I do not permit you to affect me.*'
5. If the person is being really intrusive, imagine you're whisking down that screen again a second time – and then again a third time. Now you've got three-star, triple-glazed protection.
6. Should you need to, continue to interact calmly with this person through your screen. As you do so, in your mind's eye see it glinting between you and your aggressor, protecting you completely from anything that comes from them, like (as one 11-year-old Nintendo enthusiast put it) 'a hero's shield bouncing back the rays from a villain's zap-gun'.

Your screen should prevent anything your aggressor sends out from reaching you. Spiritual law teaches that 'Energy follows thought.' And your own thoughts have just created something very powerful.

However, if you still feel you need extra backup, it's there. Call in your mind upon Michael, Archangel of Courage, Protection and Strength, and ask for his help. He is the mightiest of all the archangels, and his powerful sheltering energy is always available to those who ask.

See also Fix 138: Someone's Crowding You.

80. Be SomeBody

Body beginning to look its age? Try some gentle weights. A year of regular light weight-training can turn the body's clock back *15 years* in terms of metabolism, strength, muscle bulk, flexibility, blood pressure and levels of some hormones.[49] Loss of strength and muscle mass or tone are the underlying causes of most outward signs of aging.

See also Fix 103: Meditation as Age-Reversal and Women: Anti-Aging on page 108.

Pessimism

81. Complaining and Pessimistic Characters

There is a remedy called **Wild Violet** from Living Essences of Australia, also known as the 'essence of optimism', for when you just can't shake that 'life's a bitch and then you die' feeling.

Who is it for?
Someone who:

- moans a lot
- can't seem to find a good word to say about anyone any more
- is fatalistic, pessimistic, a kill-joy and worry-wort
- underneath it all, is apprehensive about everything
- stops you from experiencing life
- finds, later in life, that they can't feel positive any more.

What does it do?
Wild Violet gives you:

- a positive spin on life
- the ability to reach out and enjoy life again
- the capacity to trust new opportunities more, even when you don't know the outcome
- a balance between courageous optimism and caution.

Put 35 drops of Wild Violet in a 30 ml dropper bottle, then make up the rest with three-quarters brandy, one-quarter spring water and shake. Take six drops of the mixture in water morning and evening until you feel better.

You can purchase Wild Violet worldwide from Living Essences of Australia or, in the UK, from the Essence Shop (15 ml, £7.55). For contact details, see under 'Shopping' in the Directory.

Relationships

82. Drifting Apart

'Drifting apart' is now the leading factor behind divorce – even beating infidelity. In a 2005 survey of 546 UK divorces by YouGov, 'gradually drifting away' from each other was given as the main reason for nearly 50 per cent of marriage break-ups, whereas an unfaithful partner was the prime factor for 30 per cent.

For lovers, husbands and wives who find they're becoming like flat-mates or who are losing sight of each other, the emotional 'reconnecting essence' **Red and Green Kangaroo Paw** can help bring you back together and become more aware of each other once again.

Note: you must *both* take it.

Red and Green Kangaroo Paw can be purchased worldwide from Living Essences of Australia (approximately £7). For contact details, see under 'Shopping' in the Directory.

83. Cooling Off

Have you been living with your partner for a long time and have found things are beginning to falter? You may already be doing many things to help resolve this – from talking together and seeing a relationship counsellor to taking pro-sexuality nutrients and going on minibreaks – but feng shui marriage-strengthening measures are well worth trying too. The effect is not immediate, but cumulative and stabilising.

This very simple technique was recommended to me by a traditional feng shui practitioner of 35 years, a spiritual but humorous, no-nonsense Black Hat Tibetan monk named Arto, who for many years was one of the UK's foremost feng shui workers.

1. Locate the 'relationships corner' of your home. For how to find it, see Fix 423: Bagua Your Space (No. 4).
2. Find seven pink ribbons and a white one. They should be around 90 cm long and of equal length. Pin them in your 'relationships corner' where the walls meet the ceiling.
3. Place a small table beneath them. Put a loving picture of you and your partner together on there, with a small vase or pot containing real flowers with either red or pink blooms. If they are roses, ensure they have no thorns. Keep these fresh at all times, except when you are away on holiday and cannot replace them.

84. Breaking up

Going forward after a break-up can be incredibly difficult. One of the most common post-relationship problems, apart from sadness, is feeling stuck in the past. However, if you need a bit of ongoing internal support, there is a terrific mixture of two Australian Bush Flower essences from the tough red outback.

The first essence, **Bauhinia**, helps combat:

- resistance to change
- reluctance to move forwards.

It encourages:

- open-minded acceptance
- flexibility.

- The second, **Bottlebrush**, is for people feeling overwhelmed by a life-change and brings:

- serenity
- the ability to get on with the next stage in life
- the confidence to cope with whatever comes.

Place seven drops of each essence in a 30 ml dropper bottle, make up with two-thirds pure spring water and one-third brandy (to preserve it), and you have one of the most powerful but gentle 'moving-on-helpers' there is. Take seven drops twice a day until you are feeling better.

You can buy the essences direct from Australian Bush Flower Essences or Healthlines (15 ml, £8.95 each). They last a long time. Alternatively, Healthlines can make up a mixture for you far more cheaply, so you don't have to buy two separate ones, and will mail it to you within 24 hours. For contact details, see under 'Shopping' in the Directory.

For suggestions specifically for men, see Men: Women and Relationships on page 235. See also Fix 56: The Look.

Repetitive Strain Injury (RSI)

RSI is now the most common work-related illness reported in the West and it has many different names, depending on which part of the body it affects – you've probably heard of racquet wrist, golfer's shoulder, tennis elbow, and violinist's or keyboard wrist? The latter two are also known as carpal tunnel syndrome.

The carpal tunnel is the narrow passageway through the wrist down which your nerves and tendons travel into your hand. If the tunnel's tissues become swollen and inflamed by injury or overuse, they can squash the nerves running through the area, causing pain, numbness and tingling.

If you have RSI of any type but don't deal with it promptly, it will worsen, eventually meaning you can't play that sport you love without pain, or if it's developed as a result of keyboard work, that you might have to give up your job. So it's crucial not to ignore the sysmtoms, becasue they won't go away on their own.

Medical treatments: what helps?
Seeing your GP, who will probably give you painkillers and anti-inflammatory drugs and recommend resting the joint(s) for many weeks. May also offer supportive strapping.

Seeing a good sports physiotherapist as soon as possible. There is usually one based at or affiliated to major sports or health clubs; word of mouth is a good way to find a reputable sports physio, but in the UK you can also try the Sports Injury Clinic; in Canada, try the Sport Physiotherapy Canada website for your nearest one. For contact details, see under 'Therapies and Therapists' in the Directory.

85. Complementary treatments: supplements

As this is a condition caused by inflammation, one of the very best things you can do is to *take a temporary rest* from whatever brought it on and take a good natural anti-inflammatory. For suggestions, see General: Pain (Chronic) on page 67 and Fix 12: Herbs and Spices.

Also take **cod-liver, flaxseed** or **borage (starflower) oil** to help derail those enzymes producing ongoing inflammation. Nature's Best do a good range: try their Flaxseed Oil (90 x 1 g capsules, £8.95) or Borage Oil (100 x 100 mg capsules, £9.95). For contact details, see under 'Shopping' in the Directory.

Some people with carpal tunnel syndrome are short of **vitamin B6**, which supplementation can correct, says neurologist Dr Shreyas Patel of the Queen Elisabeth Hospital and also formerly of the Marino Center for Progressive Health, Boston. Vitamin B is available from any health food shop. Dr Patel adds that 100 mg twice daily helps his RSI patients reduce the amount of painkillers they need.

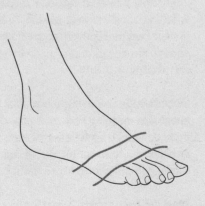

Other Things to Try

86. DIY reflexology

You can also help relieve pain from RSI with simple self-reflexology. Press gently but firmly on the relevant area (see picture) five times daily for three minutes at a time to help stimulate the release of anti-inflammatory substances in the body and soothe the discomfort.

> **87. Cut the coffee**
> Coffee can make the pain of RSI worse. Try switching to other hot drinks like herb teas flavoured with honey, a caffeine-free tea like **11 O'Clock Rooibosch** (though any caffeine-free brand will do fine), plain water, milk and hot juices. Research shows that instant coffee blocks the opiate (painkilling chemical) receptors in the brain, which makes you more sensitive to all types of discomfort.[50]

Restless Leg Syndrome (RLS)

Restless leg syndrome can be a puzzling condition and is not always easy to treat. There seem to be two different sets of symptoms:

1. shooting pain or cramps in your lower limbs that are usually worse at night and often accompanied by numbness
2. periodic spasm in your legs and they sometimes seem to have a life of their own (hence the 'restless' bit).

88. Nutrition Route
RLS is often caused by a biochemical imbalance: something that you are eating that doesn't agree with you or a vital vitamin, mineral or nutrient you are lacking. A classic cause is a shortage of **folic acid**.[51] Some drugs can interfere with the amount of folic acid you absorb, including H2-blockers for stomach problems, the Pill and even ordinary aspirin, which is ironic if you are taking it to ease the pain of cramping.

What helps?

- **Take supplements of folic acid.** Sufferers may sometimes need doses up to six times higher than is usual, so it is important to check with a nutritionist, who would also need to supervise you while you were using this amount.

- **Keep your blood sugar steady: don't skip meals.** In one study of 350 people with RLS, nearly all were found to have low blood sugar levels.[52] Eat plenty of complex carbohydrates as they release energy slowly and steadily into your body (e.g. baked potatoes, pasta, porridge, muesli and wholemeal bread).
- **Give up caffeine** – that includes not only coffee but tea, colas and anything with cocoa in it, like chocolate.[53]
- **Get your iron levels checked.** Studies suggest a quarter of people with RLS don't have enough iron in their blood.[54]

Ringworm

Ringworm is not a worm at all but a contagious fungal infection – the same one that causes athlete's foot – affecting the scalp, skin and nails. It tends to start as a small round itchy spot, then develops into a scaly mark that heals from the centre, spreading outwards to its edge, giving the appearance of a ring.

89. Propolis & Probiotics

If it is proving hard to get rid of, **bee propolis** works well – one Eastern European study in 1989 found that of 110 people with hard-to-shift ringworm, 97 were cleared when they used a cream containing 50 per cent propolis. For more information about the healing power of bee propolis, see Fix 64: Bee'ing Herpes-Free.

If you have ringworm, it is well worth cutting out yeast and sugar for six to eight weeks as fungal infections love them. Also take **probiotic** supplements (capsules of beneficial bacteria, e.g. by Bioforce) for six to eight weeks. For more information about probiotics, see Fix 7: After Antibiotics and Young Children: After Antibiotics on page 242.

See also Athlete's Foot (Tinea Pedis) on page 25.

Scars

90. Reducing the Appearance

Rosehip oil can help reduce the appearance of certain types of scarring, according to American research carried out in 2002, including scarring from acne, surgery and burns, and may even help stretch marks.[55] The oil contains fatty substances that are thought to work by supporting the regeneration of the skin's collagen scaffolding. For the best results, rub it in twice daily for several months.

Pure rosehip oil is available in most health shops. If it is hard to find in your area, you can buy it via Medshop or, in the US, through Zooscape. For contact details, see under 'Shopping' in the Directory.

91. Sore, Red Scars

For sore, red post-operative or accident scars and stitching, an excellent tip – once the wound has closed properly and so long as there is no infection – is to use a mixture of **arnica cream** and **Angelsword** (from Australian Bush Flower Essences). To make 'Angel Cream', mix a 5p-sized blob of arnica cream with two drops of Angelsword and apply topically twice daily. It speeds healing, soothes soreness and reduces the angry appearance of recently sutured areas. Arnica can be bought in most chemists. Angelsword can be purchased direct or from Healthlines (15 ml, £8.95), Flower Sense and IFER. For contact details, see under 'Shopping' in the Directory.

Note: if your scars are inflamed or puffy, check with your doctor as the area is probably infected and may need additional medical treatment.

See also Teenagers: Scars on page 368.

92. Cold Sores

Pierce a capsule of vitamin E and squeeze the oil on to a cotton bud or tissue, then dab at the cold sore. Or, better still, soak a bigger piece of cotton wool well in the oil and hold it over the sore for 10–15 minutes twice a day. This brings topical relief and can clear up the sore (they can be pretty persistent sometimes) within a couple of days.[56]

See also Fix 64: Bee'ing Herpes Free on page 59.

Sciatica and Nerve Inflammation

Want an easy, drug-free treatment that relieves pain in minutes? Try a professional therapist's frozen gel pack on the area.

93. Cool Tip

Called the **TheraFlex**, it takes the heat out of nerve inflammation (which is what is causing the pain) and also acts as a local anaesthetic and painkiller. Pliable and comfortable, it takes an hour to get cold enough to work well and moulds itself to your body shape, unlike the lumpy packets of frozen peas usually suggested.

Do not put against bare skin as this could give you a cold burn, but wrap in a thin, clean tea towel – or a cotton T-shirt, even a pair of men's cotton-jersey boxers. The TheraFlex is available from osteopaths and chiropractors. You can also buy it from Natremed (30cm x 9cm, £6.95). For contact details, see under 'Shopping' in the Directory.

If the sciatica is very sore, you can use it for 5–15 minutes once an hour: it stops any pain and inflammation building up so you are both far more comfortable, and your body can heal more easily. Often, it's the build-up of inflamation over several days or even weeks that can make sciatica so difficult to either treat really effectively, or get rid of altogether – but these cool packs can prevent that happening.

If you're having treatment

If you have just had osteopathic or chiropractic treatment for the problem (or indeed any other sort of back, shoulder or neck pain), put the TheraFlex on as soon as you get home, then at intervals for the rest of the day to reduce post-treatment pain. If you have been given any exercises to enhance recovery but they make you sore, the TheraFlex is useful there too.

Baths

Use the TheraFlex if you have just had a hot, soothing bath. Baths are bliss for sciatica and backpain sufferers because the heat both relaxes the spasmed back muscles, which are causing pain by squeezing the nerve fibres threaded through them, and also soothes pain by stimulating the release of endorphins. However, hot baths unfortunately also exacerbate inflammation so the area needs to be cooled down again promptly when you get out.

See also General: Pain (Chronic) on page 67 and Women: (Mothers) Backs on page 127.

Seasonal Affective Disorder (SAD)

94. Treatments for SAD
Try:

- a **lightbox** (£100–£280), which weigh 3.5–4.5 kg.
- a **light visor** – similar to a tennis visor and not that much heavier, these have a powerful little battery-powered light unit in the brim. They are similar to those worn by astronauts in an international space station. You can potter about the house wearing them or they can be worn on aeroplane journeys. They were developed by the National Institute of Health Research in America, the organisation that first diagnosed and validated SAD. Contact Outside In for products and for a detailed practical explanation of how to use them.
  Note: Outside In's Solarmax visor is as effective as a bulky 10,000 lux lightbox and provides 100 times the amount of light you'd get in the average home (£160).
- **eicosapentaenoic acid (EPA)** – the new nutritional approach for mild to moderate depression, also effective for SAD and apparently side-effect-free. See General: Depression on page 45.

St John's wort
Trials in 1994, 1997 and 1999 all confirm that St John's wort extract (hypericum) is as good as the popular full-spectrum light treatment for beating SAD – and that's saying something.[57] Even Edward Ernst, the notoriously picky professor of complementary medicine at Exeter University's School of Postgraduate Medicine says, 'St John's wort seems to be as effective as light therapy for SAD.'

It also takes less time (pill-popping two to three times daily instead of 45 minutes in front of a special light unit) and is considerably cheaper than the average £200 lightbox unit – though costs would even out over a couple of years' seasonal usage. One good, powerful source is Solgar's St John's Wort (50 capsules, £12.35). Take twice daily, preferably with meals.

Note: St John's wort is not compatible with certain drugs, including tricyclic antidepressants, SSRI inhibitors like Prozac and the Pill (so check with your doctor first if you are taking any regular medication), and might possibly, in some cases, cause photosensitivity and skin rashes.

For all contact details, see under 'Shopping' in the Directory.

See also Fix 72: Bright Light, Fix 298: Light Therapy and Notes on page 548.

Sex

95. Sex Boost

Interested in boosting your sex life by 10 per cent for free? The usual response to that question is along the lines of 'Is the Pope Catholic?' Not only is the boost free, it requires no complex study of Tantra, expensive 'herbal Viagra' or awkward pelvic exercises. It's . . . um . . . volunteering.

A 2005 study by the New Economics Foundation, which introduced Time Banks (a means of reciprocal volunteering), argues that most people 'have a serious need to make what President Kennedy called a "cause beyond self"' and that volunteers reap benefits ranging from improved confidence and employability to inches lost round the waist, reduced chocolate consumption and a better sex life.

The phenomenon is backed by 2004's 'happiness league' of UK cities: chart-toppers Bristol, Chester and Aberdeen reported the highest levels of happiness and contentment in the country and also did the most voluntary work.

If you'd like to get involved in helping your local community and see if it enhances your bedtime, see under 'Useful Helplines, Websites and Contacts' in the Directory for companies who will match you up with local initiatives.

96. If You're Too Stressed to Want It

If this is the case for you, you aren't alone. Lovemaking has become the latest casualty of our 24/7 culture, and the TINS (two incomes, no sex) syndrome is now a common phenomenon among couples. In fact, according to recent research by a British organisation called the Chartered Institute of Personal Development, over half of all young to middle-aged adults say their sex lives are suffering because both partners work such long hours: they are simply too tired and stressed to feel like making love at the end of the day.

Hormonal downturn

Tiredness is an anti-aphrodisiac in its own right, but stress hormones also hit sexuality hard. Higher-than-usual levels of substances like adrenaline, noradrenaline, cortisol and prolactin (which triggers the making of breast milk in lactating mothers but is also produced when we are up against it) interfere with the production of sex hormones – testosterone for men, and both oestrogen and small amounts of testosterone for women – because it's the same gland, the pineal, that makes them.

Stress also decreases the production of another hormone called dehydroepiandosterone (DHEA), which has a role in regulating sex hormones and appears to slow many of the signs of aging.

So if you want your libido back, it helps – in addition to looking at sexuality-stimulating substances – to spend a bit less time working (not always possible) *and* address those elevated stress-hormone levels. One way to do so – apart from cutting back working hours and taking up an exercise, relaxation or meditation programme – is with the non-sedative anti-anxiety plant extracts *Phellodendron amurense* and *Magnolia officinalis*, which are available in a herbal combination called **Relora**. Try it with a libido-boosting supplement such as **Libilov** (for men) or the Peruvian herb **maca** for women.

In the UK, Relora is available direct from the manufacturer or through Victoria Health (90 capsules, £19.95); in the US, try Food and Vitamins (180 capsules, $22.98). In the UK, Libilov is available from Victoria Health (30 tablets, £17.95); in the US, you can buy it direct from makers Nutrica (30 tablets, $29.99). Maca can be bought in the UK through Victoria Health (120 x 750 mg capsules, £14.95); in the US, direct from Life Time (120 capsules, $16.99). For contact details, see under 'Shopping' in the Directory.

97. Sexy C

Forget pricey herbal aphrodisiacs: taking extra **vitamin C** can *triple the amount of sex you have*.

A trial of 42 healthy twenty-something adults with a steady sexual partner involved taking either 3 g vitamin C a day or dummy pills – though they weren't told which group was taking the real thing. The vitamin group started having sex ten times a month compared with three times a month for the other group – interestingly, however, it affected the women but not the men.

Note: if you try this at home, it is worth knowing that 3 g vitamin C is a high dose and may cause temporary stomach upset or mild diarrhoea. You can only really absorb 500 mg at a time – the rest is peed out and lost. So, either use a time-release product, such as Nature's Best Time-Release Vitamin C (60 x 1,500 mg tablets, £7.50), or try True Food C from Higher Nature (30 x 100 mg tablets, £5.20): most vitamin-C supplements are lost fairly rapidly from the body, but research shows this one can last up to eight hours so it's more effective. In the US, try Vitamin C With Bioflavonoids and Rosehip Extract (for easier absorption) from Greatest Herbs on Earth (90 x 500 mg tablets, $11.40). For contact details, see under 'Shopping' in the Directory.

For more suggestions specifically for women, see Women: Sex on page 185. For advice specifically for men, see Men: Sex on page 230.

Shingles

98. Homeopathic Help

A quarter of a million people develop the painful viral rash shingles every year in the UK. If an attack is just beginning, homeopaths say you can often cut it short with the right remedy. Top British medical homeopath Dr Andrew Lockie suggests taking the following every two hours for up to ten doses while waiting to see the GP:

- **Apis 6c** if the skin burns and stings
- **Arsenicum 6c** if the burning is worse between midnight and 2 a.m. or if more blisters are appearing and merging together

- *Rhus tox* 6c if warmth and movement help, if the person is young, if the skin is blistered, itchy and red or if the scalp is affected
- *Ranunculus scleratus* 6c for nerve pains and itching and if even small movements or the lightest touch make it worse.

It is felt to be good medical practice to treat shingles with a powerful antiviral agent the minute it shows itself in order to avoid a complication called post-herpetic neuralgia (PHN), which can be really miserable. It causes such skin sensitivity that even the touch of light clothing is painful and this may last for months or years. So even if the homeopathic remedies cause the shingles to die down, it is still a good idea to be checked out by your GP. Some of the above (e.g. Apis) will be available from local health shops or independent chemists; others, like Ranunculus, are less common, but you can get them via homeopathic pharmacies that offer mail order, like Helios's. For contact details, see under 'Shopping' in the Directory.

Recommended reading: *The Family Guide to Homeopathy* by Dr Andrew Lockie.

> **Comfort Tip**
> If it hurts when your clothing touches the shingles rash on your skin, try wrapping cling film over the area.

Sinusitis

99. Clear it the Yogic Way

Called sinus irrigation, this traditional technique takes a little getting used to, but it is safe and immensely effective for miserably blocked sinuses. Its traditional Indian name is *jala neti*, and it is one of the major cleansing practices in yoga. *Jala neti* involves the use of a little pot with a spout filled with boiled salt water to both clear the nasal passages and protect them from infection.

The device is simple and very easy to use. Just add some coarse sea salt to warm (not hot) water, fill up the *jala-neti* pot, then:

1. lean over the sink or basin and gently tip the salt solution into one nostril.
2. tilt your head, allowing it to trickle out of the other nostril.
3. blow your nose gently – you'll need to keep a box of tissues by you as you have to blow after each nostril cleanse.
4. repeat for the other side.

According to a six-month trial of *jala neti* with 200 yoga-class members in western Sydney, Australia, initial reactions when first told about the treatment ranged from '*Yuck, no way!*' to '*But I'll drown.*' However, many found benefits after just one session, especially those who were suffering sinusitis, asthma and hay fever. People who had long-term respiratory problems reported an 80–90 per cent improvement. Interestingly, all 200 trial participants found their sleep quality much better too. Later comments included 'relaxing', 'tingly', 'like swimming', 'I miss it if I don't do it every day' and 'I could breathe properly again at last.'

Jala-neti pots are available in the UK from the Sivananda Yoga Centre in London or, in the US, Japan and India from Health and Yoga. For contact details, see under 'Shopping' in the Directory.

For further information on the practice, visit www.jalaneti.com.

See also Young Children: Colds and Flu on page 257, Teenagers: Colds on page 334 and Fix 48: (Office) Coughs, Colds and Flu.

Shyness

100. Overcome it with essences

Most us feel shy sometimes, but for some, the feeling can make almost every day excruciating. Maybe we feel deep down that it's somehow big-headed to be confident? Yet true self-confidence isn't arrogance: it's a quiet but unshakable belief in your own value, and accepting yourself for just who you are. This can take years to achieve, but once you have it, nothing – and no one – will ever take it away from you.

All sorts of holistic approaches can help alleviate shyness by supporting someone to develop strategies to overcome or circumnavigate their doubts and fears while still remaining very much themselves, rather than encouraging them to try and 'change' their personality to become as up-front and socially resilient as an alternative comedian on newcomer's night. These approaches range from drama therapy and dance, to hypnosis, autogenic training and behavioural therapy.

Essences can be a terrific adjunct to any of these – or used on their own as a first-base 'try it and see how you get on' strategy, working gently from within to slowly but surely help develop someone's natural, innate self-confidence. And gentle though these remedies may be, they can be so effective that they're starting to be used in state hospitals worldwide, including the Texas Cancer Care Center in Fort Worth, the University Hospital of Sao Paulo and the Royal Perth Hospital in Australia.

For combatting shyness, the following are some of the very best:

- **Monkey Flower** is a gentle essence made in the spiritual community of Findhorn in Scotland and, like its surroundings, is straightforward, direct and deeply grounded. This essence can be of particular help to women, especially if they feel over apologetic.
- **Mountain Lion** from Wild Earth Animal Essences. Men especially may like this. Go roar!
- **Five Corners** from Australian Bush Flower Essences is for those who cannot seem to help giving away their power and knowledge to others for no return; being overly appeasing and on the defensive; worrying about being bullied or making the other person angry; feeling timid, nervous, afraid of criticism, put-downs or ridicule; and for those who have trouble saying no.

Monkey Flower is by Findhorn Flower Essences (15 ml, £6.90); Mountain Lion is by Wild Earth Animal Essences, available from Healthlines (30 ml, £8.95); in the US, it can be bought direct ($8.99). Five Corners is by Australian Bush Flower Essences, which can also be bought via Healthlines (15 ml, £8.95). For contact details, see under 'Shopping' in the Directory.

See also Women: Assertiveness and Confidence on page 116, Men: Shyness on page 233, Young Children: Confidence on page 261 and Teenagers: Self-Esteem on page 373.

Sleep

101. The Aromatherapy Approach

Lavender oil can be a great sleep aid, especially if you have difficulty dropping off or tend to wake frequently and find it hard to go back to sleep. Put 10–12 drops of organic lavender aromatherapy oil on your pillow or on the neckline of your nightwear so you breathe it in till morning. The oil appears to sedate lightly and steadily all night long without producing the morning 'hangover' that you get from many sleeping pills.

For lavender oil, try Baldwin's (organic, 10 ml, £4.95) or, a little cheaper but perhaps not such good quality, Holland & Barrett (10 ml, £3.99).

Who says it works?

In 1995 the University of Leicester carried out a six-week trial with a small group of elderly people who all had problems falling asleep and had relied on sedative drugs. According to the study, which appeared in *The Lancet* (an august doctors' journal not usually noted for its sympathy towards complementary therapies), the researchers found that being in a room scented with lavender oil ensured the elderly men and women 'slept like babies'. More recently, a month-long study in 2005 by the University of Southampton of ten volunteers found the same – with especially good results if you were either female or a younger candidate with *mild* insomnia.[58]

Sleep-promoting pill

One of the newest natural sleep-promoters is the gentle but effective **Seditol**, which contains extract of *Magnolia officinalis* and *Zizyphus spinosa* (used in traditional Chinese medicine). Stress-calming and muscle-relaxing, this natural medication also seems to produce mild sedation: independent trials in March 2005 found that more than 90 per cent of the 45 subjects slept soundly after taking it and woke feeling refreshed.

Seditol is available in the UK from Victoria Health (30 capsules, £12.95); in the US, try Special Gifts (30 capsules, $20). Take one an hour before bedtime.

For all contact details, see under 'Shopping' in the Directory.

102. The Sleep Shake

If pills, herbs and potions don't appeal to you, why not try the **Sleep Shake**?

1. Crush an eighth to a quarter of a cup of walnuts in a blender.
2. Add half a cup of full-fat or semi-skimmed milk.
3. Walnuts alone will do the trick, but it tastes good if you can add a teaspoon of ground flaxseed or sunflower seeds, one of lecithin granules, a pinch of powdered cinnamon, a dash of vanilla extract and a little soft brown sugar or maple syrup to taste.
4. Whizz in the blender and serve.

Drink this 30–45 minutes before bedtime to enhance sleep. Walnuts are one of the richest dietary sources of serotonin, the neurotransmitter that encourages relaxation and feelings of well-being. The milk and seeds help you to feel fuller and more satisfied.

See also Fix 451: Restoring Sleep and Relaxation and Work and Office: Sleep on page 529. For sleep advice specifically for children, see Young Children: Sleep on page 299 and Teenagers: Sleep on page 380.

103. Meditation as Age-Reversal

Forget pricey rejuvenation programmes – it's regular meditation that can knock 12 years off your age.

When a 1982 study compared a group of people with an average age of 50 who practised regular **transcendental meditation** with a similar non-meditating group and measured indicators of biological age like blood pressure and sight acuity, it found those who'd been meditating for five or more years were scoring what you'd expect to see in people whose average age was under 38.

For a class near you, contact Transcendental Meditation Independent UK. For anyone who is unemployed or a student, they have a scale of course fees from £90. For contact details, see under 'Training Courses' in the Directory.

See also Fix 80: Be SomeBody and Women: Anti-Aging on page 108.

Sore Throat
104. Tea time

Speed healing and reduce pain immediately with **red sage tea**. It is quick and easy to make, and it is not only antiseptic but when gargled with is blessedly anaesthetising on a throat that feels like it's lined with grit and glass. Red sage is also far cheaper than the cocaine-containing numbing sprays from the chemist.

To make:

1. Put two teaspoons of dried sage in a cup of boiling water.
2. Let it steep for six to ten minutes.
3. Gargle with it three to four times, keeping the mixture bathing your throat for as long as you can each time. Try not to swallow: it is very bitter.
4. Repeat three to four times daily, depending on how sore your throat is.

Any unused tea can be kept covered in the fridge for up to three days to save you making more several times a day. Red sage herb is available from some natural health and herbal stores, and from Neal's Yard. For contact details, see under 'Shopping' in the Directory.

105. Bee Better

Honey is traditionally used for sore throats and all honey types are healing to some extent, but the best and most effective antibacterial variety, according to trials by the Department of Biological Sciences in New Zealand's University of Waikato, is **unpasteurised manuka honey** from Australia and New Zealand, with an AMF, or active manuka factor, potency of ten or more. (Lower-rated honeys are cheaper but not so effective.) The dosage is a neat teaspoonful (half for a child) three times daily.

Manuka honey is available in some health shops. Look for MediBee Active UMF 10+ from Goodness Direct (250 g, £8.92) or the Comvita brand. You can also visit Manuka Honey's website. In the US, you can buy it from GloryBee. For contact details, see under 'Shopping' in the Directory.

For more information about the healing power of manuka honey, see Fix 63: Wound, Ulcer and Sore Healing.

Stress and Stamina

106. Calm the Herbal Way

Stressful job? Got a major push coming up? Party season? Everyone's got their favourite energy enhancers. But one of the best is *Rhodiola rosea* herb (also known as golden root, roseroot or Arctic root) because it's an adaptogenic herb that helps you stay calm *and* ups your energy output – most substances will only do one or the other.

Rhodiola is also a good mood-booster: a welcome plus if you're finding stress and tiredness are really getting you down. This is because it disrupts the enzyme that would otherwise be busy breaking down serotonin, your body's natural happy chemical. It has no reported side effects, but be careful how you use it as more isn't better: it will stimulate your system at lower doses but sedate you at higher ones. And it's best not to use it long term – try Astralagus instead (see page 37).

Research suggests that supplementing with *Rhodiola rosea* can significantly up your concentration levels, mental performance, athletic endeavours and infection-fighting quotient, making it the herb of choice for party animals, shift workers, sportspeople and anyone who needs to keep calm while they gear up to high-performance mode (like exam candidates). Doctors working the night shift have used it to good effect, and students' capacity for revision, sense of well-being and exam scores have been enhanced by taking it.[59] The suggested dose is 200–600 mg daily (in the form of standardised 3 per cent rosavins and 0.8–1 per cent salidroside – the active ingredients).

In the UK, check out Rhodiola and Ginkgo Complex from Home Herbs (60 tablets, £11.45); in the US, try Herbal Remedies (the common name for this herb in the US is Arctic Root). For contact details, see under 'Shopping' in the Directory.

Note: don't take this if you are pregnant or breastfeeding.

107. Energy Boost – the Vitality Colour-Breath

You don't need to see or wear a colour to benefit from it – it can work equally well if you imagine it. When you want a bit of extra energy, try the simple three-step **Vitality Colour-Breath**, devised by Theo Gimbel, founding president of the International Association of Colour Therapy.

1. Close your eyes and feel your feet firm on the ground.
2. Take a deep breath in and imagine you are breathing in a wonderful vibrant *red* colour. Hold it in for a count of five.
3. Breathe out softly and imagine the breath leaving you is *turquoise*.

Repeat this five times. When you are finished, open your eyes, stand up and stretch.

For more suggestions on stress, see Women: Stress on page 89, Work and Office: Burnout on page 488 and Work and Office: Stress on page 530.

Sunburn

For prevention, try and keep out of the sun when it's at its hottest in the four middle-of-the-day hours (you'll know all about that one already) and make like the Australians' old safe-sun campaign with **Slip, Slop, Slap** – slip on a big white T-shirt, slop on waterproof sunscreen and slap on a shady hat (not a baseball cap).

108. Essentially Soothing

If you still get a bit sunburnt, add two drops of **lavender essential oil** to a palmful of pure **aloe-vera gel** and dab it gently on the affected areas. Both are used to treat burns and have clinical trials backing their efficacy[58] and both are widely available from health shops. If you can't find any locally, try Higher Nature's Ultimate Aloe Skin Gel (60 ml, £9.20). They will also deliver to the US. If you need a good-quality mail-order organic lavender-oil supplier, try Star Child (10 ml, £5.95); in the US, try Neal's Yard website (0.34 fl oz, $32). For contact details, see under 'Shopping' in the Directory.

If the skin is blistering, swelling or you feel unwell, go to the doctor: you may have a more serious, second-degree burn that needs treating medically.

> **Paste it on**
>
> Nothing in the medicine cabinet? Head for the kitchen instead and see if you can find some **tomato paste**, as that can reduce the sting of sunburn too. This is because tomatoes contain a particular nutrient (a carotenoid called lycopene) that can be anti-inflammatory.[59]

109. Pull Away Sunburn Pain

A good DIY acupressure first-aid trick for soothing sunburn anywhere on your body is to massage both earlobes, pulling them down slightly as you do so, then massage the bridge of your nose (so long as it's not too sore to touch).

110. Take Out the Sting

To help take away the sting immediately, apply **Microvita Pain Cream** (Living Essences of Australia), which contains healing plant essences and is used by 16 pain clinics in state hospitals throughout western Australia. Microvita is sold in the UK as Body Soothe Cream and is available from Victoria Health (125 ml, £9.99) and The Essesence Shop.

If the skin's starting to feel sore and glow like a beacon, take seven drops of Australian Bush Flower 'fire' remedy **Mulla Mulla** under your tongue twice daily. You can also add ten drops to a pint of cool water and dab on gently with cotton wool to soothe. Mulla Mulla is even used for patients who have sore patches on their skin from radiotherapy treatment for cancer. It can be bought from Healthlines (15 ml, £8.95).

For all contact details, see under 'Shopping' in the Directory.

See also Fix 208: Driver's Arm.

111. Stomach-Bug Drink

Sip strong **green tea** throughout the day. Russian doctors use it successfully for a wide range of gastric infections including dysentery, and the stronger the better because American and Indian research confirms that green tea's tannins (which give that astringent taste) are both antibacterial and antiviral.[60]

Green tea is available in most health stores and good supermarkets, but if you have trouble finding some in the UK, try Grey's Teas, who have over a dozen types (125 g, from £4.80); in the US, try Green Tea Lovers. For contact details, see under 'Shopping' in the Directory.

Teeth

112. First-Aid for Toothache

When someone's got toothache but is having to wait a little to see their dentist, apply some pure **aloe-vera gel** to wherever it's hurting. According to Seattle dentist Rick Chavez, this will temporarily relieve certain sorts of toothache in 15 minutes flat.

Try to get 100 per cent pure gel, which is available in many good health shops. In the UK, try Higher Nature's Ultimate Aloe Skin Gel (60 ml, £9.20); they also deliver to the US, or you can try 1001 Herbs (8 fl oz, $13.45). For contact details, see under 'Shopping' in the Directory.

113. Acupressure While Waiting for Dentist

Toothache doesn't usually go away on its own for long, so it is best to see a dentist as soon as you can arrange it. However, while you are waiting, try gently stimulating what traditional Chinese doctors call the **ying xiang** acupressure points on each side of the nostrils. Do so for two to three minutes three times daily.

For extra effect, also work the **di cong** points for the same amount of time three times daily. These are on the edge of the mouth. See picture.

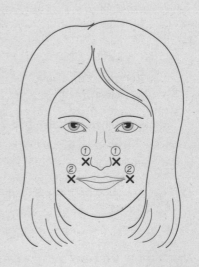

114. Homeopathy for Dental Extraction

Need to have a tooth out? There is a general homeopathic treatment for calming post-extraction pain, swelling and bleeding that works better than arnica alone. According to Professor Henri Albertini, assistant dean of the Faculty of Odontology in Marseille, it's **arnica** plus **hypericum**.

Take both remedies at potency 30c three times daily the day before, three times on the day of extraction and for up to four days afterwards, depending on your reaction to the tooth removal.

Arnica is available from most good health shops and some chemists, but for tooth extraction you need the 30c or, in some cases, even 200c potency. Taking it in potency 6, which is the most widely available in shops, won't help sufficiently. Contact one of the specialist homeopathic pharmacies like the Queen's chemist, Ainsworths, as they can make a remedy up for you containing both arnica and hypericum in the right strength (approximately £3.50–£4.50). For contact details, see under 'Shopping' in the Directory.

115. Too Many Fillings? Keep Your Mouth Shut

If your filling count's going up despite the fact you're keeping up the oral hygiene, find out whether you keep your mouth open or shut when you sleep. If it's shut, saliva will be bathing your teeth and gums all night, helping protect the area against bacteria and promoting re-mineralisation. Leave it open and this doesn't happen.

Ask your partner (if you have one) to check whether your mouth is open or shut when you sleep (perhaps they night-wake, as we all surface two to four times nightly, or come to bed later than you). If it's open, ask them to nudge you to make you roll over – when we change position in bed, we will often instinctively close our mouths too. They could also try running a finger along your lips and saying quietly, 'Close your mouth!' People are highly receptive to positive simple instructions when asleep.

Mercury ('Silver') Amalgam Fillings

If you have 'silver' mercury amalgam fillings in your teeth, mercury leaks into your body after those fillings begin to break down. This is not good as, after plutonium, mercury is the most toxic substance on the planet.

After eight to ten years mercury amalgam tooth fillings begin to break down and mercury is discharged. (Amalgam fillings are made up of 50 per cent mercury, 35 per cent silver and 15 per cent tin and other metals.) 'Mercury vapour leaches out into your fillings and body all the time, when you eat, when you drink – especially something like hot tea or coffee – when you brush your teeth or chew gum,' says Jack Levenson, former president of the British Society for Mercury-Free Dentistry. 'It is also used in root-canal treatments and may leak out of them too as the protective covering begins to break down.'

> What colour are your metal fillings, if you have any? If they are silvery still, OK; if they are going grey or darkening, watch out. This means they've started degenerating and are releasing mercury into your body.

So what?

Excess mercury lodged in the body's tissues has been provisionally linked to a slew of health problems including Alzheimer's, ME (or chronic fatigue syndrome), arthritis, mood disorders (including anxiety and depression), heart problems, allergies, weakened immune system, recurrent miscarriage and infertility, though the most common problems seem to be lack of energy and feeling permanently below par.

One of the biggest studies on the subject was carried out in 2000 by Tübingen University's Institute of Organic Chemistry on 20,000 people who suffered from ME and possessed an average of nine mercury amalgam fillings each. The researchers found all participants had raised levels of mercury in their systems, some considerably higher than the World Health Organization's recommended safe limit for humans. A good overview specialist resource listing several hundred trials looking at mercury-related health problems is *Infertility and Birth Defects: Is Mercury From Silver Dental Fillings an Unsuspected Cause?* by Sam Ziff and Dr Michael Ziff. Also see *It's All in Your Head* by Dr Hal A. Huggins.

On another subject, infertility, a rapid Net search today through some of the standard medical sites such as MedLine produced around 70 clinical trials whose quality varied, but which all linked the issue with mercury. See also 'Malicious mercury' on page 144.

What to do

If you feel you would like to get your mercury fillings taken out and some white resin or porcelain ones put in instead, it is vital to see a dentist who is specially trained. Do not, under any circumstances, allow a dentist who has no specialist knowledge of this area to take out your 'silver' fillings.

First, ask your chosen dentist to arrange a test to check whether you do have mercury in your body. If they can't suggest anywhere (though they ought to be able to), you may want to reconsider letting them remove the fillings – see 'Help and advice' below. If you have the test and it confirms there is no mercury present in your system, you feel well and your fillings aren't yet discolouring, you may want to consider waiting a while as the process can be expensive (£250–£400 for each molar) or at least going for gradual removal.

If your test comes back positive and you decide to have all the fillings removed, the dentist will use either a special suction device or a dental dam. You will also wear a mask during the procedure. If the fillings are taken out in the ordinary way, you risk ingesting a big dose of mercury in the process instead of getting rid of it all, because:

- The metal is highly reactive to heat, which is why it is used in thermometers. It vaporises at relatively low temperatures and will certainly do so on contact with a high-speed drill, meaning you'll breathe it in.
- You may swallow some fragments of old filling material as they are drilled out. And a one-off hefty dose of mercury could make you feel worse than the gradual leakage.

Note: Canada has long recommended against mercury amalgam fillings being used for pregnant or breastfeeding women. Sweden, Denmark and Austria have banned the use of 'silver' fillings for all young adults as well as for pregnant women and nursing mothers. In Switzerland and Japan, dental students are no longer taught to use amalgam as a first-choice method of filling teeth, whilst the US is experiencing growing disquiet among consumers – and many in the medical and dental professions – about this traditional dental mercury mix. As a result, its use is tapering off in favour of the white resin fillings, but (perhaps fearing the possibility of mass litigation) the FDA has not yet actually gone so far as to ban amalgam ones. In the UK, the official line from, for instance, the British Dental Association is that apart from 'a tiny number of people who have localised reaction to mercury sensitivity', the substance is safe so protected removal is not something you'd be able to get on the National Health Service.

Help and further information
For further information, including lists of mercury-free dentists (i.e. those who use no mercury products in their practice, all of which are private) in the UK, contact the British Society for Mercury-Free Dentistry or Patients Against Mercury Amalgams. In the US, contact the Foundation for Toxic-Free Dentistry; in Canada, try Canadians for Mercury Relief. For contact details, see under 'Therapies and Therapists' in the Directory.

What Doctors Don't Tell You magazine has an 80-page booklet on dental health, which amongst other things gives details of the relevant toxicity tests, how and where to get them done, and lists of mercury-free dentists in both the UK and US. For contact details, see under 'Shopping' in the Directory.

116. Sorting Mercury Toxicity
Some of the common symptoms of long-term, low-grade mercury poisoning are thought to include:

- constant fatigue
- aches and pains in the joints and muscles
- irritability and moodiness
- depression, anxiety, panic attacks and insomnia
- swollen lymph glands behind the ear, in the jaw and at the back of the neck
- worsening memory and poor concentration
- recurrent candida (thrush) infections
- bad breath, bleeding gums and oversensitive teeth
- menstrual problems, fertility problems and low libido
- poor immune system
- heart and circulatory disorders.

Note: as with other 'syndrome' illnesses like ME or candida infestation, many of the above can be symptoms of other conditions too, so it's sensible to check with a mercury-free dentist or reputable holistic physician before deciding whether it is definitely mercury deposits causing you the problems or whether it might be something else and you need some specific diagnostic medical tests to get to the root of the matter.

How to get rid of mercury

If you had mercury-amalgam fillings but they have been safely removed, the next step is to clear the rest of your system. If you've still got mercury fillings and are suffering symptoms of subclinical mercury poisoning, get them taken out safely first, then move along to removing any lingering deposits from the rest of your body tissues.

Getting any mercury deposits out of the tissues of the body usually takes 3–18 months, depending on how many fillings you had and how long you'd had them for, with about six months as the average. This sounds like a long time, but those who have done it say it is well worth it.

The process of pulling mercury, or indeed any other poisonous metal such as lead and cadium from your body tissues, is called chelating. It involves using certain minerals, vitamins, amino acids and other nutrients to encourage the body to let go of the poisonous metal, then excrete it via the usual channels (in sweat, urine and faeces). The other important part of the programme involves drinking plenty of pure water (1.5–2 litres daily). One of the most effective, though expensive, chelation agents is based on *Chlorella microalgae* and called NDF. However, in some cases, just taking very high doses of vitamin C over a few months can do the trick, and works more gently.

A good nutritionist needs to choose the chelating agent or programme for you and monitor you while you are using it. Your mercury-free dentist should be able to suggest one in your area, or, alternatively, contact a help association for advice on how to find one. For contact details, see under 'Therapies and Therapists' in the Directory.

You can initially feel unwell when you start pulling the mercury out of your tissues (fluey and tired, aching in head, joints and muscles). Some people need to take the process very gradually.

117. Tooth Powder – DIY and Fluoride-Free

If you ever run out of toothpaste, you can make your own teeth-cleaning, breath-freshening mix in 60 seconds from the contents of your kitchen cupboard with this old-fashioned natural recipe.

2 tablespoons dried lemon or orange rind (dried if you've got it, or grate a little fresh)
¼ cup baking soda
2 tablespoons sea salt

Put the rinds in a food processor and grind them to a powder. Add the baking soda and salt, and give the mixture another quick whizz. That's it.

Store in an air-tight jar. To use, simply moisten your toothbrush, dip it in and brush. Rinse out your mouth well afterwards. The baking soda and salt clean and whiten; the rind is a flavourer and astringent.

If you don't have time for all that but like the idea of a natural tooth powder, try **Dental Miracle**: it's herbal-based, and though it costs £17.99, it lasts ages, does a great job of removing teeth stains and keeps gum disease at bay. It's available from Victoria Health. For more information, see Teenagers: Teeth on page 382.

Don't fancy fluoride?

If you have fluoridated water at home and don't want to drink any more, add milk to your tea: the calcium content will balance the effect.[61]

For more suggestions on fluoride, see Fix 288: Fluoride – Fearful? and Fix 289: DIY Toothpaste.

Wake Up!

118. The Smell That Cheers & Sharpens

Need to stay on the ball? Sniff a little **Melissa aromatherapy oil** (lemon balm, or *Melissa officinalis*) straight from the bottle. Student volunteers found that this both lifted their mood and sharpened their mental performance. And according to a recent study in *Pharmacology, Biochemistry and Behavior*, less was more – the 18- to 24-year-olds did better on 300 mg a day than on 900 mg.

Melissa can also help older people concentrate better: one double-blind placebo trial found 71 elderly patients with dementia were less agitated and withdrawn and more constructively active after being treated with it for just a month.

For stockists, try Revital or Neal's Yard, which does a standardised extract, Melissa Essential Oil (2.5 ml, £35.75). For contact details, see under 'Shopping' in the Directory.

Weight Loss

There are dozens of natural slimming aids out there that offer to help you burn up excess fat, keep your appetite under control and gee up your metabolism, often all in the same handy pill. But which ones are any good? And what about side effects?

Here are some of the most effective natural fat-fixers.

119. Green-Tea Extract

Available in capsule form from many different companies, **green-tea extract** acts as a metabolism-booster if you take enough of it. Its active ingredients are catechins, and one American study found taking the extract with every meal upped the daily number of calories burnt by more than 40 per cent.[62] Another strict double-blind placebo trial carried out in Japan in 2005 found that after 12 weeks of taking the extract volunteers' weight, waist sizes and body mass indexes (BMIs) were all reduced; the group that was taking fairly high doses – 690 mg a day – got the best results.[63]

Green-tea extract is available in the UK from Healthy Direct (60 x 300 mg capsules, £4); in the US, try Thermo Green Tea Capsules from Green Tea Lovers, based in New York state. For contact details, see under 'Shopping' in the Directory.

Note: side effects from drinking much more green tea than usual may include gas, upset stomach, nausea, heartburn, abdominal and muscle pains, headache and dizziness, so it doesn't suit everyone.

120. Hydroxycitric Acid (HCA)

This compound is derived from the Malabar tamarind fruit (*Garcinia cambogia*) and is found in many popular slimming supplements as an appetite suppressant. In fact, in south-east Asia, where it's often used in cooking, they say it makes the food more filling.

Several strict placebo-controlled studies confirm that **HCA** does suppress appetite and increase weight loss,[64] and further research suggests if you supplement it with chromium the weight-loss effect is enhanced.[65] The suggested dosage is around 500 mg three times daily with a glass of water, 30–60 minutes before each meal.

However, not all HCA-containing products are the same. Dutch scientists report that some of the more effective ones for reducing food intake are **Citrin K** and **Regulator**, as opposed to the promising-sounding Super CitriMax HCA-600-SXS, despite the hefty doses it contains.[66]

In the UK, try the combination capsule Citrin and Chrome from Alternative Medicines (90 x 500 mg/100 mcg tablets, £6.80); in the US, try Appetite Suppressor, which contains Citrin K, from the Michigan-based N B Nutrition. For contact details, see under 'Shopping' in the Directory.

121. Do Breakfast, Stay Slim

Eat breakfast if you want to be slimmer. A study in the *Journal of Nutrition* showed that those who eat breakfast consume fewer calories a day than those who skip it. If you can make it high in unrefined carbs, like wholemeal cereal and bread, with fresh fruit, then that is even better because it will keep you motoring without snacking until lunch.

122. Secret of the Non-Fattening Dessert

If you cannot live without chocolate mousse or cream slices (most of us, right?), the **Three-Bites Rule** is a very simple technique that can help you eat treats without putting on weight. The rule is simply that you can go right ahead and have your favourite pudding, but stick to three forkfuls, place them in the middle of your prettiest plate and pass the rest to someone else to remove immediately. Eat your serving *slowly* and with pleasure. Dietary experts say that we only really taste those first three mouthfuls anyway, and finishing off the rest is merely a 'positive-feedback loop reaction' – i.e. automatically repeating an action to reproduce the initial hit of pleasure, even though the returns diminish fast.

123. Fill Up, Lose Weight
If you want to eat filling meals but lose weight, check out a substance called **phaseolamin** (available as Freecarb from Higher Nature). It's an extract from the white kidney bean that seems to block the absorption of calories from up to a third of the starch you eat, and recent research at UCLA's School of Medicine by medical director Jay Udani found it produced a steady 2.7 kg weight loss over four weeks. Testers who ate the *most* carbohydrates lost *most* inches round the waist.

124. Spray Away Hunger
A quick support for a dieter's resolve, the nasal spray **NoSnax** contains, among other things, a botanical appetite suppressant and mood enhancer called **hoodia gordonii**, derived from the hoodia cactus, which African tribesmen have used for centuries to subdue their hunger during periods of famine. Taking any substance nasally is fast and effective because of the thin skin and rich network of tiny blood vessels lining each nostril.

NoSnax is used by spraying between meals. It is made by Salcura and is available from Victoria Health (30 ml, £9.95). For contact details, see under 'Shopping' in the Directory.

See also Men: Weight Loss on page 235 and Men: Exercise on page 211.

125. Carrots for Smokers
If someone in your family is a smoker, try and get them to eat a raw **carrot** a day. American research suggests this could cut their risk of lung cancer by half.[67]

Women

Women are powerful, nurturing, creative and astonishing. And we're all those things despite having to handle so many (often conflicting) demands on our energy. We also have to cope with many challenges to our health and peace of mind that men don't, because their hormones aren't permanently fluctuating under the influence of menstrual cycles or the menopause, and they don't usually have the main responsibility for any children.

The information in this section is intended to support and help women with as many different issues as we could possibly pack in, and not only the Big Stuff but the Small Yet Invaluable Stuff as well.

So start reading right here for the inside track on everything from how to thicken your hair immediately, get rid of frown lines the ten-second French way and talk to your unborn baby telepathically to how to become (and stay) pregnant after a series of miscarriages, banish PMS for ever and get hold of the best low-dose herbal pill for smoothing away the menopause.

Anti-Aging

126. Creams, Serums and Supplements

For a pot that will last four to six weeks, decent anti-aging **creams** usually start from around £40 and average out at £60–£80 for Lancôme, Helena Rubenstein or an indie premium brand like the splendid Dr Sebagh Pure

Vitamin C Powder Cream, available from Space NK (£72). Of the less expensive creams, Olay's Regenerist (£22.50) is rated highly by professional beauty editors.

Beauty **serums** rather than creams are now on the up – they are a similar price but are better absorbed.

Natural face creams that rock
If you want a holistic face cream that genuinely does seem to combat the signs of aging, doesn't cost the earth and reduces any inflammation (e.g. the odd juicy spot, which women often start getting again during the peri-menopause or menopause; spots *and* lines together – very unfair), try **Mega Mushroom Face Cream**, formulated by Dr Andrew Weil, from Origins (50 ml, £45). If you can afford it, the accompanying **Mega Mushroom Face Serum** is well worth getting too (30 ml, £55).

Try also **Hyaluronic Acid (HA) Day Cream** (Derma E Skin Care, £24.95, 56g , via Victoria Health. They also have a Night Cream, same size and price). HA is a terrific skin plumper-upper, as in solution, it can hold a lot of water. It's a top joint-improver as well as it helps retain more water in joint fluid, so lubricating them and improving their shock-absorption rating (see Arthritis, page 14).

One to watch
It doesn't come in a designer jar, wasn't made by a famous cosmetics multinational and has no ad campaigns shot by top photographers (better and better), but look out for **NBG Cream**. Made by Norwegian biotech company Pharmacon and originally developed to help heal stubborn wounds, it blazed a trail during its research trial at Russia's City Hospital Number One at Arkhangelsk (an international leader in wound management), where it didn't just cure the diabetic skin ulcers it was meant for: when the medical and nursing staff saw further possibilities and began using it them-selves as a health and beauty cream on their faces, necks and backs of hands, it seemed to leave ordinary aged or sun-damaged skin 'soft, supple and crease-less'.

NBG Cream is now being marketed to the public as **Immuderm;**

a tube lasts about four months if used on the face twice daily. You can have it shipped via Immunocorp (6 oz tube, £55.95, plus £8.95 postage). Pleasingly, you can try it for a month and if unimpressed, send the unused portion back in its tube and get all your money back.

Beautiful skin from the inside

The successful holistic approach to beautiful skin, however, is also *from the inside out* – i.e. putting the right things in your mouth, instead of just on to your face.

And while sufficient sleep, healthy eating and drinking at least six to eight glasses of pure water daily all help greatly, softer, dewier, less lined skin can also come in a handy capsule at half to a third of the price of a good-quality replenishing face cream.

For a not-to-be-sneezed-at improvement of up to 20 per cent, new independent German research in the *International Journal of Cosmetic Science* suggests you can just take inexpensive **evening primrose oil** capsules, which have the additional benefits of helping alleviate PMS and soothing premenstrually tender breasts. In fact, they do the latter so well they are available on the NHS for cyclic mastalgia – see also Fix 148: Breast Pain – Cyclical. Evening primrose is clinically proven to add lustre to skin, hair and nails, and reduce arthritis and eczema. The double-blind placebo-controlled study of 40 men and women (with an average age of 44) found participants had 'better moisturised, firmer, more elastic facial skin' after 12 weeks taking six 500 mg capsules of evening primrose oil a day.

Evening primrose oil boosts skin quality because the gamma linolenic acid (GLA) it contains is an essential constituent of all cell membranes and is vital for skin structure. Check out Holland & Barrett stores, which often have budget special offers on decent-quality evening primrose oil (120 x 1 g capsules, £9.97); in the US, try Web Vitamins (100 capsules, $22.05).

GLA is present in even larger amounts in **borage (starflower) oil**. Take a 1 g capsule six times daily (three in the morning and three in the evening) for two months. You can buy them from Nature's Best (360 x 1 g capsules, eight weeks' supply, £35.80).

Antioxidant nutritional supplements are also really starting to come into their own. The combination capsule **Imedeen** was perhaps the first of the 'beauty capsules'. The most popular Imedeen product is Time Perfection, but prices (for 120 capsules) vary from £71.50 (from Boots) to over £80, so it pays to shop around. The dose is two capsules a day.

Imedeen contains pro-skin nutrients like vitamin C, zinc and marine extracts, was developed in Sweden and researched in Europe and the US. One paper presented to the American Academy of Dermatology in Washington in 2004 reported 'impressive results' when taken for 12 weeks.

But top of my own skin anti-aging list are:

1. **Organic linseed oil**, a deep-golden liquid rich in the pro-skin omega-3 and -6 fatty acids. I originally used linseed as an effective re-energiser following acute fatigue syndrome, and though I cannot find any skin-benefit research – only anecdotal evidence from users – I remember that after eight weeks not only was my energy coming back but it was doing for my face what liquid linseed oil does for wood. Terrific.

   In the UK, try the high-quality and great-value High Barn Oils (100 capsules, £13.50); in the US, look for Barlean's Organic Flaxseed Oil on Livespan Nutrition's money-saving site (90 x 1 g capsules, $12.65).

   Note: do not take linseed oil if you are pregnant or breastfeeding. And never use linseed oil intended for animals or woodcare on yourself (not that you would, would you?): it's of a very different quality and purity.

2. **AgeLoss tablets** – known to those who take them in London as the 'Get out of my way, I'm fabulous' tabs, AgeLoss is packed with powerful anti-aging ingredients, including the antioxidant GliSODin (a new form of superoxide dismutase, which, unlike the original, isn't destroyed in the human gastrointestinal tract), alpha-lipoic acid (another good antioxidant), N-acetyl cysteine (a popular anti-aging supplement in its own right), plus copper and zinc, both of which are co-factors in free-radical elimination. AgeLoss is available from Victoria Health (60 tablets, a month's supply, £24.99), and the dosage is two a day. For maximum good effect if you are in your late thirties or older,

combine with **MenoHerbs2** (twice a day), also available from Victoria Health (90 tablets, six weeks' supply, £14.95).

For all contact details, see under 'Shopping' in the Directory.

127. Take Ten Years Off Your Face – Now

'Pluck your eyebrows. It takes ten years off your face immediately,' says Nicky Hambleton-Jones, presenter of TV series *10 Years Younger* and MD of British style consultancy Tramp2Vamp. But as many of us tend to pluck away too much or don't get them even at first, it pays to get a good beautician to do it the first time round: in five minutes they will have established the most flattering shape for you to simply keep in trim.

128. Top Treat for Tired Skin

Try the **egg and olive oil treat**. This is one of the best and most moisturising face masks there is – and you can make it yourself from wholesome natural ingredients in seconds. Add a beaten egg to a teaspoon of olive oil, use cotton-wool balls to pat all over your face and neck. Rinse off with warm water when dry. It leaves skin soft, supple and with a healthy sheen.

129. Sagging Face – Try the Natural, Free Facelift

Surgical facelifts cost from £3,000 and involve a general anaesthetic, while face creams tone the skin but not what's holding it up underneath and are pricey. And if you wanted to firm up flabby upper arms, would you rub a cream on them?

No, you'd probably exercise. The same holds true for your face, as when the muscles beneath the skin are toned, they support everything far better. **Facial exercise (facercise)** can take ten years off you, and, encouragingly, you may start seeing results within two to three weeks.

You can facercise passively with a special Slendertone machine, which can be bought direct from Slendertone (approximately £190). For contact details, see under 'Shopping' in the Directory. But you can also facercise naturally and actively. Check out programmes of videos, DVDs, tapes and books such as Carole Maggio's system, used by celebs like Trudi Styler and Queen Noor, whose sculpted faces at 50-plus and remarkable contoured cheekbones show just what this method can do.

Natural DIY

Eva Fraser's system is also good. Not only does it work, it's easy. Try one of Fraser's beginner facelift tricks for 14–21 days and start to see the difference. The one below strengthens your upper cheek muscles, and once they're toned and strong, they give a face real lift for free.

1. Sit in front of a mirror, elbows resting on a table and looking straight ahead into it. Take a slow, deep breath, and as you let it out, relax.
2. Place the flat side of your thumbs in each side of your mouth, between teeth and cheeks.
3. Hold on outside with the side of curved index fingers, letting your knuckles face in towards each other.
4. Now curve your thumbs slightly outwards, keeping your hands steady and holding them down.
5. You're in position. This is it: lift the muscles on each side of your nose in three little movements, *pausing after each one for a count of five* and working against the resistance of the hold exerted by your fingers and thumbs.
6. Release in three movements, taking rests for a count of five between each.
7. Relax. Breathe calmly.
8. Repeat three times.

Recommended reading: *Eva Fraser's Facial Workout* for the full system.

For contact details for both Carole Maggio and Eva Fraser, see under 'Useful Helplines, Websites and Contacts' in the Directory.

130. Instant Icy Facelift

Fill a sink with ice and cold water. Soak a clean flannel in it, then press the freezing cloth on to your face several times, suggests make-up artist Charlotte Tilbury, who says she uses this for models who've just come off long-haul flights. Pat gently dry after a few minutes.

131. Drooping Jowls

Drooping jowls are unfairly aging, even if they're only going a little bit and even when the rest of your face still looks pretty good. But this simple

face-sculpting jowl-eliminator (also
devised by facercise queen Eva
Fraser) can produce great results
if you do it daily for just six to eight
weeks (better still, twice daily).

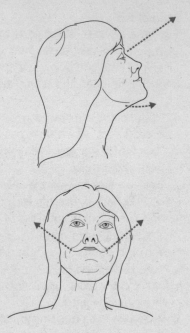

1. Sit or stand in front of a mirror,
   tilt your head up and jut your
   chin forwards.
2. Slide your lower lip up over
   your top lip. Feel the stretch
   around your jaw-line and
   throat?
3. Smile slowly, upwards and
   outwards in five slow stages.
4. Hold that for a slow count of
   five, stroking gently upwards
   along your jaw-line.
5. Release in five gentle stages and
   return lips to usual position.
6. Relax. *Breathe*. Many people find they are concentrating so hard they
   hold their breath.
   Repeat three times.

132. The Ten-Second Frown-Fighter

French mothers have passed this one on to their daughters for generations;
it may be one reason why you don't see so many deep V-shaped frown
lines between the eyebrows of women in France.

1. Place the tip of each index finger on the inside end of each eyebrow,
   the bit closest to the bridge of your nose.
2. Using the little muscles under the skin around an inch below your
   third eye (the centre of your forehead), move the ends of your
   fingertips apart slightly.
3. Hold for the count of ten, then release gradually rather than 'letting
   go' all at once.
4. Repeat three times, twice a day.

Frown-smoothing muscles can be hard to locate to begin with (just like when you first do pelvic exercises – 'I've got to squeeze what, where?'). If at first you can't identify the frown-smoothers, try scowling lightly with a fingertip resting between the ends of your eyebrows and feel the muscles move.

You can repeat the exercise up to ten times a day, or as often as you remember. For just a minute or so a day, this exercise will help fade lines already there and reduce the chances of them forming. It's said to save a fortune on collagen infill.

133. Hands Looking Old?
Hands show age even more clearly than a face. Make your mitts look better fast with the **Kitchen Cure**: mix a pinch of sea salt with a blob of decent-quality olive oil and rub gently all over your palms and the backs of your hands in small circular motions. Rinse in warm water and pat gently dry. You could also check out **Miracell**, a fabulous mixture of plant oils (£9.95 for 15ml from Victoria Health).

See also Fix 80: Be SomeBody and Fix 103: Meditation as Age-Reversal. If you are over 35, see also Women: Peri-Menopause on page 163 and Women: Menopause on page 151.

134. Spotty T-Zone Sorter
Milk of magnesia (that old-fashioned chalky medicine from the chemist's that has settled generations of upset stomachs) makes a good, and very inexpensive, anti-inflammatory face mask. Dab on with cotton wool, allow to dry and leave it for five to ten minutes, then gently rinse off with warm water. Repeat every other day as necessary to help calm the complexion. (Do not use on areas of broken skin.)

Anxiety

135. . . . about Your Children

If you feel that you are worrying too much about your children, or are aware that you're overprotecting them but just can't seem to get things in perspective, try **Heart Mother**. It's a remarkable essence made from clear quartz and the cyclamen plant by Suffolk healer, teacher and essence-developer Rose Titchiners, and it embodies the balanced archetypal mum in all of us – the one who is gentle, strong and wise, who respects her own needs and can nurture her young without smothering them.

Heart Mother is also great for *loving, supportive mothers who need to stand back a bit* because they are becoming so involved in their children's problems they're wearing themselves out.

Perhaps your son or daughter is having painful relationship problems, is long-term unwell, differently abled, has learning difficulties or is being bullied. These are all challenges that from a spiritual-development point of view are essentially their own to learn from but which pull loving parents in deep and cut them to the quick.

It can be easier to help a child (or indeed anyone else), however, if you do not jump into the pit with them but are able to stay a little bit detached so you're grounded enough to lean over the edge and help pull them out. Heart Mother, taken in water four times daily, can help you do that. It is made by Light Heart Essences and is available direct (10 ml, £5.15). For contact details, see under 'Shopping' in the Directory.

See also General: Anxiety on page 11.

Assertiveness and Confidence

136. Increase Your Personal Power Now

Do you ever find that as a female it can be more difficult to be heard and taken seriously than if you were male? Just the smallest bit? Especially, say, at work? If so, try this:

The Purple Power Breath

The **Purple Power Breath** is a *right-now* fix and a half.

For many thousands of years purple has been the colour of royalty, power, dignity and respect, which is why emperors, church dignitaries and spiritual or ceremonial leaders all traditionally wear it. If you imagine yourself filled with purple light, you will also absorb some of its qualities.

First, sit somewhere quiet (the loo will do if you're at work and cannot get any peace elsewhere) and take five 'power breaths' as follows:

1. Imagine you are surrounded by light that is a wonderful bright, clear, imperial purple.
2. Breathe it in for a steady count of five, taking it right down into your lungs, saying to yourself, 'I am breathing in *power*.'
3. Hold it for five, then breathe that glorious purple light out for five, saying as you do so, 'I am breathing out *strength*.'
4. Repeat Steps 2 and 3 five times (*in* power, *out* strength).
5. Send the fifth and final out-breath down through your chest, through your tummy, legs and feet, and let it stream deep down into the ground, holding you steady.
6. Now, say to yourself, '**I have all the power and all the strength. I need to be respected and heard.**'
7. Stretch, open your eyes, have a quick drink of water, then go and say your piece firmly, calmly and clearly.

They'll listen all right.

137. R.E.S.P.E.C.T.!

Because women tend to be rather more accommodating and placating than most men, usually preferring 'to cooperate rather than annihilate' (as one Texan psychologist put it) when they encounter problems or resistance at home and at work, they are more likely to be seen – most unfairly – as a soft touch.

However, if you find people aren't respecting or taking notice of what you say, or you find it hard to assert yourself effectively, there is an essence that's subtle dynamite – start taking it and others may not know what's hit them.

Justifiably called **Inner Fire** (often referred to as the 'Enough is enough' essence), it is made from red fire agate, red sandstone and eagle feather, and is the one to use when you need to say, calmly and in a way that brooks no argument, 'Hey, you, the line in the sand is *there*.'

To make up a bottle is easy: just place as many drops of the original tincture as you instinctively feel is right for you – this can be anything from 3 to 30 or more – in a 25–30 ml dropper bottle from the chemist. Fill half of it up with spring water, add a teaspoon of brandy or vodka as a preservative, replace the dropper lid and shake gently. Inner Fire is taken for three days, three times a day. Each time you take it, think about what you wish to say or do first.

It is available direct from Light Heart Essences (10 ml, £5.15). For contact details, see under 'Shopping' in the Directory.

Note: it's not a good idea to use the essence for more than three days at a time (this one's a true focus fix) or you may find you start getting too driven and agitated.

138. Someone's Crowding You

Sometimes you may find that a person close to you is crowding you mentally and emotionally, draining you, giving you no space. Women, since they are the natural givers, nurturers and mothers of this world, are especially likely to have such a person (or even a succession of them) in their lives.

Typically, this person seems to want your attention and help all the time. They ignore your boundaries, tug constantly at your consciousness, are too often in your thoughts and demand more than you wish to give. They are often someone you love dearly – a lover, a child – a close friend or a family member, like a sibling or parent.

If you would like to re-establish the strong, healthy boundaries between the two of you – a case of saying kindly but firmly, 'This is *me* here; that is *you* over there. And though I love you and will always support you, that's the way it needs to be' – there is a gentle but powerful spiritual technique that will help you. It is a version of a method taught to trainee healers by the UK's National Federation of Spiritual Healers.

I call it the **Healthy-Distance Ceremony** and have made use of it a few times over the past few years, once with one of my own children.

Remember, you are not rejecting the person – merely re-establishing some necessary positive distance in a clear but compassionate and loving way.

1. Find some beautiful flowers (just a couple will be fine if you can't find more) and a white candle or tea light. Arrange them next to each other in a place in your house where you will not be disturbed for a while.
2. Now light the candle, asking as you do so 'in the name of Light' that the angels of love and Archangel Michael's angels of courage, protection and strength come to help you. If the ceremony concerns one of your own children – which for many people it does – ask, too, that Mary, Queen of Heaven and protector of mothers, homes and children, also comes to help you, as her energy is soft, nurturing and gentle but also firm and balancing.
3. Sit or lie down quietly for a few moments. Breathe easily and regularly – in for five, hold for five, out for five. Feel your heartbeat slow and your entire system calm down.
4. Still lying down, imagine you are sending roots down from the backs of your feet into the earth. See the roots spreading deep and wide like those of a beautiful tree. Ask that you be grounded securely by them throughout the ceremony.
5. Close your eyes. Imagine a golden ball of light growing around you. See it spreading several feet:

   • above your head and below your feet
   • to your left and to your right
   • in front of you, and
   • behind you.

   You are now enclosed in a golden globe. Ask in your mind that this be an inviolate protection from all negativity throughout the ceremony.
6. See both the person you have in mind and yourself enclosed together in a ball of soft-pink light. Pink is the colour of love and also has a very reassuring, calming effect. Greet the person by name, either out loud or in your head. Tell them gently but firmly that you love them very much (or are fond of them, if more appropriate), you'll always

be there for them (if that is what you wish. If it isn't and you feel you need to go your own way instead, leave that bit out!), but you need to have your own space back now.

7. Now see that beautiful pink ball of light dividing down the middle until it looks like a figure of eight, with that person in one circle of the eight and you in the other. Next, see those two circles separating so they sit close together but have some clear space in between.

8. Bless or send love to the person, then say goodbye three times.

9. Gently 'blow' the person's pink globe, with them sitting comfortably inside it, off and away from you. See the globe getting smaller as it floats away gently. Continue to blow the pink ball of light until it is as far away as feels right. Some people will do so until it has disappeared out of sight; others, until it appears to be, for instance, on the opposite side of the room. Do whatever feels right for you.

10. Now bring your full attention back to yourself and your own pink ball of light. See the ball growing larger and stronger around you. Feel those roots you created earlier, strong and deep. Enjoy the feeling of security and peace.

11. When you're ready, take a deep, easy breath and open your eyes.

12. Say thank you to the angels, Archangel Michael and anyone else you asked to help you. Request that the loving boundaries and healthy distance that you just created should hold firm *always*.

13. Stretch, rub your hands together and maybe stamp your feet on the floor a little to ground yourself.

14. Sit quietly for a few moments, then get up and, if you are feeling a bit spacey, have a drink or a snack.

How you may feel immediately afterwards

Some people report initially feeling a bit tearful or quite tired after the Healthy-Distance Ceremony. This is quite normal because while it is straightforward and anyone can do it, it is also a profound exercise and you may have 'undone' a very strong and long-standing (but no longer appropriate) connection that someone had made to you.

Be nice to yourself if this is the case. Go for a calm walk, have a warm, peaceful bath, curl up in bed for a while with a hot-water bottle and a milky drink, and take it easy. Ask the angels for help and support if you feel you could do with some. They will give it to you.

The Law of Three

Sometimes people find they need to repeat this ceremony on three separate occasions if the inappropriate connection with the other person was very deep or long-standing. However, the Universal Law of Three is that if you ask, with loving, kindly intent, for something to be done **'in the name of the Light'** three times, if it is for the best and harms no one – it will be.

139. Under-Confident and Over-Spending

Many of us are not totally happy with the way we look. When the first international survey about how women feel about their appearance was carried out in 2005 by Dove, with British eating-disorders expert Dr Susie Orbach (author of *Fat Is a Feminist Issue*) and Dr Nancy Etcoff, an American psychologist who teaches at Harvard Medical School (author of *Survival of the Prettiest*), they found that only one in five of us actually believes we are attractive.

And that's only 'OK attractive', not even pretty and certainly not beautiful. No matter what we see in the mirror or what our friends and partners say.

If you find you are spending more than you want to on beauty treatments, clothes, cosmetics, even cosmetic surgery and are constantly unhappy with how you look, or if you cannot help seeing your body negatively, there is a deep-acting but gentle essence remedy that may help you recover your confidence and balance. Called **Salvia**, it has been developed by Dr Judy Griffin, an aromatherapist and fourth-generation essence-maker who is trained in Native American, Western herbal and Chinese medicine. Dr Griffin also works with the Baylor Medical Center in Dallas and the Texas Cancer Care Center in Fort Worth, and says Salvia operates gently but surely to help anyone who:

- feels overly self-conscious about their appearance
- has a real thing about a particular aspect of their appearance that others don't see as a problem (e.g. feeling that their nose is too big, when others genuinely see it as just fine)

- spends heavily on clothes, beauty treatments and cosmetic operations
- lacks self-esteem in general
- may have difficulty with anorexia, drugs or alcohol.

Salvia:

- encourages strong, healthy self-esteem and real belief in your own worth
- helps you change your self-image for the better
- supports you in feeling truly comfortable with the way you look
- brings in sheer joy.

It is available in the UK via mail order from IFER (3.8 ml, £7.50) and from the Nutri Centre; in the US, from Petite Fleur Essences in Texas ($18). For contact details, see under 'Shopping' in the Directory. Another good one to use, which helps us feel happy about being who we are and know that beauty is more about the love you give and receive from others than being dependnant on designer clothes, ruinously expensive hair salons and cosmetic surgery, is the subtle but deep-acting **True Beauty** from Light Heart Essences. This is known as 'the one that lets your light shine' and is available direct from Light Heart at £6.50.

Babies: making them

141. Choose Your Baby's Sex . . .
. . . without Paying a Fortune
It is already possible to ensure you have a boy or a girl. Clinics like the Fertility Institute in the US use a method called pre-implantation genetic diagnosis (PGD), which virtually guarantees the baby-sex of your choice, but the price tag is over $18,000 plus travel (at 2005 rates). Also, the Genetics and IVF Institute in Fairfax, Vancouver, is currently calling for participants to try its flow-cytometry method, which involves staining and sorting DNA, and while a handful of commercial centres are beginning to offer this (they call it MicroSorting), it's not yet widely available.

Medically assisted sex selection is banned in Europe – and $18,000 is a lot of money – but there are some fairly effective holistic methods you can try at home if it's not *essential* that your baby is of a particular sex.

Unborn babies are of indeterminate sex until they reach six weeks of age in the womb, after which their hormones kick in and they begin to become either male or female.

1. Mamas and Papas

The first method, claimed to have an 80 per cent success rate in the 5,000 pregnancies in which it was used that were tracked by the Port Royal Hospital in Paris, is based merely on the food you eat. The **Papa method** was developed there in the 1980s by a French obstetrician called, appropriately enough, Dr Francois Papa. Basically, a woman must eat plenty of foods rich in sodium and potassium if she wants a girl, and high in calcium and magnesium for a boy. Its popularity is in no way reduced by the fact that if you'd like to try for a girl baby, the Papa system tells you to eat plenty of chocolate.

Food for a boy baby
Eat lots of meat, pasta, rice, salty foods, fish, milk-free puddings, fresh fruit, sugar, milk-free butter substitutes and all vegetables except those on the girl-food list.

Avoid milk and milk products, pastries, shellfish, brown bread, salad vegetables, chocolate and nuts.

Food for a girl baby
Eat lots of dairy products, eggs, jam, honey, chocolate every day, foods containing cornflour, unsalted nuts, carrots, beans, turnips, onions, leeks, peas, peppers and cucumbers.

Avoid salty foods and foods with added salt (check labels on packaged food).

Suggested reading: for further information, read my book *Natural Fertility*, which contains information on holistic sex selection.

2. The Pavlovec method

The second is the **Pavlovec method**, a more complex but very workable natural-selection programme based on the timing of biological rhythms. It claims a 90–95 per cent success rate. Meli Pavlovec worked at the famous Sloan-Kettering Institute in New York for many years and has written more than 20 clinical papers in respected peer-review scientific journals like *Nature*. Her co-author, Dr Ivette Vazvary, is head of clinical psychology at the Hospital of St Cyril in Bratislava.

Suggested reading: *You Can Influence the Sex of Your Unborn Child* by Meli Pavlovec and Dr Ivette Vazvary. This is available as an e-book via info@chooseyourbaby.com or through Bergen e-Books. For contact details, see under 'Shopping' in the Directory.

3. Timing ovulation

If you like to keep things holistic and want to check out some more options, the **Shettles method** is also worth looking at. This one relies on ovulation time, timing of intercourse *and* specific sexual positions. It claims a 75 per cent success rate.

Suggested reading: *How to Choose the Sex of Your Baby* by William Shettles.

It is also worth visiting the Baby Hopes website, www.babyhopes.com.

141. Find Out Your Baby's Sex

If you're pregnant and have a scan, as most mums-to-be do, the radiographer can tell the sex of your child but is not usually meant to let you know. Some clinics offer a 'which is it?' service for around £60, but in fact you can find out for free – *because you already know*.

Just sit down quietly where you won't be disturbed, calm yourself by breathing slowly for a couple of minutes (the old 'breathe in for six, hold for six, out for six' works fast), then concentrate on your baby.

1. Say hello to your baby.

2. Send them loving, calming thoughts.
3. Next, just ask gently in your mind, 'Are you a boy, or a girl?'
4. Wait and see what impression comes back.

Don't try too hard, or allow the answer you may be hoping for to get in the way. All you need to do is wait peacefully, concentrate but keep an open mind.

An American study by a researcher called Dobrovolsky in 1995 found that under light relaxation hypnosis 25 out of 26 mothers could accurately identify the sex of their unborn baby. Chances are, you can too.

142. Calmer Baby – Three Ways to Have One

If you want to give birth to an 'easy, peaceful' baby who grows up into a calm, coping child, the three most important things you can do while you're pregnant are:

1. Keep as calm as possible yourself.
2. Avoid stress wherever you can.
3. Really want your baby and look forward to meeting them.

Your baby will pick up powerfully on all three.

What unborns know

According to San Diego-based Dr David B. Chamberlain, pioneer in foetal emotional research and past president of the Association for Pre- and Perinatal Health and Psychology, what most pregnant women have always suspected is true – unborn babies feel most of what their mother feels, it has a permanent effect on them, and 'Time in the womb isn't a free period where there are no consequences for anything.'

There is a growing body of work in Europe and the US suggesting pregnant women's emotions do affect their babies' physical and mental development, because strong feelings can pass through to unborns both biochemically (via hormones crossing the placenta) and psychically, or telepathically.[1] This is why a fraught, over-busy pregnancy can result in what Professor Hans Lou of Denmark's John F. Kennedy Institute calls foetal stress syndrome (FSS).

Foetal stress syndrome

FSS is thought to occur when throughout the pregnancy the unborn baby's system has been constantly awash with stress hormones such as cortisol and noradrenaline, which can make its developing neurological network system 'twitchier' and over-reactive for life.

This may produce a wide range of effects for the baby (and for you) after they are born – some major, some barely noticeable – ranging from mild attention deficit hyperactivity disorder (ADHD) and left-handedness to chronic insecurity, emotional instability, difficulty coping with stress and learning difficulties.[2]

Staying calm for 40 weeks is often easier said than done. However, one of the quickest and easiest ways to help mitigate tough times is regularly to take a minimum of 20 minutes a day for *focused peace and relaxation* (such as in an evening bath). A gentle massage can also be really relaxing.

The other three must-dos-if-you-possibly-can are:

1. Cut back at work (or at least don't take on extra).
2. Flex your hours to avoid the commuter crush.
3. Say no to moving and major redecorating or building work on your home.

Suggested reading: *The Miraculous World of Your Unborn Baby* by myself and Dr David Chamberlain; *The Secret Life of Your Unborn Child* by Dr Thomas Verny.

---

143. Personalise Your Perfume

. . . with essences: the holistic way to give your fragrance personal originality and oomph.

Combination essences are great for this. Try some of the Australian Bush Flower mixes, like **Confid** (for confidence-boosting and raising self-esteem) or **Dynamis** (for sheer energy and enthusiasm). Add seven to ten drops to your usual bottle of perfume, shake gently, then apply in the usual way. They are available from Australian Bush Flower Essences, via Healthlines (30 ml, £7.95 each) or Neal's Yard (£8.50 each). For contact details, see under 'Shopping' in the Directory.

(Mothers') Backs

144. Baby Backache

Both sexes may get bad backs, but two-thirds of all new mothers have a very specific and persistent sort that, according to the huge ongoing UK midwives' Avon Longitudinal Study, is still going strong eight weeks after they've had their babies.

It's often exacerbated by having to carry about not only a baby but a jealous toddler as well, and the pain tends to come from the sacroiliac joint (where the spine joins the pelvis). It varies from a gnawing ache with a few sharp twinges to downright immobilising.

While doing gentle strengthening exercises for the back and perhaps seeing a good osteopath or chiropractor with a special interest in post-natal health, it's very helpful to also use high-quality arnica cream – try Helios Arnica Cream (100 ml, £3.99) – or essence-containing **Microvita Pain Cream**, which is available worldwide by Living Essences of Australia, to help keep the soreness at bay. This cream's so good it's used in 16 of Australia's state hospitals. Microvita is sold in the UK as Body Soothe Cream from Victoria Health (125 ml, £9.99) and The Essence Shop.

The **TheraFlex** gel packs from Natremed are also invaluable to keep the joint inflammation down (30 cm x 9 cm, £6.95). For more information, see: Sciatica and Nerve Inflammation, page 84.

For all contact details, see under 'Shopping' in the Directory.

The Japanese way

As a further option, how about a traditional cotton maternity sash for extra support? Many modern Japanese new mothers still use these. Called **hara-obis**, they are often worn from the middle of pregnancy to a month or so after the birth, both for the good of a pregnant woman's back and as an honourable sign of new or approaching motherhood.

Birth educator and natural-childbirth guru Sheila Kitzinger suggests making your own using a piece of cotton material 15–20 cm wide: it needs to be long enough to go round you three times with enough left to tuck in securely so it doesn't come undone. Wind it round your lower abdomen and the small of your back either under or over your clothes so it supports you firmly but not too tightly. The idea, says Kitzinger, is to feel 'neatly packaged, without being squashed'.

145. Back Protection for Toddler-Carrying Mums

If you have to carry a heavy baby or toddler – or, as frequently happens, both – about, there is a supportive back-belt called a **Hipseat**, which has a small seat that clips round your waist. It helps to ensure you can carry your child *without* kinking your back (the primary cause of back problems for two-thirds of women later in life).

Recommended by osteopaths and chiropractors all over the UK – you'll even find leaflets advertising it in many of their practice reception areas – it's black, washable and suitable for carrying children from six months to three years. You can buy it from Hippy Chick (£34.95). For contact details, see under 'Shopping' in the Directory.

See also General: Backache on page 26.

Bloating

146. Food Intolerances

Often a side effect of PMS (see pp 165-72 for anti premenstrual techniques that work on bloating – and the rest!) your stomach blowing out can also be a sign that a particular food – most commonly wheat or dairy – doesn't agree with you. And while full-blown food allergies aren't that common, food intolerances are, so try the following:

1. Cut out first wheat, then dairy for a month and see if things improve.
2. Try taking a **probiotic** (see Fix 7: After Antibiotics), which you can get in the form of a small capsule taken once or twice daily for four to eight weeks, since an imbalance in gut bacteria is another major reason for bloating.
3. Try **gentian** – many herbalists swear by it for bloating. It is thought to work by stimulating the release of gastric juices, which help break down fat during digestion. The best way to take it is in the form of an easy-to-make herbal tea: add half a teaspoon to half a cup of boiling water in a saucepan and let it bubble gently for five minutes. Strain and drink half an hour before you are going

to eat. If it's too bitter, sweeten with a little manuka honey (which doesn't just taste good; it's antibacterial, probiotic and an excellent remedy to keep in your fridge for other things too – see Fix 105: Bee Better and Fix 62: Wound, Ulcer and Sore Healing) if you can get it – if not, use ordinary honey. You can get gentian from herbalists like Napiers.

4. **Kill candida overgrowth**: Ask a good nutritionist or AK practitioner to check whether you have a candida overgrowth in your gut: another very common bloat-inducer. If so, go for an anti-candida regime (see pp 191–2) plus supplementation with a good candida-killer like Citricidal (grapefruit seed extract: (see p 44)

For all contact details, see under 'Shopping' in the Directory.

If none of these work, see your GP, as bloating, especially if it comes on suddenly, can very occasionally indicate a more serious underlying condition (like ovarian cancer).

Also visit a good nutritionist, preferably one who is experienced in applied kinesiology (AK) testing, to see if they can pinpoint the trouble. For how to find a professionally qualified nutritionist in the UK, try the British Association of Nutritional Therapists; in the US, try the American Dietetic Association, which can put you in touch with a state-approved trained nutritionist. To find an AK practitioner in the UK and US, try the International College of Applied Kinesiology. In the UK, you can also try Kinesiology Connections; and in the US, the Touch for Health Kinesiology Association of North America. For contact details, see under 'Therapies and Therapists' in the Directory.

Breasts

147. Breast Pain – Immediate Relief
Press for painkilling
To soothe breast pain with DIY reflexology, press and smooth your thumb down along the areas shown in the picture, beginning just below your toe joints, for up to three minutes at a time once an hour.

Calming compress

If your breasts are swollen and sore, a cool compress of **lavender essential oil** is immensely soothing. Add ten drops to a half-full handbasin of lukewarm (not cold) water. Soak two clean flannels in it, wring out lightly and apply one to each breast. Repeat as necessary, as the flannels warm up with your body temperature. Lavender (*augustfolia* type) is both an anti-inflammatory and an analgesic – so effective it's used in childbirth.

In the UK, you can purchase lavender oil from Neal's Yard (organic, 10 ml, £8.95; non-organic, 10 ml, £5.75); in the US, buy it via Neal's Yard's American website (organic, 0.34 fl oz, $32; non-organic, 0.34 fl oz, $20). For contact details, see under 'Shopping' in the Directory.

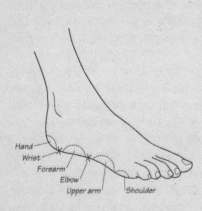

Hand
Wrist
Forearm
Elbow
Upper arm
Shoulder

Abscess action

If it's a breast abscess that is causing the pain, a GP will treat this with antibiotics – usually at least two types – to ensure it hits all possible bugs as an internal infection like this can often, as with, say, a pelvic infection, make you feel really rough, as if you have flu.

However, you might need more than one consecutive course, and possibly when the infection has gone, the fluid inside the abscess may need to be drained (aspirated with a syringe). This *ought* to be guided by ultrasound: just doing this by hand is not accurate enough so request the latter, or there is a risk that some material may be left behind that will re-infect easily.

While you are waiting for the antibiotics to kick in, which, depending on their type and the severity of the infection, can take anything from 24–72 hours , use an ice gel pack wrapped in a T-shirt for up to 15 minutes at a time every hour on the area. Blissful relief! You can buy **TheraFlex** gel cold packs from Natremed (30cm x 9cm, £6.95). For more information, see Sciatica and Nerve Inflammation on page 84.

After the course of antibiotics is over, so long as it has done the trick and you do not need to take any more, it's a very good idea to now take a good probiotic capsule of friendly bacteria like Bioforce's, as your 'good' gut bacteria will have been decimated, leaving you prone to digestive problems, stomach bloating and bad-smelling wind (see After Antibiotics, p 10).

148. Breast Pain – cyclical
What helps?
If the pain seems tied in with your periods, and tends to start after the half way point in your cycle:

- cut out caffeine altogether.
- reduce fatty and full-cream foods to the bare minimum.
- take **evening primrose oil**. The usual amount is six to eight 500 mg capsules every day. Ensure this amounts to 320 mg gamma linolenic acid (GLA) daily as different products contain different amounts, warns the Nigel Porter Breast Care Unit at the Royal Sussex Hospital.

How quickly will it work?
You may notice an improvement in as little as two to four weeks, but you'll get the greatest benefit after taking it for three months. Sometimes you can gradually reduce the dose after taking the full amount for three to six months, but many women find the problem recurs when they stop taking evening primrose oil.

Other positive benefits include improved skin, shinier hair and better nails, so it's not a bad idea to take it all the time anyway.

Evening primrose oil is available in the UK from most chemists and health shops – e.g. Holland & Barrett (120 x 1 g capsules, £9.97); in the US, a good budget source is Web Vitamins (100 capsules, $22.05). For contact details, see under 'Shopping' in the Directory.

149. Stopping Breastfeeding

There's lots of advice about starting and maintaining breastfeeding, but precious little about stopping.

The old advice used to be, 'Bind up your breasts, stop suckling your baby and put up with being bl**dy uncomfortable for several days,' because yes, those poor breasts certainly do get sore and overheated ('volcanic,' as one mother described them. 'Like having two hot rocks strapped to your chest.') Your GP might offer you a drug such as Parlodel (which contains bromocriptine and blocks the release of the milk-stimulating hormone prolactin) and suggest you take an ordinary over-the-counter painkiller. But there is also a gentler, more natural and altogether nicer option: **jasmine oil**.

Traditionally used in India to suppress lactation (women tape the flowers to their breasts to stop milk production), in 1979 one particular study compared using jasmine with bromocriptine and found both worked equally well.[3] The effect's also been confirmed by other experiments in which lactating mice had their cages lined with the flowers, so their mammary glands brushed against them as they passed by.

If you can't find enough of the fresh flowers – and most of us aren't going to have a convenient jasmine hedge at the bottom of the garden – the easy answer is to use a drop or two of **organic jasmine aromatherapy oil** in a carrier oil, like almond or safflower, and rub gently into your breasts two to three times daily.

Baldwin's supplies jasmine diluted in jojoba (5 ml, £5.89) to both UK and US customers. For contact details, see under 'Shopping' in the Directory.

Cellulite

150. The LowDown

If you're going out shopping for anti-cellulite products, first repeat the mantra: 'I will not be conned. I will not expect thighs like an undernourished pubescent girl's. I will not be conned.' Next, know that nothing on earth except liposuction can actually *take away* cellulite. Nothing.

However, the good news is that there are many products that may improve the look of the skin overlying the cellulite and some measures that will aid the removal of waste products that exacerbate it:

- creams, albeit pricey ones – e.g. Leirac Sensorielle Draining Cream (200 ml, approximately £30) is well spoken of
- 'drainage' tablets – e.g. the French Oenobiol Aquadrainant supplements (approximately £17)
- specialist salon treatments – e.g. wraps, rubs, massages and thalassotherapy (£35–£140)
- free DIY strategies – e.g. exercise and body-brushing.

Here, 'improving' means firming the skin up, smoothing, softening and reducing puffiness. All of which will make the whole area, whether it be thigh or bum, look better.

If you're buying
Ingredients to look out for in a product are those that encourage fluid drainage from the upper layers of skin and that also gently stimulate or tone. The best include:

- butcher's broom
- horse chestnut
- ginkgo biloba
- horsetail
- seabroom (brown seaweed that may also be called *Haloperis scoparia* on the packaging)
- caffeine (in topical cream)
- essentials oils such as rosemary, cypress, juniper and geranium.

Looking for a new approach? Try Tibetan Goji wolfberry juice, a powerful antioxidant packed with vitamins and minerals that has also been referred to as the 'cellulite assassinator'. You can buy it from Victoria Health (1 litre, a month's supply, £19.95). It's also good as an anti-aging supplement (your face may soon be showing its benefits) and all-round feel-good-booster. For contact details, see under 'Shopping' in the Directory.

If you're DIYing

Take regular exercise at least three times weekly, avoid caffeine in food and drink, have plenty of pure water and eat a healthy diet low in sugars and chemical additives but high in fresh and raw foods.

Also try body-brushing daily in the shower with a long-handled natural bristle brush. Leslie Kenton gives lots of information about this. If you'd like to see several entire books on the subject written by Kenton, bursting with useful information and suggestions, tap into her website (www.lesliekenton.com) for titles and purchase information.

151. The Simple Anti-Cellulite Soak

This is a holistic low-budget favourite. Two to three times a week, exfoliate all over – and you don't need a punishing loofah, a rough flannel will do fine – working in small circular motions. Then soak in a warm bath with a handful of Epsom salts to encourage your body to sweat and cleanse itself naturally.

Note: rinse flannel well after each session or it will start to smell because of the dead skin cells and the toxins you've efficiently sweated out through your skin.

Craving Sweet Stuff

152. Riding the Appetite Roller Coaster

That *'Gimme sweets! Chocolate! Biscuits!'* feeling is often caused by unstable blood sugar levels that dip and soar, sending your mood and appetite roller-coastering along with it. This is especially common premenstrually, when 40 per cent of women report typical low-blood-sugar symptoms, such as craving sweet foods, particularly chocolate, getting headaches and feeling thoroughly irritable, dizzy or faint.

What helps?

- Take **chromium** supplements, plus a **glucose tolerance factor** (GTF) product. The body makes GTF from, among other things, chromium. GTF is important because it balances blood sugar and 'normalises hunger', as top UK nutritionist Patrick Holford puts it. Try Blood

Sugar Gymena, which is a combination of vitamin B3 and the amino acids glycine, glutamic acid and cystine, plus GTF from Nature's Way (90 tablets, approximately £7.50/$12) or Sugar Factor, available from Lamberts. For contact details, see under 'Shopping' in the Directory.

- Eat plenty of **chromium-rich foods**. Dried brewer's yeast is the best by far, followed by wholemeal bread, then rye bread, oysters, potatoes and wheatgerm, which is widely available from most health food stores and chemists.
- Eat **complex carbohydrates** (e.g. baked potatoes, porridge and pasta) every three hours.

See also Anti PMS strategies pp 165–72.

Top Anti-Craving Tip
Never, ever skip a meal.

Endometriosis

Endometriosis occurs when fragments of womb-lining tissue end up in places other than the womb but go on reacting to hormonal change – i.e. thicken and bleed every month. The most common sites include the Fallopian tubes, around the ovaries and the ligaments supporting the womb, causing a variety of problems from infertility to miserably painful periods.

Endometriosis is thought to have many contributing factors, ranging from the dioxins used in bleached sanitary products to stress. Different treatments, often complementary and self-help, seem to improve matters for different people. The website www.endometriosis.co.uk offers some useful information and support.

Medical options include hefty hormone-moderating drugs like Danazol (which can have some unpleasant side effects) and laser surgery.

Complementary Treatments

There are several natural treatments, but two of the most successful are supplement-based.

153. Saw Palmetto

Traditionally used for prostate problems in men (well documented and tested – see Fix 204: Natural Remedies), a low dose of the herb **saw palmetto** helps by blocking the action of a sex hormone called follicle-stimulating hormone, the biochemical that encourages the production of womb lining-thickening oestrogen. The suggested daily therapeutic dose for women with endometriosis is 250–300 mg.

One of the best-value brands I can find is from Healthy Direct (60 x 1 g capsules, £3.95), but they'd need to be cut into quarters or thirds. Or, more expensive but less awkward to use, try Holland & Barrett's own-brand capsules (30 x 320 mg capsules, £10.95). For contact details, see under 'Shopping' in the Directory.

154. Essential Fatty Acids (EFAs)

One reason endometriosis can be so painful is because it is an *inflammatory* condition. Reduce this aspect of it with **essential fatty acids** (like evening primrose, borage, linseed and flaxseed oils), which also help reduce the inflammation of arthritis (see Fix 11: Nutritional Supplements). To begin with, try and take 1 g daily for six weeks and see how you go.

Linseed oil also has a useful knock-on effect, as Hilary Swank found when she used it in her training for Clint Eastwood's box-office hit *Million Dollar Baby*, which pitted her against real women's world boxing champion Lucia Rijker: she found it enhanced stamina and energy levels, which are often lower in women with endometriosis. For the same reason, it's also used to speed recovery from ME.

A terrific organic source of EFAs – good value too – is linseed oil from a small family-run company called High Barn Oils (100 capsules, £13.50). For contact details, see under 'Shopping' in the Directory.

155. Lusher Lips

One of the most effective, simple and quick ways to moisturise dry lips isn't good old petroleum jelly (Vaseline); it's **vitamin-E oil**. Just pierce a vitamin-E capsule, squeeze some oil on to both clean index fingers and stretch your lower lip a little as if about to apply lipstick. Beginning in the middle, work out towards the corners of your mouth in small, gentle circles, massaging the oil in without tugging at the thin, delicate skin. Repeat on your upper lip.

Exhaustion

156. Feeling Drained

Because of the huge amounts of emotional energy most women give out day after day – to our children, partners, friends and work – we tend to feel drained more often, and to a greater extent, than men who (generally speaking) seem to be able to compartmentalise and detach a little more easily.

And while feeling tired or drained is the most frequently reported physical symptom (and has several hundred different medical causes, from untreated diabetes to the onset of flu), one of the most common recurring *physical* reasons for women of menstruating age is their periods – see also Women: Periods on page 165. Peak times include the one to three days before a period starts, the day any cramps begin and the second day – when blood loss and any clot-passing (especially among peri- and pre-menopausal women) is often at its most intense.

However, there is a quick mental exercise that will power you back up again temporarily whenever you need a lift. It is directed towards your solar plexus, the seat of your energy reserves.

The Instant-Energy Breath

This is a fast technique for re-energising and is especially useful if you need to keep going but feel pretty hollow. You can do the **Instant-Energy Breath** at your desk, on public transport or the loo – anywhere you can have a few moments' quiet.

1. Sit with feet planted squarely on the floor, one hand on each knee with palms facing upwards. Close your eyes.
2. Take a slow, deep breath – in for a count of six, hold for six, out for six. Repeat three times.
3. Now, in your mind, ask the universe to send you some powerful, positive energy. Ask politely, but like you know you will be heard and expect it to happen (and it will).
4. Take another deep breath and, as you do so, imagine that the energy you asked for is pouring down over your head like a shower of soft, golden light and that you are breathing this in.
5. On your out-breath, send that energy down to your solar plexus (just above your tummy button, but deep inside your body). Imagine a *comforting orange glow* developing in there. Feel it warming and energising you.
6. Repeat three times. You can do it many more times if you'd like to, but three is the minimum.
7. Say thank you for the energy boost. Stretch, yawn and open your eyes. Rub your feet on the floor to ground yourself.

Better? The Instant-Energy Breath will get you through, but it's still important to take some rest as soon as you can.

157. Carer Fatigue and Maternal Burnout

Carers of all types can feel a grinding fatigue and sheer discouragement that goes way beyond physical exhaustion, especially if they don't have enough support or resources to back them up, or have been doing it all for too long.

And these carers are more often women than men, perhaps mothers of very young or differently abled children, daughters or partners looking after a sick or elderly loved one. However, there is a great essence that not only helps revitalise you but also enables you to look at the way you're using your energies ('*How did it get like this?*'), reassess and recover a bit of healthy balance in your life. Often, say those who've used it, it helps by empowering you to say 'no' more often and to create much-needed boundaries.

The essence comes from the tough red outback of Australia, is called **Alpine Mint Bush,** and its positive effects can be felt within days. It is from the Australian Bush Flower range and can be bought direct or, in the UK, from Healthlines (15 ml, £8.95). For contact details, see under 'Shopping' in the Directory.

Note: it is also helpful for professional carers for whom things have become too much – e.g. medical staff, therapists and charity volunteers. For beleaguered mums, try also **Heart Mother** – for use and dosage details, see Women: Anxiety on page 116.

158. Protective Earrings for Mobile Users

If you use a mobile often or tend to stay on it for long periods, try wearing a pair of little diamond stud earrings, or at least one in your listening ear. According to Judy Hall, a gem therapist of thirty years' experience and author of several international books on the subject, a diamond (of any size – it can be a small chip) offers a measure of protection against the radiation mobiles emit. See also Teenagers: Mobile Phones on page 356.

Feet

159. Bunion Bliss-Out

Bunion is the lay term for what doctors call hallux valgus – the protrusion of the first joint of the big toe at an angle. Covering the joint is a fluid-filled sac called a bursa, which generally gives some protection against friction, but too much makes it inflamed and painful. The prime culprit is fashionable pointy shoes, especially stilettos.

Fast, simple relief from bunion pain: dissolve a tablespoon of Epsom salts in a washing-up bowl of warm water (not hot, as it will increase the inflammation) and soak your feet.

If your bunion has swollen, make an easy healing compress as follows:

1. Add a drop of homeopathic **arnica** tincture, one of **calendula**, plus, if very sore around the bone, one of **Symphytum** (wonderfully soothing and used for many painful bone conditions) to 1.2 litres of cold water.
2. Add a tablespoon of **distilled witch hazel**.
3. Soak a clean flannel in the healing liquid and apply. Put your foot up while it's on and relax.
4. Leave on for five to ten minutes, then when the flannel has warmed up, repeat as necessary.

You can store spare poultice liquid in a covered jug or bowl in the fridge, which makes it beautifully chilled. It will keep for a couple of days.

To find the tinctures, try a well-stocked health shop or a homeopathic pharmacy that also does mail order. The advantage of a pharmacy is that they can make up a mix for you so you don't have to buy three separate tinctures. In the UK, try Helios (£3.75 each); in the US, try the listing website, USA Homeopathic Pharmacies. For contact details, see under 'Shopping' in the Directory.

160. Hard or Cracked Skin on Feet

Derma E's **Cracked Skin Relief Cream** does what it says on the packet and does it very well. It contains homeopathic remedies, skin vitamins and herbs, and is also great for chapped lips. It is available from Victoria Health (56 g, £11.95). And the best hard-skin removing file I've so far come across (shaped to hold so it's easier to twist and turn slightly as you use it, and flakes off the dead skin fast without leaving what's left rough and 'fluffy' as many similar devices do, is the Alida Foot File, £9.95, also from VH.

Or try the budget holistic favourite for no-fuss softening of hard skin on heels and soles: add 10–15 drops of olive oil to warm water, stir and soak your feet for ten minutes. If your feet have been having hard usage, feel 'beaten up or abused', add four to seven drops of Bach Rescue Remedy too. It is available from Healthlines (10 ml, £3.99).

For all contact details, see under 'Shopping' in the Directory.

Fertility

161. Conception – the Best Positions

There are (unsurprisingly) no definitive studies on this one, but most gynaecologists, obstetricians and fertility specialists agree that the following positions may maximise the chances of conception because they encourage deep penetration. This ensures the man's sperm is ejaculated as close to the cervix entrance as possible, and the closer they are to their goal (a ripe egg waiting in one of the Fallopian tubes a few inches further up), the better their chances of reaching it.

- the **missionary** – man on top, woman on her back
- the **pillow-talker** – place a pillow beneath the woman's hips before lovemaking
- **from behind** – the man enters the woman's vagina from behind her, especially if she is kneeling in front of him, knees apart, with her head down (similar to the cat position in yoga) so that her bottom is higher than her head.

Post-coital possum unnecessary

According to Dr Steve Brody of the Advanced Fertility Institute of San Diego, women can ignore tedious traditional advice about lying still for half an hour after intercourse with their legs up the wall to maximise the chances of conception. As long as you don't leap up immediately afterwards, 'The best-quality (fastest) sperm will have got to the egg in five minutes flat, and those are the ones you want fertilising it.'

162. Low Fertility

More women are leaving it until 35 and over to start a family (in 1989 it was one in ten British women, now it's nearing one in six), but pollution levels in food, air and water are rising, nutrient levels in foods are dropping, and the average sperm count has plummeted by 42 per cent since 1940, according to a *British Medical Journal* report in 1995. No wonder one in five Western couples is having trouble conceiving.

IVF

Assisted conception is expensive and has limited success. A single cycle of IVF – usually three are undertaken – costs £2,000–£7,000, plus at least £1,500 extra each time for the drugs (treatment is often no longer available on public health programmes). On average, IVF's take-home baby rate (not the same as pregnancy rate, which can be as high as 35–50 per cent) is usually around 10–15 per cent though some clinics claim higher rates, especially if they're selective about which couples they'll treat.

The holistic approach

Fortunately, there's also a whole raft of 'can-do' holistic techniques and a wide range of complementary therapies that can maximise your chances of conception, especially acupuncture, professional herbalism and nutrition.

Preconceptual care

If you would prefer to tackle fertility problems holistically, one of the most successful and certainly the most affordable approach – unless there are specific clinical issues that require specialist medical intervention – is a good preconceptual-care programme undertaken *by both partners three to six months before they begin trying for a baby*. It works because it gets you both into the best possible shape for conceiving and (for women) carrying the pregnancy to term.

One study carried out with the University of Surrey followed 367 couples who went on a Foresight preconceptual programme. The group included those who couldn't get pregnant at all, those who had experienced repeated miscarriages (sometimes as many as five in succession), parents who had previously given birth to babies with deformities and parents whose previous babies had been very underweight, premature or victims of cot death. The findings? Results any IVF clinic could only dream of: 327 of the 367 couples went on to give birth to healthy full-term babies within 18 months of completing the programme.[4] This compares with the fact that only about half of those undergoing traditional medical fertility treatment are successful. There were also no twins or triplets – a common, and not always welcome, result of IVF.

Several different programmes are available worldwide, but not all are equally good. If I needed preconceptual care, I would opt for the one run by Foresight – and not only because they helped my younger sister have a healthy baby after four early miscarriages in succession. This charity, which began pioneering this approach back in the late 1970s, uses a three-pronged approach:

1. Check for infection and treat it if found.
2. Check toxicity and detox if necessary.
3. Advise on pro-fertility nutrition and also suggest relevant supplements.

Using data from analysis of samples of your hair, sweat and blood, *both* partners are:

1. Assessed for any genitourinary infections like chlamydia, which can ruin fertility for both sexes but are often without symptoms, and referred for appropriate treatment.
2. Prescribed an individualised health-supplement regime of pro-conception nutrients.
3. Put on an organic, wholefood eating plan.
4. Told to stop smoking, drinking or taking any recreational drugs. According to consultant andrologist (male-hormone specialist) Anthony Hirsh at the UK's Whipps Cross Hospital, a man can wipe out his entire sperm count for the next three months with a single heavy drinking session. Smoking reduces sperm count and the sperm's ability to move – for more details, see Men: Fertility on page 218. And according to the latest research from Holland's Radboud University, published in *Human Reproduction*, smoking puts ten years on a woman's reproductive age: the fertility of a 30-year-old female smoker who has five to ten mild cigarettes a day is that of a 40-year-old non-smoker. Considering a third of UK women in their twenties smoke and the fact that fertility declines so fast anyway between 30 and 40, this effect is quite something. Smoking also increases the risk of miscarriage by about a quarter.
5. Checked and cleared of any toxic substances like lead, cadmium and mercury, including having their mercury amalgam fillings checked out.

> **Power Tip**
> The two most important things that both partners can do to maximise their chances of pregnancy are to stop smoking and drinking for three to six months before they start trying for a baby.

Malicious mercury

If your fillings used to be silvery but are now grey or, worse, black, beware – that means that they are degenerating and leaking mercury into your system. If you can possibly afford it, get them taken out safely by a specialist mercury-free dentist – *never, ever let an ordinary dentist do this* – and replaced with non-toxic white fillings.

Mercury residues in the body, usually the result of amalgam fillings, may cause or contribute to both infertility and miscarriage. In fact, mercury is so deadly to sperm (it makes them start 'head-banging', ensuring they cannot penetrate an egg) that until the early 1970s, it was still being used most effectively in contraceptive gels and pastes. And when used to treat syphilis in women 50 years ago, it was also found to induce spontaneous abortions.

There's a considerable amount of published clinical research examining the harm mercury can do – see *Infertility and Birth Defects: Is Mercury From Silver Dental Fillings an Unsuspected Cause?* by Sam Ziff and Dr Michael Ziff. It has more than 500 clinical references. Or the more recent and reader-friendly *Let the Tooth Be Known* by Dawn Ewing. Both can be mail ordered from Natural Dentistry in Florida. For contact details, see under 'Shopping' in the Directory.

If you're interested in finding a mercury-free dentist or seeking advice, contact the British Society of Mercury-Free Dentists. In the US, contact the International Society of Mercury-Free Dentists. For details, see under 'Therapies and Therapists' in the Directory.

See also: Mercury ('silver') Amalgam Fillings on page 90 and Fix 116: Addressing Mercury Toxicity.

Further information

Foresight is based in the UK, with advisers (mostly doctors and nutritionists) countrywide, but there are also some Foresight-trained professionals in the US. Telephone advice is free, their recommended battery of tests is £70 per couple, supplements cost extra. For more information, send a stamped, addressed envelope to Foresight or visit their website. In the US, you can also check out the Center for Occupational and Environmental Medicine (COEM), which offers a similar programme. For contact details, see under 'Useful Helplines, Websites and Contacts' in the Directory.

163. Idiopathic (Unexplained) Infertility

Idiopathic infertility is one of the most frustrating diagnoses a couple can be given when they want to have a baby and it's just not happening. It gives you no clues, no pointers, and, to many, this can mean no hope. According to UK fertility guru Professor Robert Winston, it is also one of the most common verdicts, since 40 per cent of the time doctors aren't sure what's the matter or with whom.

Stress connection

Stress is, however, a common culprit for both sexes. There are sound biochemical reasons for this. Stress hormones such as cortisol, nora-drenaline and prolactin can play hell with the balance and production of sex hormones and have a wide variety of concrete, measurable results ranging from stopping ovulation, 'spoiling' the womb lining so the egg cannot implant successfully and reducing sperm count or quality to sending Fallopian tubes into spasm so the egg can't get down them.

Fortunately, stress levels can also be highly responsive to **focused relaxation** (not the same as sitting down with a cuppa to watch TV). In 1986 researchers at the University of Dublin found that when a group of women who'd been told they had idiopathic infertility (and high prolactin levels) were given relaxation training, the elevated levels of stress hormones dropped and their periods (which had been all over the place) normalised. Many top teaching hospitals now offer anti-stress programmes in their fertility units: one of the first was Boston's famous Beth Israel Deaconess Medical Centre, which has done so for 25 years.

Focused relaxation: how to do it

Use any form of meditation that relaxes you quickly and completely, getting your brain into a state where it will willingly 'receive and obey' feasible instructions.

Good options include **yoga** (contact the British Wheel of Yoga) and

autogenic training (a quick form of deep meditation, ideal for those who reckon yoga takes too long!). It requires short training, usually eight group sessions, and has been widely researched clinically and found to be effective. Contact the British Autogenic Society or the British Association for Autogenic Training and Therapy (BAFATT).

Self-hypnosis tapes help too, but a short course of 'proper' training (sometimes a session or two will be enough) with a teacher is usually far more effective if you want serious results, so well worth the money. Contact the National Register of Hypnotherapists and Psychotherapists.

For all contact details, see under 'Training Courses' in the Directory.

Amazing affirmations

For conception, the most successful affirmations to repeat calmly and confidently when you are at your most deeply relaxed point include:

- 'I can and will get pregnant easily.'
- 'I am very fertile and can carry a pregnancy to term.'
- 'I will get pregnant very soon and give birth to a beautiful, healthy baby.'

Former University of Liverpool fertility researcher Paul Entwhistle, who used the above affirmations plus hypnosis and self-hypnosis for couples with unexplained infertility, then measured their stress-hormone levels before and after sessions, reported that 40 per cent conceived within four months.

See also Men: Fertility on page 218.

Hair

164. Serious Hair-Moisture Treatment
This is a lovely, lush fix and a treat for dried-out hair, suggests Charmaine Yabsley, editor of *Allergy* magazine. It uses bananas, which are full of

minerals and vitamins that help restore hair vitality, and olive oil to boost softness and shine.

Mash up one ripe banana with a tablespoon of cold-pressed virgin olive oil, pile on wet hair from roots to ends and massage in. Next, wrap your head in cling film, wind a warm towel round it and leave for 10–20 minutes. Wash out well in warm water, shampoo lightly and dry as normal.

165. Serious Hair-Thickener

This is the best and cheapest instant thicken-and-shine treatment there is, and it comes from UK massage and aromatherapy pioneer Clare Maxwell-Hudson.

1. Add a sachet of powdered gelatine from the supermarket to double your usual amount of hair shampoo in a mug.
2. Mix together and immediately work the resulting paste into damp, newly washed hair. If it's too thick to use easily, thin it a little with tepid (not hot) water.
3. Leave in for five to ten minutes, then rinse out well.

Note: sorry, but there isn't a vegetarian version of this fix.

166. Hair Loss

Nearly 40 per cent of women under the age of 60 have experienced some degree of noticeable hair loss, one in two report having had thinning hair, and in 2005 the often dramatic alopecia areata affected one in 50 Americans. Common causes for women include post-childbirth, stress, the Pill and certain medications including some blood-thinning products, chemotherapy drugs and certain antidepressants. Treatments vary, depending on the trigger.

There are so many potential 'cures', both medical and complementary, that it can be immensely confusing. This is not helped by the aggressive marketing techniques of some of the private clinics and product companies. However, the best one-stop resource I've found as an informed starting point on almost everything and anything that may help – from self-hypnosis to having your amalgam fillings removed – is a book called *Regrowing Hair Naturally* by UK kinesiologist and hypnotherapist Vera

Peiffer, who used to suffer from hair loss herself. It also comes with a useful relaxation CD.

Labour

167. How to Stay Calm – the Fast Natural Fix

For an immediate calming effect on a woman in labour, shake a single drop each of lavender, rose, clary sage and melissa essential oils on to a tissue and ask her to breathe it in, recommends Dr Vivian Lunny, former pathologist at London's Harefield and Mount Vernon Hospitals, now a medical aromatherapist. The scent works fast by stimulating the olfactory centres of the brain (hippocampus and thalamus), which are linked to the hypothalamus, the part of your brain that controls mood.

For good-quality essential oils, try Baldwin's, a leading traditional UK herbalist and natural-products supplier: Rose Maroc Oil (5 ml, £24.95) or even better, but pricier, Rose Absolu, Melissa in Jojoba Oil (5 ml, £9.99; undiluted, £47.95), Clary Sage Oil (5 ml, £4.65), Lavender (10 ml, £4.09). For contact details, see under 'Shopping' in the Directory.

168. Childbirth Doesn't Have to Hurt

Thinking about an epidural but don't fancy a needle in your spine? Want to try and avoid having a Caesarean now rates are at a record high (23 per cent in the UK and 30 per cent in the US)? Consider having a **doula** with you in childbirth.

Doula power

A doula (the name means 'woman helping women' in Greek) is a sympathetic, informed lay person who supports you by giving practical, non-medical help throughout labour – e.g. massage, fetching drinks, supporting you in positions like squatting, helping you walk to and fro or change position, encouraging you and protecting your privacy. Usually an older mother or youngish grandmother who has plenty of positive experience of normal childbirth, she does not leave your side – unless there is a major medical emergency – from the moment labour begins until your child is safely born.

Analysis of six controlled medical trials on what doulas can do for women in childbirth carried out over the last ten years in America, Britain and Guatemala confirms that just having a doula with you during labour will:

- reduce the pain by a third to half
- shorten labour time by between a quarter and a third
- lessen the likelihood of a Caesarean by around 50 per cent
- reduce the likelihood of a forceps delivery by 40 per cent.[5]

And no drug on earth can do all that.

The magic of doulas is that they give you reassurance, confidence and relax you, 'all of which have a major effect on the amount of pain you feel, how smoothly your labour goes and how long it lasts', explains natural-childbirth and water-birth pioneer Dr Michel Odent, who strongly supports the doula movement in the UK. Doulas also get to know you and your partner before your due date and will often help you at home afterwards too, with everything from establishing breastfeeding to food shopping, for up to several months.

To help you find a doula, see under 'Therapies and Therapists' in the Directory. They cost from £300 to attend a birth and £10–£20 an hour afterwards.

Recommended reading: for further information on the 20 different medical and complementary ways to reduce labour pain and side effects, and for research and pros and cons, see *Childbirth Doesn't Have to Hurt* by myself and Professor Geoffrey Chamberlain.

169. Perineal Tears and Episiotomies

In the UK, 60–70 per cent of women need stitches after having a baby, and 85 per cent of them are pretty sore from general childbirth wear and tear, sometimes for weeks after their baby's birth.[6] In the US, seven in ten women who are taken care of by private obstetricians are given an episiotomy – a sterile cut in the vaginal exit to make more room for the baby's head to come through.[7]

However, there is an invaluable herbal mix that will both soothe the discomfort and heal any stitches or tears fast. It was recommended to me by Caroline Flint, an independent British midwife of 30 years' experience and former president of the UK's Royal College of Midwives.

1. Take a handful of the dried herbs uva ursa, comfrey and shepherd's purse.
2. Add to a warm bath, sit in there and soak. To ensure the bath's not left looking like you just trimmed a privet hedge in it, put the herbs in a cotton handkerchief or a muslin wrap and knot it closed.
3. Repeat daily for seven days or more, with new amounts of the herb mixture each time. It is very comforting and soothing, and will help to heal birthing scars and tears quickly.

For quick mail-order herbs delivered internationally, try Baldwin's Shepherd's Purse (100 g, £2.09), Uva Ursa (100 g, £2.49) and Organic Comfrey (100 g, £3.89). All these herbs are also available from Baldwin's in tincture form if the herbs seems a bit fiddly.

> **170. No Time to Exercise but Feeling Stressed?**
> Do a short ten-minute burst that slots easily into your day (like a fast walk down the road to get a sandwich at work or a swift steam round the block with the baby buggy). Short bursts are just as effective for calming and de-stressing as a prolonged session, say sports-science researchers at the University of Loughborough.
> See also Men: Exercise on page 211.

Men – Mixed Feelings About Them

If you like male company and affection and wish you could enjoy men's physicality more but are not comfortable about sexualised or sensual contact with them, there is an essence that could be helpful.

Horse Chestnut Leaf Bud (which bears a staggering resemblance to a small erect penis) encourages women's attraction to, and enjoyment of, men's bodies and male sexuality, and also helps support taking real pleasure in good sex. This remedy is homeopathically dilute and very gentle, but it can be powerful and someone who takes it may start to feel its effects within a few days.

It is available direct from Light Heart Essences (10 ml, £5.15) and is taken as a few drops (as many as you feel is right, rather than a strict recommended amount). People will begin with, say, six at a time from a 'made-up' dropper bottle two to four times daily for three to six weeks, or longer if you feel the need.

Note: if you are not sure where the ambivalence towards men stems from, Horse Chestnut Leaf Bud can be very helpful, but if you feel it could be explained by a history of abuse, then in addition to sympathetic counselling, support, patience and love, you would need a different essence.

For instance, a combination of the Australian Bush Flower remedies **Wisteria** and **Fringed Violet** can be immensely healing and is often given to both women and men who have been abused physically, emotionally or sexually to help them during counselling. The remedies are available individually direct and from Healthlines (15 ml, £8.95 each), or the latter can make you up a combination, which saves money.

For all contact details, see under 'Shopping' in the Directory.

Menopause

Going through the menopause is not unlike being pregnant, in that well-meaning people *will* keep on giving you 'it-worked-for-me' advice as to how you can overcome this particular aspect or that until you're drowning in suggestions, don't know what to try first and very possibly wish they'd mind their own damn business.

The menopause usually starts in a woman's late forties (as opposed to peri-menopause, which tends to begin from 35 or so – see Women: Peri-Menopause on page 163) and may last for anything from a few months to, if you're less lucky, ten years. Fortunately, there is a wealth of tried and tested strategies from both the complementary and the clinical sectors that can help with everything from vaginal dryness to lack of energy.

171. The Menopause Top Five
Five of the very best things you can do for the menopause are:

1. Read

Your Change, Your Choice by Sarah Stacey, health editor of the *Mail on Sunday*'s '*YOU*' magazine, and Michael Dooley, consultant gynaecologist at the Lister Hospital, London, and initiator of the pioneering integrated women's healthcare programme at the Poundbury Clinic, Dorset. A comprehensive, sympathetic and highly readable résumé of the truly integrated (medical and complementary) approach to menopause. It's the best book on the 'big M' I've come across in years.

2. Try

- **Chaste berry (*Vitex agnus castus*):** one of the top hormone-balancing herbs in the business. A good form to use that doesn't involve stewing up herbal teas three times a day is **agnolyt**, a liquid tincture of *agnus castus*, which a herbalist can supply. See also 'Chaste berry' on page 169. Stop taking it if it causes you headaches, gastric upset or nausea. If you were experiencing depression with your menopause and the herb makes it worse, reducing the dose tends to maintain the herb's positive effects but also deals with the 'extra' depression. To find a professional herbalist, contact the National Institute of Medical Herbalists. For contact details, see under 'Therapies and Therapists' in the Directory.
- **Black cohosh** is another favourite of herbalists and may well suit you if chaste berry doesn't. Try it in convenient herbal tincture form taken as drops in water from Baldwin's (50 ml, £3.15).

> A great menopause-banisher is **MenoHerbs2**, a terrific mix of just about every plant extract helpful for menopause including black cohosh, wild yam and squaw vine. MenoHerbs2 has an awful lot of fans – with good reason. It is made by Victoria Health (90 tablets, £14.95) and is usually taken twice daily.

3. Pop

A mix of **evening primrose oil** and **flaxseed oil** in handy capsule form: these are great for lubricating the vaginal lining, moisturising drying external body skin (such as the face), balancing out mood dips or swings and for tackling cyclic mastalgia (premenstrual breast pain) which can worsen around this time – see also Fix 148: Breast Pain – Cyclical.

4. Use

Essences for gentle emotional, physical and spiritual rebalancing during menopause: homeopathically dilute, these energy remedies are nevertheless so effective that state hospitals in Australia and South America are using them. One of the best ones is **She Oak** from the Australian Bush Flower range (15 ml, £8.95). It is particularly good for hot flushes – see 'Side-effect-free things to take' on page 154.

Recommended reading: see my book *Heal Yourself With Flowers and Other Essences* for which essences work best for anything from sleep problems and low libido to stress and PMS.

5. Eat

Eat right for a healthy menopause. Check out which types of food will help you feel best and healthiest at present and whether you need any additional nutrients to help you sail on through. A good nutritionist could be invaluable here. See 'Finding a good nutritionist' on page 13. The Natural Health Advisory Service (incorporating the Women's Nutritional Advisory Service) also provides professional nutritional help. For contact details, see under 'Therapies and Therapists' in the Directory.

For all supplier contact details, see under 'Shopping' in the Directory.

172. Hot Flushes

These are one of the standard, expected (ha!) symptoms of approaching menopause and by far the most common. Sometimes they are the only one women experience. Though different countries and cultures vary in the level of symptoms women have, in the UK, according to a survey by the Menopause Awareness Alliance, 68 per cent of all women have hot flushes during their menopause years.

However, there is a very easy, deep, slow-breathing technique that, according to work by Robert Freeman, professor of psychiatry and behavioural sciences at Wayne State University School of Medicine, can stop a hot flush in its tracks and, performed daily, reduce their frequency by 50–60 per cent.

Flush patrol

The second you feel a flush coming on:

1. Deliberately slow your breathing rate.
2. Take deep, slow inhalations that fill up your whole belly and allow long, smooth exhalations.
3. Try to reduce your breathing rate to seven or eight breaths a minute.

This breath-slowing is thought to reduce temperature because, according to Dr Mosaraf Ali of the Integrated Medical Centre in London, this is the rate at which your pituitary gland, which controls (among other things) the body's thermostat, works best.

Practising this slow breathing twice daily helps limit the number of flushes and sweats, and also helps you deal more easily with stress and anxiety.

Recommended reading: the excellent *Your Change, Your Choice* by Michael Dooley and Sarah Stacey.

Side-effect-free things to take

Treatments for menopause as a whole will also address hot flushes. However, if it's *just* those flushes you want soothed and the breathing technique has not totally tackled them but you don't want to take herbs or hormones, there is a gentle, subtle alternative that women anecdotally report reduces the strength and number of hot flushes. **She Oak** is being used in a three-year double-blind placebo trial for female hormonal rebalancing by gynaecologists in Australia; results will be available by the end of 2007. Anecdotal reports from my own patients, and from other UK users, suggest She Oak can halve the intensity and frequency of hot flushes within 10–14 days. It is available direct from Australian Bush Flower Essences (15 ml, £8.95).

To strengthen the anti-flush effect, add seven drops of **Mulla Mulla** to your treatment bottle. The mulla mulla plant grows in the blazing-hot, red Australian outback and is also the cooling and healing remedy for 'trauma associated with fire and heat'. Mulla Mulla is available direct from Australian Bush Flower Essences (15 ml, £8.95).

The excellent **MenoHerbs2** complex by Victoria Health can do the trick with hot flushes too, and help take care of any other menopausal symptoms you are getting – see the box on page 152.

For all contact details, see under 'Shopping' in the Directory.

Miscarriage

Miscarriage is the medical term for the loss of an unborn baby before the 20th week of pregnancy – after that point, doctors call it a stillbirth. It is the single most common complication of pregnancy and is thought to occur in 50 per cent of all of them – usually before a woman even knows she is pregnant. Of very early confirmed pregnancies (within a few weeks of conception, usually detected via a DIY home test done around the time of the first missed period), the rate of miscarriage is one in six. This tends to show up as a heavy menstrual flow a couple of weeks later than usual. Of all later confirmed, but still fairly early, pregnancies (i.e. when someone is 6–12 weeks pregnant), the rate of miscarriage is about one in eight. After that the likelihood drops very dramatically.

In two-thirds of miscarriages, the cause is a chromosomal abnormality, or perhaps abnormal cell division at a very early stage (i.e. first few days) which may often be prevented by good preconceptual healthcare and positive nutrition next time around. For the remainder there can be a wide range of contributing factors, but, frustratingly, doctors usually cannot tell for certain what happened. Women who conceive as a result of fertility treatment have a higher rate of miscarriage.

According to Dr Richard Aubry, professor of obstetrics and gynaecology at the State University of New York, the chances of a woman having a miscarriage after she has confirmed her pregnancy are, in general:

Under 35: 10–12 per cent
35–40: 15 per cent
40–45: more than 25 per cent
Over 45: more than 45 per cent

There are many different important nutrients that may affect a woman's ability to carry a pregnancy to term, including **selenium**[8] and **folic acid**[9]. However, a substance called **homocysteine** has also been causing interest recently. It's produced when we break down methionine, itself a by-product of protein from the food we eat.

When homocysteine's present in the right amounts, it can do its job of helping build up and maintain the body's tissues. However, having too much of it can damage the lining of the arteries. Studies suggest women who have had recurrent miscarriages have high levels of homocysteine, and an increasing number of specialists reckon that this sort of damage may cause problems with the blood supply to the developing embryo or foetus, resulting in the loss of that pregnancy. Homocysteine can also thicken the blood, causing clots, and this may be a factor as well.[10]

173. Five Anti-Miscarriage Action Points

1. **Keep up your levels of B6, B12 and folic acid,** suggests top GP and nutritionist Dr John Briffa. They help convert homocysteine into a harmless substance called cystathionine. The suggested level of B6 is 10 mg, B12 is 400 mcg, and for folic acid it's 800 mcg daily.
2. **Cut down caffeine** from tea, coffee and colas. One particular study showed that women who drank 100 mg or more of caffeine (that's just two cups of tea or one of coffee a day) were more likely to lose their babies before 12 weeks of pregnancy than those who drank no caffeine at all.[11]
3. **Avoid aspirin and NSAID painkillers** like ibuprofen around conception time: there is some evidence that they increase the pregnancy loss rate by up to 80 per cent.[12] Paracetamol does not seem to be a problem, however.
4. **Contact Foresight before you try to conceive again.** Foresight is a very sound preconceptual advice and assessment organisation. Its success with couples who have had either repeated miscarriages or difficulties in getting pregnant in the first place is considerable, and research by the University of Surrey over a three-year period backs up Foresight's results. See also 'Preconceptual care' on page 142.

5. **Reduce stress** – often easier said than done. A lot easier. But some of the suggestions in this book might offer a starting point. See General: Stress and Stamina on page 95, 'Focused relaxation: how to do it' on page 145 and Women: Stress on page 189. It's well worth doing it if you can. Huge international research projects like Europop 2000 identify psychologically stressful work to be a major cause of both miscarriage and premature birth. This is partly because high levels of stress hormones like noradrenaline and cortisol can affect the amounts of oestrogen and progesterone your body makes, meaning they may not be produced in sufficiently large amounts, or in the right balance, to maintain a pregnancy.

174. Soothing and Rebalancing

If you have had a miscarriage recently, there is a very gentle essence that can help soothe the distress and trauma. Called **Candystick**, it's taken by mouth, diluted in water and made from an unassuming but effective little plant growing on the shores of the wild Canadian Pacific coast.

Candystick is made by Pacific Essences and is available in the UK on 24-hour mail order from Healthlines (7.5 ml, £6), who also have many more essences that may help; in the US and Canada, Candystick is available direct from Pacific Essences ($11).

For more information about other gentle, inexpensive but powerful essences which may help you, see *Heal Yourself With Flowers and Other Essences*.

Nails

175. Natural Nail Tricks
Tip 1
You're usually told to 'push your cuticles back', cut them or even remove them (as some products say they can do), but according to the Natural Nail Company – and any manicurist worth their salon fee – the truth is that cuticles need to be pushed back as little as possible, because they're protecting and sealing the living nailbed below.

Tip 2

Massage **cold-pressed olive oil** into your cuticles every night: the ultimate low-maintenance holistic tip for keeping them supple and healthy so they don't split and snag. This also encourages good blood flow to the area, bringing oxygen and food with it for cell division and taking away cellular waste products.

Tip 3

Buff your nails regularly. Again, it increases blood flow to the living part, encouraging healthy cellular replenishment and growth, and promoting waste removal. It also gives them a soft, healthy, natural shine, which beats clear nail polish hands down.

Osteoporosis

There is a huge amount women can do to slow, or even to some extent reverse, this gradual age-related slide towards bones that are brittle and break easily. Osteoporosis affects one in three women, and one in five men in the UK and US, and yet, as Sandra Reynold of America's National Osteoporosis Foundation says, 'Most of these could be prevented.'
    Your bone strength is determined by four main factors:

- what you eat (especially your calcium intake during your growing-up years)
- how active you are (particularly how much weight-bearing exercise like walking, running, racquet sports, dance or keep-fit routines you do)
- hormone levels (especially that of oestrogen)
- genetics (which predetermine the sort of bones you have).

176. Do-It-Now Action

A conventional doctor is likely to suggest a drug such as etidronate or alendronate, both synthetic compounds based on phosphorous, which combine with the calcium still in your bones to help prevent its loss, plus a calcium-rich diet or supplements. Holistic measures you can undertake yourself include:

- Eat a calcium-rich diet.
- And depending on how much you're getting through diet, **take calcium supplements** that contain the other minerals and vitamins vital for bone-building and calcium absorption, including **phosphorous, sodium, magnesium, boron,** and **vitamin D**. All these minerals and vitamins are important for helping the body use the calcium you take in: calcium taken alone often passes straight through you. It is worth consulting a good nutritionist to find out how to add them in separately in the right ratios with single-supplement capsules. See under 'Therapies and Therapists' in the Directory.
- If you are over 40, **arrange through your doctor for a bone-density test** to see just how solid your bones still are, or aren't. This is non-invasive and doesn't hurt, but will show what's going on and indicate the precise treatments you will need to keep your skeleton strong.
- **Get regular sunlight** on your skin: it will react by producing vitamin D. Full-spectrum sunlight is essential for bone health as well as helping you feel good psychologically (as anyone who suffers from seasonal affective disorder could confirm). See also General: Seasonal Affective Disorder (SAD) on page 85 and Fix 298: Light Therapy.
- **Take essential fatty acids (EFAs).** One study carried out at South Africa's University of Pretoria suggests that taking EFAs improves the absorption of calcium through the gut wall, reduces the amount lost through peeing and helps transport calcium into the bones where it is needed.[13] Try Efamol, available from Boots, Superdrug, Holland & Barrett and other health shops in the UK (90 capsules, £9.99); in the US, you can purchase it from Academy Health (90 capsules, $16.50).
- **Go for weight-bearing exercise** – every day if you can. This is defined as anything that puts extra pressure on your bones, so it also includes stay-in-one-place activities like press-ups, weight-training and sports activities that require you to stand upright and keep moving – like racquet sports or running. Swimming is not a weight-bearing activity, neither are stretch classes or yoga. However, a daily no-fuss, no-frills, fit-it-in-when-most-convenient

30-minute pavement-pound round the block certainly *does* qualify.

- **Cut out fizzy drinks, alcohol and smoking** – they're all calcium-robbers, and the latter accelerates the loss of a wide variety of other vital nutrients as well. Women who quit smoking and drinking around the time of their menopause may cut their risk of hip fracture when they're older (commonly caused by osteoporosis) by 40 per cent. See 'Advice on stopping smoking' on page 218 and Men: Smoking on page 234.

Suggestions for things to take

Try **Osteoguard** by Nature's Best (90 tablets, £9.50), which contains calcium, magnesium, boron, vitamin D and vitamin K, or Healthspan's **Osteo Plus**, which contains chelated calcium – the easiest form for the body to absorb – zinc, magnesium, copper, boron, vitamin D, digestive enzymes and a particular bioflavonoid that helps increase bone density. In the UK, Osteo Plus can be purchased direct from Healthspan (180 tablets, £6.95); in the US, purchase it through Inate Source (60 capsules, $22.75). For contact details, see under 'Shopping' in the Directory.

Note: don't take this or any other calcium supplement if you have kidney stones or kidney disease without speaking to your doctor or specialist first.

Worth the money

If you possibly can, it is well worth seeing a good nutritionist who's also properly trained in applied kinesiology (AK). Using AK and, if necessary, sending a sample of your sweat, hair or blood to a reputable testing laboratory like Biolab in London should be able to tell you the amounts and ratios of extra nutrients you'll need according to your age, health profile and skeletal status. One size doesn't fit all.

In the UK and the US, try the International College of Applied Kinesiology. For contact details, see under 'Therapies and Therapists' in the Directory.

The best sources of calcium from food are milk, yoghurt, cheese, white bread, bony fish like mackerel and, though it's not so good for the insides of kettles or plumbing pipes, hard water. For vitamin D, eat fortified cereals, margarine, butter and eggs.

Vital time

Something every woman in her late thirties should know is that if she wants to avoid osteoporosis, one of the most vital times to take plenty of weight-bearing exercise is *from the time menopause first begins to around ten years afterwards.*

This is because the rate of bone loss during that time is triple what it is in your mid-thirties. Numerous clinical studies consistently show that the gravitational stress weight-bearing exercise exerts on your skeleton as you walk, jump, dance or jog stimulates bone regeneration. The fact that at least 30 minutes' exercise four or more times a week also helps keep your figure looking good, your weight down, your legs and bottom toned and stress levels lower doesn't hurt either.

Pelvic-Floor Muscles

177. Weak Pelvic Floor

If, like most women over 35, you ever, even occasionally, leak a fraction when you cough, sneeze, laugh or climax, or if you'd like what the Japanese call a 'glove of velvet and steel' to maximise both your own orgasm power and your male partner's pleasure, this is the ten-second exercise for you.

It's an incontinence-avoiding and sex-enhancing squeeze that strengthens that sling of muscle (pelvic floor) holding up your guts, womb, stomach and bladder, and is called the **Pelvic Lift**. Ideally done every day, for life – OK, we know we should, but who actually does? – especially vital times are:

- when you are pregnant from about week eight (that early, since muscle and ligaments soften as your level of progesterone rises)
- post-natally for six months
- approaching, and while going through, the menopause
- after the age of 65.

Though the Pelvic Lift is just a simple but effective pelvic-toner (the sort of thing you may have been shown after you have a baby), it is being mentioned in this book because many women are not taught to do it right: they report being told to just pretend they are trying to stop themselves passing water. But that's only part of it. The full pelvic monty as recommended by the Royal College of Midwives, and some-times called the Pelvic Smile because that is the shape it makes inside you, is this:

1. **Squeeze the front** (your urine-stopping muscles) for a count of ten. Release slowly.
2. **Squeeze the back** (your bowel-movement-stopping muscles) for ten. Release slowly.
3. **Squeeze the middle** (your vaginal muscles) for ten. Release slowly.
4. **Front, back, middle, pull UP** (squeeze all three sets together, then lift the lot) and hold for ten. Release slowly.

Start with just three repetitions of the above three times daily: a good time is when brushing your teeth in the morning and at night and as soon as you get into bed.

Work gradually up to ten repetitions, then 20, 30, 40 at a time. You can do this four, five, even six times a day if you get the odd opportunity and because this is an internal exercise, it can be done waiting in queues, on hold on the phone, stuck in traffic jams, standing up and cooking.

Do the lift
It's front, back, middle, pull *UP*.

178. Brilliant Body Oil
Mix **extra-virgin olive oil** with ordinary **Nivea Creme** and slather over your body, suggests designer Caroline Herrera Junior. Having used this one for years, two-thirds Nivea to one-third oil seems to be a good mix.

Peri-Menopause (PM)

If you're between 35 and 50 and three or more of the symptoms below sound familiar, you may well be peri-menopausal ('peri' means 'around' or 'in the area of'), since they are all telltale signs that you are developing a perfectly natural, age-related hormonal imbalance:

- weight gain when you've not been eating more or doing anything differently
- forgetfulness and difficulty concentrating
- more erratic periods
- heavier periods and passing some heavy clots
- sleep problems
- mood swings and general anxiety
- changes in sexual desire and response
- skin changes – it may be drier.

In the 10–15 years or so leading up to the menopause, women's hormone levels start dropping. At first this is so slight that the changes this causes are barely perceptible, but they become increasingly noticeable (and often troublesome) as time goes by. Yet most women have never heard of the peri-menopause even when they're going through it, despite the fact that it is normal, natural and, best of all, fixable with both orthodox and complementary medicine.

If you think you may be peri-menopausal, it's a good idea to go to your GP for a check-up to rule out any other condition (to ensure, say, it's not fibroids that are causing your heavier periods, or mild to moderate clinical depression that's producing the anxiety and sleep problems).

179. Things to Take

Many women feel peri-menopause is too early to go the 'full' hormonal route, whether HRT or substantial doses of oestrogen-moderating herbs like black cohosh (the latter can, incidentally, sometimes actually increase heavy period bleeding), and may prefer effective gentler approaches. These include:

- **Embo Ruda essence**, which was developed in Brazil and has been used by many progressive doctors and gynaecologists there for some years. The remedy seems to bring with it some of the sensuality and exuberance its country of origin is famous for and can be a lovely one to use if, in addition to your PMS or period pains worsening as your get older, you are also feeling irritable and gloomy by turns, and not as sexual as you used to. It is available direct from Araretama Rainforest Essences (30 ml, approximately £8), which is based in Brazil, or through Healthlines, who can order it by special request.
- **Evening primrose oil** and **flaxseed oil** are both good for hormonal balancing and for moisturising the skin (both on the face and the vaginal lining). They are also helpful for mood moderation and are so effective at reducing breast tenderness that EPO is prescribed (as Efamol) on the NHS. Aim to get around 320 mg gamma linoleic acid (GLA) a day: check on the side of packaging for how much of this is in each capsule as amounts vary depending on the manufacturer. See also 'Gamma linoleic acid (GLA)' on page 170.
- If you are not feeling sufficiently better after eight weeks of taking the above, try adding the splendid **MenoHerbs2**. This is an increasingly popular combination of the herbal remedies (including red clover and wild yam) traditionally given for menopausal symptoms. It is available from Victoria Health (90 tablets, £14.95). If, as some women find, these work really well for a few months, then symptoms begin to return, the advice is to up the dosage temporarily to three a day for a couple of months, then drop back down to two a day every other day, gradually tailing off to two every day again and see how you go.
- Try taking **AgeLoss** capsules (see page 111) with MenoHerbs2 to help combat the cosmetic signs of aging (i.e. drier, less resilient

skin and less life in your hair), though MenoHerbs2 on its own also seems to help.

For all contact details, see under 'Shopping' in the Directory.

Period Pain

180. Immediate Relief
Press here for DIY pain relief: soothe with the **shousanli** acupressure point.

1. Place your index finger on the crease on the inside of your elbow.
2. Slide your finger down a couple of inches on the outside of that arm.
3. Feel around gently until you find an area that's especially sensitive.
4. When you've got it, rotate the ball of your thumb there gently for around four minutes.
5. Repeat every 20 minutes as necessary.

Calming cuppa
Try to drink **chamomile tea** instead of a PG Tips-style brew throughout the day (that vital morning wake-up mug of tea is still OK). A recent German study in which volunteers drank five cups a day for two weeks found that not only did their menstrual cramps calm down, their immune systems became stronger.

As to why something as gentle as chamomile can relieve something as robust as period pain, it's glycine, an amino acid proven to act as a nerve relaxant and reduce muscular spasms of most types, that does the trick. The chamomile drinkers' urine showed an increase in this substance.[14]

Premenstrual Syndrome (PMS)

Premenstrual syndrome is a collection of up to 150 different symptoms that appear regularly in the second half of a woman's menstrual cycle, before the start of her period. The most common ones include irritability, tension, mood swings, anxiety, depression, water retention, tender breasts, lack of energy, skin and hair changes (spots and greasiness) and food cravings (especially for sweet things).

PMS affects nine out of ten women who have periods, and for a sizeable minority it has a very negative effect in all areas of their lives from personal relationships to jobs. Research by the UK's Natural Health Advisory Service (incorporating the Women's Nutritional Advisory Service), which specialises in helping women with conditions including PMS and the menopause nutritionally, suggests that 40 per cent of women have pretty unpleasant PMS symptoms and another 10 per cent report theirs are really severe or incapacitating. It's thought that the condition is triggered by changes in the ratios of oestrogen and progesterone.

PMS positives
It's not all bad. Research in 1989 at Canada's University of Toronto found that 18 per cent of women said they have more energy premenstrually, 11 per cent were more creative, 29 per cent had an increased tendency to get things done, and 37 per cent said their sex drive rose.

There are many different treatments offered for the negative aspects of PMS, ranging from dietary control to flashing light, from natural progesterone and the Pill to Prozac. Finding the best approach to help you personally is partly a question of trial and error, as different things help different women, but if you prefer the natural route, the following holistic approaches have the best all-round track records.

Exercise
Exercise reduces the water retention that often goes with PMS and also helps keep your mood stable because it boosts the production of the body's own feel-good chemicals, endorphins. But which sort to choose? Try to find something you like that fits very easily into your timetable or you might not be doing it for long. Exercise regularly (three times a week): women who do so rarely suffer from premenstrual mood swings, and their physical symptoms of PMS are much reduced too.[15]

Which sort?

Anything active that you enjoy: tennis, martial arts, cycling – you name it. Swimming and yoga are both inexpensive and calming; running and brisk walking are free, flexible and can fit easily into a tight routine. Any type of dance from jazz to bellydance, or Bollywood to ballroom are great whole-body exercise and good fun with it. Weight training gets pretty swift body toning results but not everyone finds it relaxing . . . gardening's another good one (see Green Gyms, on page 211.)

Stress reduction

Stress may be an overused and often non-specific term, but it is technically a permanent state of biochemical alert and the physical effects are as real as the chair you are sitting on.

It can affect the regularity of your menstrual cycle, the heaviness and painfulness of periods, the likelihood and severity of PMS, and your fertility – because when you are up against it, your pituitary gland orders up the release of stress hormones, such as adrenaline, noradrenaline, cortisol and bromocriptine, from other glands in the body. This can impact on many different physical things from the strength of your womb contractions during a period to the quality of the womb lining prepared for a possible fertilised egg – if it's not right, the egg won't implant itself and you won't get pregnant.

However, the pituitary is also the control centre for sex hormones. So if stress-chemical levels are too high, this interferes with the balance of oestrogen and progesterone, which can then produce PMS.

Things to try

Exercising three times a week or more is one great way to stress-bust; besides exercising, regular (e.g. weekly or fortnightly) treatment sessions with relaxing complementary therapies such as massage, aromatherapy, reflexology, reiki and healing are great if you have time and can afford them. Used regularly, focused DIY relaxation techniques such as autogenic training, self-hypnosis, visualisation and meditation can also be terrific for stress reduction and, once you have been taught to do them, are free because you can DIY at home.

Less stress = less PMS.

Eat smart

What you eat when you are premenstrual – actually what you eat all month long – makes all the difference. And though natural therapists urge, *'Just listen to your body – it'll tell you what you need,'* when it come to PMS days, they're wrong. Research shows that women in the PMS zone crave things *that make them feel worse*. For instance, we eat more sweet, salty and rich, fatty foods – to be exact, nearly *three times as many sugary things* (which definitely worsen symptoms), 62 per cent more refined carbs, 78 per cent more salt (some will demolish entire chicken stock cubes and Oxo cubes like sweeties) and 79 per cent more saturated fat dairy products.[16]

Positive Eats
In a nutshell, go for:

- slow-release carbs every three hours
- lots of fresh fruit and vegetables three or more times daily
- wholefoods (i.e. non-refined ones such as brown rice, wholemeal bread, nuts and seeds, wholemeal pasta, baked potatoes and oatcakes)
- dairy products low in saturated fat (semi-skimmed milk, yoghurt, reduced-fat cheese and olive-oil spreads instead of butter)
- lean meat, fish and chicken.

Also, bear in mind these not-so-good-for-you foods:
  Try to avoid/strictly limit

- junk, convenience and fast foods and takeaways
- meat products high in saturated fat (e.g. burgers, sausages and pork pies) and fattier red meat like lamb, pork and steak[17]
- caffeine (American studies in 1989 and 1990 show it makes PMS worse)[18]
- high refined-sugar foods (which give you a rapid high followed by an equally rapid low)

• salty foods: don't add salt to food when cooking or at the table unless absolutely necessary.

See also Women: Craving Sweet Stuff on page 137.

Snack attack

In the week before your period starts, according to clinical nutritionist Dr Alan Stewart, who has long pioneered the nutrition approach to PMS, you need *an extra 500 calories a day* (yes). Divide that into two 250-calorie healthy snacks – one for mid-morning and one for mid-afternoon (good slow-release snacks include oat biscuits with peanut butter, small packets of unsalted nuts, a slice of wholemeal toast and Marmite, a banana etc) to avoid the shakiness, irritability and the *'Gimme me chocolate, buns or biscuits now, now, now'* craving that accompanies plummeting premenstrual blood sugar levels.

For detailed advice including consultations, leaflets and books about controlling PMS with food and nutrition, check out the Natural Health Advisory Service (incorporating the Women's Nutritional Advisory Service). For contact details, see under 'Therapies and Therapists' in the Directory.

Anti-PMS herbs
Chaste berry (Vitex agnus castus)
Chaste berry is one of the most important traditional remedies used by herbalists to ease women's hormonal problems of all types. It relieves many PMS symptoms by balancing out oestrogen and progesterone levels, and is found to be particularly useful for women who find they also suffer from heavy periods and breast tenderness.

Two large surveys in Germany of 1,542 women found that, according to patients and their doctors, 90 per cent of cases of PMS found relief with a standardised liquid form of chaste berry called **agnolyt**, with improvements taking an average of 25–26 days to kick in.[19] The suggested dose is ten drops morning and evening, and women tend to use it for about six months before taking a rest from it. It is available from the Nutri Centre (100 ml, £24.95).

If you're using non-standardised extracts in capsule form, take around 250 mg daily; but it's best to stick to standardised doses because you know where you are with those – e.g. try Nature's Best Vitex (60 x 100 mg of 10.0 dried extract each, £9.95).

Note: potential side effects may include nausea, headache and gastric irritation. Do not take alongside the Pill or HRT, as it can interfere with their action.

Black cohosh

Black cohosh is state-approved in Germany for treating PMS. Try Nature's Best Black Cohosh (60 tablets, £11.95).

Anti-PMS nutrients

Gamma linoleic acid (GLA)

GLA is found in evening primrose oil. Try Efamol, the brand that has been subject to the most extensive research. Take six to eight 500 mg capsules daily. It is available from Boots, Superdrug, Holland & Barrett and other health shops in the UK (90 capsules, £9.99); in the US, you can purchase it from Academy Health (90 capsules, $16.50).

Other sources even richer in GLA include **borage (starflower) linseed** and **blackcurrant-seed oil**. Women with PMS often have low levels of omega-3 fatty acids in their bloodstream – possibly due to a genetic blip in their make-up that impairs the conversion of linoleic acid (LNA) to GLA. And GLA reduces, among other things, PMS symptoms,[20] especially breast tenderness,[21] mood swings and water retention. It may also help control your blood sugar levels, thus reducing premenstrual craving for sweet things.

Note: for breast tenderness in particular, the suggested dose of GLA, according to the Royal Sussex Country Hospital's breast unit, is 320 mg. It may take two to three months before you feel the benefits, however, and you need at least a four-month course. Many women feel so much better on it that they take GLA all month long, every month.

Vitamin B6
Many women have taken **vitamin B6** for PMS, and while if you look at *all* the clinical trials, the results seem to contradict each other, there are many that suggest it is useful.[22] The recommended dosage is under 200 mg a day, as more can cause gastric problems and very high doses have been linked with mild neurological symptoms. It may take around three months to see results from taking B6.

Magnesium
Women with PMS are often short of **magnesium**. In a 1998 trial, taking just 200 mg daily was found to reduce symptoms relating to premenstrual water retention including weight gain, breast tenderness and abdominal bloating.[23]

Potassium
Taking 600 mg **potassium** daily can help relieve bloating, irritability and tiredness. Full positive effects take about four menstrual cycles to achieve.[24]

Calcium
Women who experience PMS often have low levels of **calcium**, but American research suggests those who eat diets rich in calcium tend to have less severe symptoms and that supplementing can cut them by around half.[25] Trials at Columbia University Medical Center, in which around 500 women took 300 mg calcium carbonate, found it was helpful for mood swings, bloating, depression, headaches and food cravings.

Excellent anti-PMS essences
Gentle and subtle, these can be surprisingly effective on a physical as well as an emotional level, and they have no side effects. Used by homeopaths and other complementary therapists, but also increasingly by psychotherapists, psychologists and even some enlightened psychiatrists, essences are finding their way into the surgeries of private gynaecologists in Australia, Switzerland, Brazil and some state hospitals worldwide.

Embo Ruda

Embo Ruda is an exuberant life-loving remedy from the Brazilian rainforests and is used for PMS and period pains in its country of origin but also for enhancing female sexuality, fertility and sheer pleasure in sensuality. It is made by Araretama Rainforest Essences and can be bought direct (30 ml, approximately £8) or from Healthlines: they can get you some by special request.

Macrozamia

Macrozamia is a great all-rounder and used in western Australia for women's hormonal and sexual problems of all types. It is equivalent to the herbalist's heftier favourite *Vitex agnus castus*. It is made by Living Essences of Australia and you can buy it direct worldwide or via IFER in the UK (15 ml, approximately £8).

She Oak

Also used for the menopause and the peri-menopause, **She Oak** helps balance female hormones and is currently being trialled for PMS by a group of Australian state hospitals. Results are expected in late 2007. It is made by Australian Bush Flower Essences and is available direct worldwide or via Healthlines in the UK (15 ml, £8.95).

For all product contact details, see under 'Shopping' in the Directory.

For suggestions about breast pain, see Fix 147: Breast Pain – Immediate Relief and Fix 148: Breast Pain – Cyclical. For spots, see Teenagers: Acne and Spots on page 311.

For advice specifically for teenagers, see Teenagers: Periods on page 358.

Polycystic Ovarian Syndrome (PCOS)

PCOS produces multiple cysts on one or both ovaries. It can also cause other symptoms including irregular periods, excessive facial or body hair, acne, breast pain and fertility problems. Women with PCOS often have higher levels of male hormones, including testosterone (hence the spots and hirsuitism).

A GP would probably suggest a drug called cyproterone acetate, available as Dianette, or sometimes anti-diabetic medication because there is some evidence to suggest that PCOS may be linked with insulin resistance. Extra insulin in the bloodstream makes the ovaries up their output of male hormones – they naturally make small amounts of these anyway – which are responsible for characteristics like sex drive and assertiveness.

181. Eat the GI Way

With the insulin-diabetic connection in mind, one very useful holistic treatment for PCOS is an eating plan designed to normalise your blood sugar levels. It's essentially a diet lower in starches and carbohydrate-based sugary foods, better known as the **glycaemic index (GI) diet**, currently hitting a popularity high as the sensible new way to control your weight without actually dieting.

Recommended reading: a good, easy-read book if you are a woman looking to tackle PCOS through blood-sugar stabilisation, good health and weight maintenance, instead of straight weight loss, is *The Family GI Diet* by Dr Ruth Gallop and Rick Gallop (former president of the Heart and Stroke Foundation of Ontario).

182. Herbal Help

If you are interested in doing something more, the herbal approach is also promising. Try **saw palmetto**, as it slows down the conversion of testosterone into its even more active form, dihydrotestosterone, which is why it is also successfully used to treat prostate problems in men – see also Fix 204: Natural Remedies.

The usual dose for women with PCOS is around 320 mg standardised saw palmetto extract a day. In the UK, try Holland & Barrett's own-brand capsules (30 x 320 mg capsules, £10.95); in the US, try Active Herb. For contact details, see under 'Shopping' in the Directory.

Pregnancy

Top Five Problems and Solutions

183. Morning Sickness (No. 1)

Misleadingly named as it can occur at any point during the day, or all day, morning sickness is thought to be caused by the initial rise in progesterone (and, for the first three months, another hormone called human chorionic gonadatrophin). It usually starts around week five or six but has faded by weeks 14–16 and is usually completely over by week 20, though some women experience it all the way through their pregnancy.[26] About one woman in 100 develops a particularly severe form called hyperemesis gravidarum, which may need to be treated with fluids and nutrients by IV in hospital.

For mild to moderate morning sickness, keeping your blood sugar steady by eating small, frequent plain snacks and meals helps. So, according to American research in 1995, may supplements of **vitamin B6** at a dose of 20–40 mg a day.[27]

Top Tip

Ginger can be really effective, either drunk regularly as a tea made from the chopped root and sweetened with a little honey or, as researched by obstetrician John McGarry at the Royal Devon and Exeter Hospital, in handy capsule form – take one to four 250 g capsules a day. McGarry found this dealt with 80 per cent of women's sickness. As one woman said, 'I still didn't feel totally brilliant, but I no longer felt like I had food poisoning. Life was actually possible again.' The effectiveness and safety of ginger in capsule form is also backed up by another study in which it got rid of 28 out of 32 women's morning sickness.[28]

In the UK, try ginger capsules from Nature's Best (90 capsules, £7.95); in the US, try Nutrivea USA (100 x 500 mg capsules, $29.45). For contact details, see under 'Shopping' in the Directory.

---

184. **Pregnancy Backache (No. 2)**

There are two great positions for relieving the pregnancy-related backache that affects almost every pregnant woman. The first is the **L-Rest** (see picture), which was suggested by consultant osteopath Stephen Sandler, who set up the UK's first specialist osteopathic clinic for expectant mothers. Stay like this for as long as you feel comfortable.

The second is yoga's **Frog Stretch**, taught in Active Birth classes. You can either do position A (see picture) – i.e. rest on your elbows – or

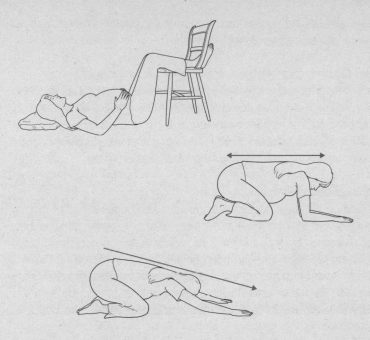

if it feels OK, slowly stretch your arms out in front of you to position B (see picture). Stay there for a minute or two, then come up just as slowly.

Note: for either the L-Rest or the Frog Stretch, be careful not to arch your back.

Also try the **hara-obis** support sash – see 'The Japanese way' on page 127.

For more suggestions, see General: Backache on page 26 and (Mother's) Backs on page 127.

185. Can't Breathe? (No. 3)

As your baby and womb grow, they take up more room and start pushing the other abdominal organs up towards your diaphragm, leaving less room for your lungs to expand when you breathe.

Apart from sitting up straight and taking slow, deep, deliberate breaths (and making sure you prop yourself up well in bed), try the **Belly Drop**, as suggested by Professor Mike Chapman, ex-head of obstetrics and gynaecology at Guy's Hospital in London. Just get down on all fours, tummy hanging down – easier breathing instantly.

186. Cramps (No. 4)

Many pregnant women are plagued by cramp in their feet, calves and legs, often at night. This is partly due to poorer circulation (the rise in progesterone relaxes the walls of blood vessels) and/or to calcium deficiency (your baby is taking someof yours to build his or her skeleton). Consider calcium supplements, but for immediate help when cramp strikes:

- Get up and walk about.
- Massage the area: supercharge this by adding three drops of **Angelsword** to a bit of oil or massage cream. It seems to halve the time it takes to get rid of the pain, which many women report can take up to 45 minutes or more. Angelsword is made by Australian Bush Flower Essences and is available direct, via Healthlines (15 ml, £8.95) and selected health shops in the UK; in the US, try Flower Vision Research. For contact details, see under 'Shopping' in the Directory.

187. Stretch Marks (No. 5)

Very light, gentle self-massaging with rich **wheatgerm oil** containing a specific blend of aromatherapy essential oils daily can considerably reduce stretch marks by nourishing the skin and maximising its elasticity – sometimes even preventing them, says Dr Vivian Lunny, former clinical pathologist at London's Mount Vernon Hospital, now a medical aromatherapist.

The mix she uses is a blend of **lavender, mandarin** and **geranium** or **chamomile**. Mix 20 drops of lavender, 20 drops of mandarin, 15 drops of geranium or 15 drops of chamomile and add to 50 ml wheatgerm oil. Use a palmful at a time. Important tips:

- Start around week six, well *before* the skin begins to stretch.
- Do all areas potentially prone to the marks – upper thighs, breasts and abdomen.
- When oiling the abdomen area, make sure you go all the way round to the middle of your back.

Note: there is no clinical evidence to back up this mix's efficacy. However, Dr Lunny, who trained at the medical school of San Andreas University in Bolivia and was the head of scientific research at the UK's Aromatherapy Organisations Council for many years, recommends it and uses it on her own patients.

For good-quality essential oils via mail order, try Baldwin's Spike Lavender (10 ml, £4.09), Mandarin (10 ml, £2.69), Geranium (10 ml, £5.15) and Chamomile Roman (5 ml, £7.85). These oils are also available at slightly different prices and in the States via Neal's Yard, which has a US website. For contact details, see under 'Shopping' in the Directory.

For avoiding varicose veins, see also 'Support Tights in Pregnancy Tip' on page 194.

Breech Baby
By the eight-month mark, most babies have turned into the 'head down' position which is easiest for labour. However, even by the time labour starts, three per cent still remain breech i.e. bottom first with their legs tucked up in front of them. It is very helpful if they can be persuaded to turn around before the contractions of childbirth begin – some will do so by themselves anyway in these last few weeks, often in the last few days – as one of the most common reasons for Caesarean delivery is that the baby is breech.

Some babies who haven't yet changed poition can be persuaded to turn round by massage or gentle manipulation from a skilled midwife, obstetrician or osteopath who has a special interest in, and good experience of, this area. Others, however, can literally be talked around . . .

The power of persuasion
. . . by using gentle but focussed and emphatic speech. In 1995, for instance, a team of obstetricians from Phoenix, Arizona, used an electronically synthesised voice machine to do so many times.[29]

Phrases midwives use include 'Sweetheart, come along now – your mother needs you to turn round and get your head down. Please begin to turn now if you feel safe to do so.' Mothers can of course do this too. In fact, though there are no studies to prove it, they may well be far more successful than a medical professional, as they are better tuned in to their own babies. If you would like to try:

1. Take a few quiet moments for deep, calm breathing and relaxation.
2. Next, send your baby love and reassurance, as if 'stroking' them with it.
3. Focus on your baby. Ask, in your head or out loud, if they can hear you.
4. Ask them to turn round for you now if they feel safe to do so, with their head down. See them doing this easily and gracefully in your mind's eye and 'send' them this picture. Successful telepathy relies on received visual impressions, as well as verbal ones.
5. Repeat three times.

Recommended reading: if you'd like to find out more about the whole area of what unborn babies really can do and understand and how to communicate with them, see *The Miraculous World of Your Unborn Baby* by myself and Dr David Chamberlain.

The breech-turner
The position in the diagram below is for encouraging a breech baby to turn round and is recommended by John McGarry, former consultant obstetrician at the Royal Devon and Exeter Hospital in Britain.

Note: only stay like this for as long as you feel comfortable. If you feel you should stop, do so right away. And if it doesn't quite feel right for you don't do it at all.

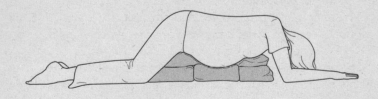

Pulling Men – and Chatting Them Up

Body Language That Works

'Good looks may appeal to the eye, but it's the sensual signals that truly pluck at the reproductive organs.' *Judi James*

Judi James knows a thing or two about body language. She has written several best-selling books on the subject including: *Sex Signals* (Piatkus), and *Body Talk* (Spiro Press). She's also got her own column in *Heat*, and the Mail on Sunday's *You* magazine, appears regularly on TV series including *Strictly Come Dancing*, *Big Brother* (and her own series *Naked Celebrity*) commenting on how contestants and celebrities' gestures, ways of sitting, standing or looking at someone unwittingly reveal – everything. James lists the following as good posing rituals i.e. the ones to which men respond best. Many (lucky) women find they do these instinctively.

Standing – the Miss World

1. Bend your right knee in towards the left one and push your right foot out to the side.
2. Let your pelvis drop down on the right, but push it out and up on your left.
3. Hold your drink with both hands at waist height – no higher or it looks like a barrier.

This one may feel a bit girlie, but it's a winner because it makes your legs look longer and slimmer, and your hips smaller and somehow sexier, so if a man's looking over at you, he'll like what he sees. An alternative involves:

1. Balance your weight evenly on both feet at shoulder-span width.
2. With one hand, hold your glass at waist height.
3. With the other, touch your chin or mouth lightly (ensuring you don't cover them, as that too is a barrier gesture).

Smiling
Smile with your lips apart but mouth not too far open. Ensure your smile reaches your eyes.

Laughing
Laughter must look and sound genuine. Make sure you're not doing it too loudly. Never slap yourself or another person while doing so, unless you are from a vast Texan ranch and Daddy's extremely rich.

Listening
Use eye contact with the person who's talking to you and look genuinely interested in what they are saying (even if you're not). Any men watching will admire your apparent ability to focus on someone without distraction. They like women who do that.

Subtle sexual touching and gesturing
. . . with the emphasis on 'subtlety'. Pick one, or at most two, of the following:

- **Mouth:** a very slight licking of the lips with the tip of the tongue, or a small touch of the tongue tip on the index finger. Practise in the mirror at home to check which bit of your finger to work with: some women perfect a tiny, sexy cat-lick on the side of the tip; others use the very end. See what looks best when you do it.
- **Neck:** stretch your chin up a little to bare the soft skin of your throat.
- **Hair:** the movement needs to be a small stroking gesture (no fringe-flipping or mane-tossing).
- **Wineglass:** stroke the stem with the tip of one finger or rub lightly round the rim *once* only. This doesn't work with lager cans, but could be adapted to small designer beer bottles (e.g. a Beck's, not a Grolsch).

Never do all of the above in turn. You'll look like Porno Barbie.

Radiating energy

We're attracted to people who radiate vitality like iron filings to a magnet. This is partly because, like success, we want some of that for ourselves and hope it will rub off on us. But it is also because vitality detonates the instinct (rooted deep in the evolutionary past of our species) that equates a high life-force quotient with being a fit – in all senses of the word – sexual partner and gestator of the next generation.

So appear energetic. Imagine you've just had a fantastic massage or workout that has left you supple, glowing, full of it. Move about a bit rather than appearing stuck or static. Your energy will transmit positive signals round the room and the men will notice.

Don'ts

- **Don't look bored.** It won't send him a message that you'd like him to come and rescue you; it just makes you look rude and as if you pass judgement on people easily.
- **Never stand with your legs bending outwards at the ankle.** It looks sad and twee.
- **Don't suck or eat any slices of fruit from your drink.** It looks greedy rather than sensual – or as if you're a wannabe extra in a budget Bond film.

Facial Expressions That Score

'Generally, men like two facial expressions in women – "fun" and "sympathetic" –because these will provide all the hints they need that they have discovered the best buddy, sex siren or mummy substitute they have spent their lives searching for.' *Judi James*

Use your eyes

These expressions need to be shown mostly from the eyes. If you place too much emphasis on mouth movement, James warns that you may end up looking insincere.

People tend to trust what they see in another's eyes, as they know unconsciously that it is harder for a person to fake emotions there than on their face. Doesn't everyone instinctively look into someone's eyes if they are searching for the truth?

It is difficult to put an emotion you don't feel *at all* into your eyes. But it is not so hard to ensure that for chatting-up purposes, they show an intensification of a feeling you already have.

- **'Interest'** in what someone is saying to you verbally can be bulked up into 'major interest for short periods' if there is a good reason for doing so (such as being sexually attracted to them).
- **'Fun'** can be shown by a slight narrowing of the eyes, although you also need to keep moving your gaze from his eyes to his mouth, as though you are amused by what he is saying. Combine this with a suppressed smile – lips held together, but one or both corners turned up – as if you are trying not to smile but this man's so engaging that you can't help it.
- **'Sympathetic'** can be put across by a slight frown of concern and by making an expression in your eyes similar to the one you'd have if he'd just told you his cat had died. Combine with leaning forwards slightly and nodding slowly.

Keep your eye expression soft rather than wide. Wide equals surprised, and surprised can suggest, 'I don't believe you,' which is not very flattering. Also avoid the expression adopted by some psychologists and counsellors: the 'neutral listening face', which in personal situations can announce, 'Chilly professional detachment!' when what you are trying to project is empathetic warmth and understanding.

See also Flirting, on page 52.

Safety

188. Threatening Situations

You're going home alone, it's night and you have to pass by a group of hoodie boys you don't much like the look of. Or maybe you're sitting on a bus, Tube or train and someone who makes you instinctively wary gets on. You'd rather they didn't notice you, but what can you do? Try the **Cloak**. It's easy, takes only seconds, and, done with firm intention, it works.

The Cloak of Invisibility

I was shown this technique ten years ago by a highly experienced – and rather glamorous – senior trainer for the National Federation of Spiritual Healers called Darryl O'Keefe when I was going to practice sessions at a place called the Helios Centre. Sited round the side of London's King's Cross Station, it was not such a great area to hang about in at night. Coming home at 10 p.m., you'd have to walk past all the small-time pimps and pushers while running the gamut of cruising cars, ignoring the looks, comments and the odd 'playfully' grabbing hand. If someone wasn't walking back to the Tube my way, I'd get a bit edgy.

'Oh, you'll be fine,' said Darryl cheerfully, when he found me hovering in the hall one evening after class because I'd been in the loo and emerged to find everyone else had gone. 'Just use the Cloak of Invisibility.' He told me how.

'Is that it?' I thought. 'Doesn't sound like much.'

But it was. It wasn't that the King's Cross regulars didn't see me – they just didn't really register me. That night not one single person accosted me, made any comments or even looked over as I went past. They didn't do it any other night after that either because I used the Cloak every time. If ever you need it, it is very easy and works immediately.

How to put on the Cloak of Invisibility

1. In your head, call quickly on Michael, mighty Archangel of Courage, Protection and Strength, for help.
2. Ask him to please wrap the Cloak of Invisibility around you *now* and

request that it hides you completely from all negative attention or harm.

3. Imagine you are slipping on a floor-length sapphire-blue cloak, draping its hood over your head to hide your face, *Star Wars*-style. See it zipping swiftly shut all the way from feet to neck.

4. Consciously draw in your own energy output, like a snail drawing in its feelers, so you are not radiating any of the 'I'm here!' vibes we usually send out.

5. Now just stay quiet, all wrapped in your cloak. If you're sitting on a bus or a Tube do not even glance their way. Perhaps read, plan the perfect holiday or have a conversation with a friend in your head to keep your mind off that person over there. If you're walking, flit swiftly and lightly by, looking past them rather than at them, and giving them as wide a berth as is practical.

6. Thank Archangel Michael for his help.

Resist the temptation to look back to see if they've spotted you. Though you can flick a quick peripheral glance at them as a safety check, a direct and possibly emotionally charged look has quite a strong energy, which they might register and so clock you after all. For the same reason, SAS commandos are trained not to stare at someone's back if they are trying to come up quietly behind them from some distance away, but to let their gaze go slightly past the person: they know that otherwise the subject of the stare or 'purposeful focus' will feel it and react accordingly. The same goes for experienced wildlife photographers trying to capture shy subjects on camera.

Important: remember to take the cloak *off* when you feel safe to do so (e.g. when you get home).

Note: the Cloak is purely a protective technique for whenever someone is feeling threatened and wishes to remain unnoticed in order to stay safe. However, it may well backfire should a person try to use it with a negative motivation (e.g. for listening in on a private conversation).

Sex

189. Libido-Boosters

The official figures are that 40 per cent of women and around 30 per cent of men are thought to be affected by loss of libido at some point in their lives. The real levels are probably far higher; in fact, I've never met any woman who doesn't recall going off sex for months at some point. Causes are usually multi-factorial and diverse – ranging from over-work, caring for young children, stress and hormonal change to the passage of time, clinical depression (plus the drugs prescribed for it), relationship difficulties and lack of key nutrients.

However, if you are looking for natural sexuality-enhancers, herbs that improve both general energy levels and blood flow tend to have the best results. Two in particular are worth a try: **muira puama** ('potency wood') from the Amazon and ginkgo biloba, perhaps better known for helping alleviate Alzheimer's disease and circulatory problems.

Muira puama is available in the UK from VitAmour, which you can buy from Healthy Direct (90 x 1,440 mg capsules, £17.95); in the US, try Zooscape (100 x 1.8 g capsules, $23).

One recent clinical trial involving 200 women carried out by Dr Sarah Brewer, who runs a genitourinary clinic at Queen Elizabeth Hospital in Norfolk, looked at the effects of muira puama combined with ginkgo; 63 per cent found their sex drive increased and that their ability to reach orgasm and the strength of their climaxes improved. Research in the *Journal of Sexual and Marital Therapy* found ginkgo alone enhanced the libido by up to 90 per cent for both men and women whose sex drives had been suppressed by antidepressants.

See also the herb **maca** for women. Organic maca is available via the Maca Company's website (100 x 800 mg tablets, approximately £18) or from Victoria Health (120 tablets, £14.95); in the US, purchase it from LifeTime (120 capsules, $16.99). Look for the maca zepidion meganii walp variety or the Peruvian chacon. This herb from the Peruvian Andes is said to increase energy, stamina and libido – research in China, Peru and Italy seems to back this up.[30] For all contact details, see under 'Shopping' in the Directory.

To some, abnormal female libido means 'not wanting it as often as their male partner'. Interestingly, recent research by international expert Alan Riley, professor of sexual medicine at the University of Central Lancaster, found that on average men seem to be on a five-day cycle when it comes to wanting sex, but women are on a ten-day one.

190. Sensual Tea

The subtle way to feel sensual: make a pot of black or, preferably, **green tea** with three to four cups of boiling water, add a drop of **jasmine essential oil**, 'serve immediately and observe', advises Maggie Tisserand, international pioneer and authority on aromatherapy.

This drink can act as a delicate aphrodisiac, and it both smells and tastes exquisite: totally different from the so-called jasmine teas you can get in tea-bag form.

Tisserand Jasmine Absolute Oil is available from Victoria's Health and Beauty (2 ml, £18.60); in the US, you can buy it direct from Tisserand (0.34 fl oz, $38). For contact details, see under 'Shopping' in the Directory.

191. Sexual Response – Strengthen Yours Instantly

Anything you take to enhance the intensity of your physical responses to sexual pleasure (such as pro-sexual nutrients and herbs) or increase your libido is likely to take four to eight weeks to kick in. If you need to do something *immediately* – perhaps your partner wants to make love and you'd like to too but are feeling a bit tired or flat – this visualisation technique only takes two minutes and works right away. Providing, that is, you are not so shattered (or so psychologically off sex) that you just need to go to bed by yourself.

1. Sit down quietly for a moment somewhere you won't be disturbed. Close your eyes.
2. Breathe calmly and deeply: in for a count of five, hold for five, out for five. Do this five times.

3. Imagine you are sending roots down from your feet deep into the earth. See them in your mind's eye spreading out deep and wide like those of a beautiful tree.

4. Now see a golden ball of light around yourself, growing brighter and stronger by the moment. Sit in it, enjoying its warmth and protection, literally breathing it in for a few moments and feeling it spread through you.

5. The next 'golden-light' breath you take, as you let it out, mentally send it down to the area between the top of your pubis and your tummy button. This is the sacral chakra region, the energy centre responsible for, among other things, sex drive.

6. Do the same with the next four breaths so you've done five in all. Feel each one fill your sacral chakra with golden energy. Sense the area warming up and energising. See it in your mind's eye glowing fiery orange.

7. Open your eyes, take a few deep, easy breaths, stamp your feet lightly on the floor to ground yourself – and go get him!

Many women report this exercise, besides helping them 'feel like it after all', increases the intensity of their sexual response and the strength of their orgasms.

192. Ardour-Cooler

So much has been written about how to turn your partner on. But what if you simply aren't in the mood tonight, while he's really up for it?

If you don't want to turn him down as such (yet don't want sex either), suggest a massage 'first', add several drops of **marjoram aromatherapy essence** to the base oil and rub him down. This is really relaxing. So relaxing, in fact, that it tends to send the receiver to sleep and dampens libido, says UK aromatherapy queen Maggie Tisserand.

Note: use the Spanish variety of marjoram (*Thymus mastichina*). The other variety, *Origanum marjorama*, is French and is generally used for relieving anxiety. You can buy the Spanish variety in the UK and the US from Tisserand (9 ml, £5.60/$11.50). For contact details, see under 'Shopping' in the Directory.

193. Sexual Cramp

Some women find that when they become sexually aroused, or immediately after orgasm, they get a bruising, crampy pain or perhaps sharp spasm in their genital area. This is usually around the perineum (the thick band of muscle that divides vagina from anus), but it may also appear in the muscles at the sides of the rectum. And pain every time you get thoroughly turned on can be enough to put even the most sensual women off sex.

Why does it happen?

Of the women who report sexual cramp, many say it developed or worsened after their second or third childbirth and report that the more quickly they orgasm (say, a rapid and efficient climax by masturbation), the worse the pain can be.

Some gynaecologists have suggested that the blood vessels supplying the entire pelvic area, front and back, may have been dilated by the huge rise in oestrogen and progesterone during pregnancy and never quite got back to their usual dimensions. This means that there is a relatively smaller (i.e. usual) volume of blood flowing through (permanently enlarged) vessels, producing localised oxygen deficiency in the surrounding muscle tissue and thus causing cramp pain – muscles really hurt when they lack oxygen (which is what angina pain is).

Medical treatments for sexual cramp include the Pill and danazol since both level out sex hormones. But if you don't fancy taking artificial hormones and especially if you have an attack of this pain and need to do something about it right away, try the **Scrunch**.

The Scrunch is ten firm repetitions of the **Pelvic Lift** – see Women: Pelvic-Floor Muscles on page 161. It works because it helps shift any de-oxygenated blood through quickly and replace it with oxygenated. If you can't do the lifts, just clench the whole area and hold for a count of ten, let go, then repeat three times. Getting up and walking about or taking a hot bath can also relieve the discomfort by bringing more oxygenated blood into the area.

See also General: Sex on page 86.

Stress

194. Stressed? About to Lose It?
Keep your cool with **Instant In-Breath Calm**. It's quick, easy and it works. Just:

1. Breathe in for a count of five.
2. Hold for five.
3. Breathe out for five.
4. Repeat five times. And that's it . . .

195. Relax
Overwrought and cross? Take a nice bath, they tell us. Light your scented candles, pour in the essential oils and just *be*. Fine, but what if you can't relax in your own tub without other people banging on the door or bellowing through the keyhole ('*Mu-uuum* . . . ')?

If you just want to download without interruption or effort – which cuts out things like exercise, yoga and weekends away – and don't wish to have to talk or relate to the means of your relaxation and pampering (ditto masseurs, talkative complementary therapists or chatty hairdressers), consider a floatation tank.

Its weightless, silky warmth and womb-like security can give both the neurological and emotional systems an intensive holiday in less than an hour. Afterwards people tend to feel rested, energised and have a fresh perspective on life without having actually 'done' anything or exchanged a single word with anyone. See www.floatopia.co.uk for information, or get in touch with the Floatation Tank Association for your nearest tank. For contact details, see under 'Therapies and Therapists' in the Directory.

See also General: Stress and Stamina on page 95.

Sweating

If your sweating is due to hot flushes caused by the menopause – an estimated 68 per cent of women have these at some point during this time – see page 153. If it's due to anxiety or panic attacks, see page 65.

Any night sweats, however, which are not connected with the menopause, or clinical anxiety, can be a sign of a shortage of **vitamin B1**, says top UK clinical nutritionist Dr Stephen Davies. Suspect this if you're also getting any numbness or tingling in your hands and feet: ask a good nutritionist to arrange a blood or sweat test to check.

Medical Treatments

Standard medical approaches to general sweating include beta-blockers (not that effective but routinely offered by GPs), and Botox injections – a more robust solution – involving about 20 injections into the sweat glands of each armpit. The effect lasts for four to six years.

Complementary Treatments

196. Herbs and Minerals
Herbs
The National Institute of Medical Herbalists suggests **sage tincture** for sweating and flushing. Try Nature's Answer's Sage Alcohol-Free Fluid Extract via Baldwin's (30 ml, £9.45).

The mineral route: fix this now
However, if you are in dire need of an effective and immediate temporary fix or, like many people, only tend to 'pour' if you're nervous (and you have, say, a major presentation or intimidatingly smart party coming up) when expending a lot of physical energy (energetic dancing), consider mineral salts. Your GP can prescribe a strong underarm roll-on called **Anhydrol Forte** (by Dermal Laboratories), which contains a higher percentage of aluminium chloride than is found in commercial brands. You put it on at night for two evenings in a row, then take a break for two nights, causing the sweat glands to close up so efficiently that you'll stay drier than Death Valley. It is best for occasional use, however, as for some people it can cause a rash or itching (for the same reason, try a patch test first and wait 24 hours to see if your skin is happy with the substance)

For all contact details, see under 'Shopping' in the Directory.

See also Fix 316: Beat Body Odour.

Thrush

Thrush isn't an infection as such, though it certainly feels like one; it's an overgrowth of the naturally occurring yeast organism *Candida albicans*. The most usual place to get it is around the vagina and vulva, though breastfeeding women can sometimes develop an infection of the nipples, which is miserably sore and itchy.

> A good anti-thrush fighter in a single oral capsule that contains no chemicals (unlike the Difucan you can get over the counter at the pharmacy) but some pretty potent natural anti-fungal plant extracts called tannins, is **Tanalbit** (by Intensive Nutrition Inc, £19.95, 60 capsules, via Victoria Health). You need to take it for 6-8 weeks, but many people report a distinct improvement after just two.

Much is written about how to get rid of vaginal thrush, including taking probiotics, wearing loose cotton underwear instead of cute, tight synthetic briefs or thongs, using sanitary towels instead of tampons and cutting out yeast, sugars and refined carbs from your diet. But there's little advice offered about what to do to make life more comfortable *immediately* while you've got it, especially if the pain or itching flares up in the middle of the night, which it often does.

197. Tea Up

> The best and fastest way to calm down rampant vulval itching I've yet come across is **chamomile tea**. Not to drink, to sit in.

Chamomile tea bags left to steep for ten minutes will do at a pinch, but it is even better if you can make it up from a handful of whole dried chamomile flowers in a pint of boiling water. Brew up a jugful. Pour it (cooled) into a bowl and squat so the tea flows into and covers your vulva.

If you can't get in the right position, just dip your hand in and keep gently sloshing the tea over the affected area for 10–20 minutes. It's very soothing.

In the UK, you can mail-order dried chamomile from Neal's Yard (approximately £2 a packet); for dried whole chamomile flowers in the US, try New York-based Mother Nature (1 lb, $9.49). For contact details, see under 'Shopping' in the Directory.

If you have no chamomile and it's an emergency, run a few inches of just-warm water into the bath and squat in that, knees apart so the inflamed labial issues aren't touching, for 20–30 minutes, perhaps with a book or magazine to keep your mind off things. When you get out, carefully slick a little Vaseline or plain vaginal lubricant like KY Jelly over it to stop the labial surface tissues rubbing against each other.

Vaginal Dryness

This can cause discomfort, itching, constant day-to-day soreness, painful intercourse, and pre-dispose you to developing vaginal and vulval infections. The dryness may be due to chemical or mechanical irritation (e.g. rubbing from tight clothing or vigorous sex) but if you suddenly become dry, especially if there is also irritation, redness or discharge, always ask your doctor to check you for possible infection.

For women over 35 coming into the peri-menopause and menopause (see Women: Peri-Menopause on page 163 and Women: Menopause on page 151), the culprit can be dropping levels of oestrogen, for which most doctors would suggest localised application of a prescription oestrogen cream. The Menopause Awareness Alliance Survey (undertaken by two menopause charities and the maker of a nutritional supplement) found 13 per cent of women going through menopause have trouble with vaginal dryness.

Relief NOW
Ordinary **lubricants** can bring immediate temporary relief. Over-the-counter brands like **Replens** or **KY Jelly** work fine; the mail-order brand **Sylk** (from Victoria Health) has many fans. **V-Gel** is a good one too – it contains

soothing, cooling alo vera gel and extract of the healing herb comfrey (the latter is accredited with, amongst other things, being able to help retain the elasticity of the vagina's walls too. (V-Gel's available from Higher Nature, £10.90 for 75ml.)

US holistic well-woman pioneer Dr Christine Northrup also suggests **cold-pressed castor oil, flaxseed, vitamin-E oil** or **sesame oil** applied locally. A capsule of any one of these can be gently inserted in the vagina, where the warmth of your body melts them and releases the soothing oil just where it's needed.

Flaxseed oil can also be taken by mouth and is sometimes helpful in the long term: it certainly improves the moisture content of external skin, not to mention hair and nails. Try organic High Barn Oils (100 capsules, £13.50); in the US, try Barlean's Essential Woman range on Livespan Nutrition (90 x 1 g capsules, $12.65). For contact details, see under 'Shopping' in the Directory.

One study in the *British Medical Journal* in which women with vaginal dryness took flaxseed oil, the phyto-oestrogen red clover and also upped their soya intake found that their vaginal tissues changed for the better in just ten weeks.

Varicose and Spider Veins

These enlarged blood vessels lying close to the skin's surface are most likely to appear in the legs and feet because of the extra pressure the blood vessels are under when you stand and walk. Pregnancy, hormonal change and lots of standing are all common causes. The appearance of the veins ranges from a thread-like spider pattern (not uncomfortable, more of a cosmetic issue) to the often aching, bulging, fully fledged varicose variety.

198. The Natural Way
One of the favourite natural treatments for veins is **horse chestnut** (*Aesculus hippocastanum*). An extensive review of 13 strict randomised controlled trials involving 1,083 people with varicose veins strongly suggests that horse chestnut works just as well as, and in some cases better than, the conventional treatments offered by your GP – i.e.

compression stockings and medicine called hydroxyethylrutosides, made from the herb rutin.[31]

In the UK, try Healthy Direct's Horse Chestnut Extract (60 tablets, £6.95). The suggested dose is once or twice daily. In the US, try Venarin capsules from Nutrica; these capsules also contain extracts of other natural circulation- and drainage-supporting plants like butcher's broom, Japanese pagoda tree and grapeseed – a topical cream is available too – both carry a 60-day money-back guarantee. For contact details, see under 'Shopping' in the Directory.

Support tights in Pregnancy

If you're pregnant and want to avoid developing varicose veins (which sometimes prove to be permanent), *wear support tights from the fourth month* – don't wait for your legs to start aching.

Caroline Flint, independent midwife and former president of the UK's Royal College of Midwives, suggests keeping the tights under your pillow and putting them on each morning before setting a foot on the floor. If you put them on when you've already got up, it's a bit late since gravity will have ensured that blood has already pooled in your legs and feet.

Walk This Way

For anyone trying to avoid or reduce varicose veins, go barefoot at home, in the garden or on the beach as much as you possibly can. Work by the University of Innsbruck suggests that this exercises the feet muscles far more than if you're wearing shoes and stimulates venous flow to the legs.

Men

OK, so men tend to be more sceptical than women about complementary therapies. Yet once they have actually tried them – often via the nutrition route for performance-enhancement (in bed or out of it) or through a few sessions of robust physical manipulative therapy like osteopathy or chiropractic for sports injury – they usually realise just how effective holistic treatments can be. An increasing number are also finding that the concrete results for complementary therapies, which are now regularly documented in prestigious peer-review medical journals, speak louder than a residual reluctance to being caught near anything remotely New Age.

In the following chapter, men will find anything from the holistic way to treat the andropause and male menopause to why vitamins plus hypnotherapy can help a balding bloke grow more hair (and who says it works?) to the traditional Arab penis-lengthening methods that involve exercise instead of surgery – not to mention how to tackle everything from farting to subfertility fast, effectively and without drugs.

Andropause (Male Menopause)

The andropause (or 'pause of the androgens'– i.e. male hormones) is a collection of both physical and psychological symptoms associated with there being a *decreasing amount of testosterone available to the body*. This is not the same as having lower testosterone levels *per se*, and, indeed, in many men, these do not fall that much with age. What it means is that the amount of available, *usable* testosterone has dropped, so there is less of it around to affect the relevant male tissues (from hair follicles and muscles to brain) than there used to be.

This happens because as a man gets older – into and past middle age – his system tends to make more of a substance called sex-hormone-binding globulin (SHBG). This, as its name suggests, binds with testosterone, so the sex hormone is still there in the bloodstream but an increasing amount of it is biochemically 'tied up' and cannot be used. You may, therefore, still have plenty of testosterone but your body can't do anything with it, so it's no help at all. The result is that you start developing symptoms of testosterone shortage even though you have plenty of it.

Why the medical cynicism?
Because there is no actual shortage of male testosterone, doctors have traditionally sniffed at the idea of a male menopause and the suggestion that, like the female menopause, it's caused by dropping effective sex hormone levels. 'Look,' they'd say, checking ordinary blood-test results, 'plenty of testosterone there in *your* bloodstream. Go home and pull yourself together.' Regrettably, there are still many doctors who reckon the andropause doesn't exist. You may even have come across one or more of them personally: 'Your symptoms are just a natural, inevitable part of getting older – get used to it'. As Professor John Mackinlay of the New England Research Institute in Boston put it, after spending ten years measuring the hormone levels of 2,000 men aged 39–70, 'Call it what you like – andropause, viropause, bullshit – there is no evidence to support its existence.' He then added that the *general* testosterone levels in men don't seem much different in late middle age than they were 10–15 years before. This is perfectly true – general testosterone levels do not differ. What he and other doctors need to check for is bio-available testosterone, by measuring SHBG levels. And this is what more enlightened physicians are now doing.

Opinion shift
However, opinions are now changing and those who feel andropause is real (and, equally to the point, treatable) include the World Health

Organization. At their 2000 conference in Geneva on the 'Aging Male', the majority of the 700 delegates voted 'Yes' to the existence of the male menopause, and 80 per cent also voted in favour of treating it with testosterone-replacement therapy (TRT).

Figures and Triggers

Andropause can affect a man at any time between the ages of 35 and 70, says British andropause pioneer, clinician and former head of pathology services at the Maudesley Hospital, Dr Malcolm Carruthers, whose work has come in for a fair bit of criticism from the conventional medical establishment. Based on a sample of 1,000 of Carruthers' andropausal patients over a five-year period, he estimated that 'Perhaps 25 per cent of 50-year-olds and 40 per cent of 60-year-olds may experience it.' According to respected UK hormonal and sexual expert Dr John Moran, ongoing emotional distress at home and stress at work can have a similar effect – see 'Hormonal downturn' on page 87. It is thought that two further important reasons why some men experience more marked symptoms of andropause than others are because their levels of bio-available testosterone dip more markedly than most or because their systems are more reactive to the drop.

Midlife crisis

Andropause is not the same as the male midlife crisis. The latter is a well-established psychological and emotional condition, primarily one of reassessment and wondering where, if and how to make changes in your life. It tends to resolve itself spontaneously, though counselling can be helpful, as can talking things through with your partner if you have one. Most men are affected by a midlife crisis to some degree, usually between the ages of 35 and 45, and it may overlap with, or lead on to, the andropause.

Symptoms of andropause

These can include:

- increased tiredness and tendency to find sleep unrefreshing
- loss of drive and determination in all areas (at work and in bed)

- the 'So what?' factor: feeling that you are not so interested in anything you used to be interested in
- increased ratty or grumpy behaviour and a lower flashpoint, perhaps partly brought on by tiredness and hormonal mood changes
- general low-level depression
- drier skin, lanker, thinner hair, body hair less thick or reduced, less of a five o'clock shadow than formerly
- potency issues: erections not so firm, not so easy to maintain, fewer early-morning erections
- less-generous ejaculations
- drop in libido
- night sweats
- stiffness in arms or legs not associated with arthritic conditions
- a degree of gynaecomastia (fatty development around the male breast area)
- thickening round the waist, increased tendency towards a beer gut and general weight gain.

Thanks for the above to Dr Adrian Visser, former general director of the International Health Federation in Geneva, Barry Carruthers, former consultant andrologist at St Thomas' Hospital in London, Dr Malcolm Carruthers, and The Andropause Society.

Medical Treatments

Medical treatments for the andropause involve giving additional testosterone in different forms – male HRT, or TRT. These were originally testosterone injections or pills, but now include implants, creams, gels and skin patches.

In fact, type 'male HRT' or 'TRT' into the Net and a flood of sites comes up, but it's not a great idea to buy male-hormone products off the Web. There's a major black market in male hormones (steroids) thought to be worth around $400 million annually (current polls indicate this is down to use by sportsmen, around 10 per cent of whom are teenagers); however, the Andropause Society, a UK-based charity that works to treat, research and raise awareness of the andropause, estimates that around half all Net-sold products are counterfeit, and purity of the substances is also an issue.

Anyone on TRT should definitely be monitored regularly by a specialist clinician, since its use is linked with a potential increased risk of prostate cancer. Furthermore, TRT is not suitable for anyone who has certain medical conditions, including liver disease, heart disease, diabetes (which, if not controlled properly, can also cause potency problems and endemic tiredness) or an enlarged prostate. Side effects include acne, excess body hair and an increase in male-pattern baldness – see Men: Baldness on page 201.

It's also worth knowing that even major TRT enthusiasts like Dr Carruthers insist that men shouldn't just be offered hormone-replacement therapy right away if they have andropausal symptoms and warn that anyone who does that is more likely to be interested in your money than in you – TRT's usually only available privately. Instead, he advocates first trying some sensible self-help measures for a couple of months, which will, if nothing else, level the playing field, and are also likely to help reduce some andropausal symptoms on their own.

199. First-Base Self-Help for the Andropause
The main self-help measures are:

- Tackle any relationship problems.
- Stop smoking and drink far less alcohol.
- Exercise regularly.
- Eat healthily.
- Make a conscious effort to take more time out and relax more.
- Have a full health check-up with your GP.

Complementary Treatments

200. Natural Alternatives to Male HRT
Originally, the andropause was treated just by giving extra testosterone, the best known of the male hormones, which governs sexuality, potency, virility and masculinity. However, specialist physicians now believe that it's a bit more complicated than that, because maintaining healthy levels of bio-available (i.e. usable) testosterone involves a vital *balance* between:

- **luteineising hormone (LH)**, which is involved in testosterone production
- **sex-hormone-binding globulin (SHBG)**, which joins with testosterone in such a way that it cannot be used by the body's tissues
- tiny amounts of **oestrogen**, which all men naturally make
- **dihydrotestosterone (DHT)**, a more potent form of testosterone.

They also believe that just giving extra testosterone can, in fact, further reduce a man's natural production of this hormone and eventually shut it down altogether. Which would result in you feeling first better – then worse.

Natural supplements

With this in mind, and if the potential side effects of medical TRT do not appeal, there is a promising-sounding natural supplement combination called **Amidren** that works on each of the above. It contains magnesium and zinc (to support sperm production and testosterone levels), a herb called *Tribulus terrestris*, which is traditionally used to strengthen male libido and sexual performance, red-clover extract (a natural low-dose source of plant oestrogens), saw palmetto (another effective male-hormone-balancing herb – see Fix 204: Natural Remedies) and *Avena sativa* (oat extract). Studies by California's Institute for the Advanced Study of Human Sexuality – the only graduate centre in America that trains sexologists – suggest that *Avena sativa* increases the intensity of male orgasm and ups the amount of free-circulating (i.e. not 'bound' and therefore available for use) testosterone in men.

Amidren, developed by Sera-Pharma, is available in the UK from Victoria Health, 60 tablets, £29.95); in the US, try VitaDigest. For contact details, see under 'Shopping' in the Directory.

Other natural multi-herbal supplements with similar ingredients working together in a similar way that are available in the US include **Stamazide** by Stirling Grant Laboratories, which also contains horny goat weed and Damiana (again, both traditional pro-sexual and pro-energy herbs for men supported by research), and **Viastat** by Optimal Therapeutics.

Further information

For specialist treatment in the UK, try the Andropause Centre, London W1. In the US and Canada, there are many clinics (the US, Canada and Germany are way ahead of the UK in this area), such as the Men's Health Center, British Columbia. For contact details, see under 'Useful Helplines, Websites and Contacts' in the Directory.

Recommended reading: *The Andropause Mystery: Unraveling the Truths About Male Menopause* by Robert S. Tan; *Understanding Men's Passages: Discovering the New Map of Men's Lives* by Gail Sheehy; *Men's Health Matters: the Complete A–Z of Male Health* by myself; and *The Testosterone Revolution: Re-Discover Your Energy and Overcome Symptoms of the Male Menopause* by Dr Malcolm Carruthers. The latter can be ordered worldwide from the Men's Health Centre, London (£10 including postage and packaging). For contact details, see under 'Shopping' in the Directory.

Baldness

There are many different types of baldness, but the one discussed here is the sort that usually affects men: the progressive disappearance of hair around the front temple or crown – sometimes both – known as male-pattern baldness (androgenic alopecia), where thicker head hairs are gradually replaced by very short, baby-fine vellus hairs. It is caused by the male hormone testosterone, which gradually affects the hair roots, so any vulnerable ones start producing vellus instead of ordinary hair.

One in 20 men will have already started to go bald by the time he reaches his 20th birthday; others keep leonine manes into their seventies and beyond.

Medical Treatments

Hair transplants

No matter what the brochures and flashy websites tell you, these are going to cost you upwards of £2,000 and can only redistribute the amount of hair you've got left, not give you more.

A series of micro-transplants are now the norm – instead of old-fashioned hair plugs, flap grafts or even scalp reduction – as the look can be more natural, but the results may still be very variable. It is probably safer to ask your GP for a referral to a reputable private surgeon specialising in this area than to go for one of the clinics that advertise so energetically in men's magazines or on the Net: while there are some good specialist clinics that do take out ads, they are few in number. If your GP's not much help or if you'd like a second avenue to explore, contact the British Association of Aesthetic Plastic Surgery (BAAPS). They are part of the highly respectable Royal College of Surgeons and a very straight avenue to go down for reliable information about reputable practitioners. For contact details, see under 'Therapies and Therapists' in the Directory.

Drug treatments

The main options here are **Minoxidil** lotion or **Finasteride** tablets. Both are available via your GP on private prescription. Minoxidil's also on sale over the counter now, and finasteride, meant to be a prescription drug, is advertised on the Net. However, one of the problems about getting it that way is that you can't check its quality and have no way of knowing whether it's the genuine article, substandard or even, as in some cases, counterfeit.

Minoxidil lotion is rubbed on the scalp twice daily. According to top UK dermatologist and hair-growth expert Dr David Fenton, a consultant at St Thomas' Hospital in London, the 5 per cent strength lotion is likely to give 'some sort of' result for two-thirds of men, a 'decent' result for a third and a 'really pleasing one' for one in ten. Dr Fenton also advises that Minoxidil can sometimes give you a drier or itchy scalp and so if you have dandruff, you'd need to sort that first (perhaps with an anti-dandruff shampoo or a holistic treatment – see page xx), and if you have eczema, perhaps consider another option. He also says, 'It's best to start using it as soon as you begin to thin a bit, rather than wait till there is noticeable loss as it won't correct the latter.'

Minoxidil is available over the counter in chemists or by mail order under the brand name Regaine. 'It ought to be called Retaine, not Regaine,' says Dr Fenton, 'because it won't grow more hair for you, but it can help keep what you have left. Unfortunately, the effect is lost as soon as you stop using it.' If you buy it from a chemist, it costs around £30, or as little as $20 for a month's supply via the Net. You cannot be sure of what you're getting if you order it on the Web, however.

Finasteride, commonly known by the brand name Propecia, is taken in tablet form. It works by blocking the development of male hormones, and for this reason is often used at higher doses for benign prostatic hyperplasia – see Men: Benign Prostatic Hyperplasia (BPH) on page 206. Finasteride is only available privately, from around £30 per month. This helps about 80 per cent of men to some extent, but unwanted side effects can include a dropping libido and temporary erection problems. If you stop using the medication, any hair you regained will be gone again within 9–12 months.

Complementary Treatments

There are three key approaches: nutritional, herbal and hypnotherapeutic.

201. Nutritional

To support healthy hair growth nutritionally, pro-hair substances in food include vitamin B6, iron, folic acid, beta carotene (in dark-green, red, yellow and deep-orange vegetables – e.g. sweet potatoes, kale, mango, sweet peppers, turnip, greens, carrots, pumpkins and broccoli), proteins (including soy, fish, meat, eggs and dairy products), nettle extract, flaxseed oil, biotin (another B vitamin, which helps the body make melanin, the substance that gives hair its colour, so may be especially helpful if you are greying) and silica.

There are many different hair-growth-encouraging supplements that combine some or all of these. In the UK, consider **Kervrans Silica for Hair and Nails**, which contains silica and can be bought from Academy Health (60 tablets, £11.95/$18), **Pil-Food**, which contains millet extract, B vitamins, biotin, pantothenic acid and vitamin E, from Goodness Direct

(100 capsules, a month's supply, approximately £25) and **Viviscal** from Only Hair Loss (a month's supply, from £49.95), which supplies customers worldwide. US products include **Hairtopia** by HairBoutique (from $39.99) and **Hair Formula 37** (from $49.99), available direct, both of which offer a money-back guarantee. For contact details, see under 'Shopping' in the Directory.

Viviscal is one of the few extensively clinically researched nutritional hair supplements of which trials have been done by proper dermatology units attached to state hospitals rather than private laboratories (much of it carried out by the Department for Dermatological Research, Helsinki). The supplement contains vitamin C, fish-cartilage extract and fish oils and its results, published in professional peer-review journals, sound promising.[1] *Note:* do not take this one if you are allergic to shellfish.

> **Tip for Budget Hair Food**
> **Brewer's yeast** from the chemist's is both cheap and useful, as it is a great source of iron and B vitamins. Another good pro-hair budget tip is adding **millet seeds** – yes, the stuff that was said to make budgies bounce with health – from the health shop into your morning cereal or lunchtime salad. Try two tablespoons daily.

202. Herbal

Herbal remedies for baldness work by blocking or reducing the action of testosterone on the hair-root cells. This usually means reducing the amount of testosterone your body is producing using anti-androgenic herbs. There are a few supplements on the market that work this way, one of the best known being **Provillus**, the main ingredient of which is **saw palmetto**, the herb clinically proven in many strict clinical studies to reduce testosterone output and thus treat BPH. Provillus also contains nettle root, minerals and vitamins such as B6, zinc and magnesium, plus extract of the herb gotu kola, which is also said to support hair growth.

You can order it direct from Provillus, which is an American company (a month's supply, $30–$40). They have separate numbers for the UK and the US. For contact details, see under 'Shopping' in the Directory.

203. Focused Hypnotherapy

Focused hypnotherapy should preferably take the form of **self-hypnosis** to use regularly at home, as this puts the control in your hands and will also save you a fortune in fees for repeat sessions.

There are no good studies (that I can find so far) proving hypnotherapy works on hair regrowth. However, many experienced, high-profile hypnotherapists use it for clients. British psychotherapist Marisa Peer, who works in London and LA with rock stars and Olympic athletes, and Beverly Hills-based Riquette Hofstein, who trained at the Schwarzkopf Institute of Hair Research in Munich and specialises in hair growth, both use hypnotherapy for their patients and claim it can be very helpful. Riquette Hofstein offers both audio tapes and CDs (standardised). Marisa Peer offers tapes to use for hair-growth self-hypnosis at home and does customised tapes for each individual client. For contact details, see under 'Training Courses' in the Directory.

Hair hypno

At the very least, hypnotherapy is a motivational tool for solving hair problems ('I can and will grow more hair'), deeply relaxing and therefore provides an excellent method of DIY stress control – both chronic and acute stress are factors known to accelerate natural hair loss, or even produce sudden hair loss (alopecia areata, as experienced by Olympic swimming champion Duncan Goodhew). For best results with hair hypnotherapy, use with a good hair nutrition supplement, a stress-reduction and exercise programme and a pro-hair healthy-eating programme.

Mind over matter

Some may smirk at the mere idea of hypnotising your hair to grow more, but the effect of hypnosis on other physiological functions is actually pretty reliably documented. For instance, both self-hypnosis and its powerful variant Autogenic Training are used clinically worldwide to help control asthma and other breathing problems, pain, digestive disorders and menstrual difficulties. The hypnotherapy message can effectively be directed at different areas of the body to produce measurable changes in biological functions, as with the Withington Hospital in Manchester's work on 'gut-directed self-hypnosis' and its 80 per cent success rate with intractable IBS that had resisted all other forms of treatment – see Fix 64: IBS – Have Words With Your Gut.

Furthermore, general mind-over-matter positive thought targeted at different parts of the body has been researched on other physiological growth processes, including muscle growth and bicep development – see Fix 21: Bigger Biceps.

For how to find a professionally – and/or medically qualified – hypnotherapist, see under 'Therapies and Therapists' in the Directory.

Thinning hair

For thinning hair, tip half a sachet of gelatine powder into your usual amount of shampoo in a cup (use a whole sachet if it's past shoulder-length). You can also, if you like the idea and the smell, add two to three drops of either **cypress** or **sandalwood essential oil** – both great scents for men – which are found in quality men's toiletries and are used by professional aromatherapists to promote calm, confidence and high self-esteem.

Massage into the hair, leave for two to five minutes, then shower out very thoroughly in warm water. It leaves the barnet shiny with an instant *30 per cent more volume*, because the gelatine has melted and is lightly coating each hair, making it thicker; it is also reflecting light, so the hair shines more.

Gelatine powder can be bought from your local supermarket (5 sachets, approximately £1.30). For essential oils, try Baldwin's Cypress Oil (10 ml, £3.75) and Sandalwood Oil (5 ml, £10.39). For contact details, see under 'Shopping' in the Directory.

Benign Prostatic Hyperplasia (BPH)

The prostate is that unobtrusive little secondary sex gland that lies down at the base of a man's bladder. It is around the size of the average walnut and surrounds the urethra (the urine-carrying tube that runs from the bladder to the tip of the penis). BPH merely means a *non-*cancerous overgrowth of the prostate tissue.

Symptoms

At least a third of men over the age of 50 have uncomfortable urinary symptoms because their prostate gland has begun to grow too large and is squashing the urethral tube. This makes it harder to pass urine and also irritates the area, causing:

- straining to pass water
- 'hesitancy' – i.e. difficulty getting started even when you want to go quite badly, which can be embarrassing in public urinals
- a start-stop flow
- uncomfortable urination
- the urge to pass (small amounts of) water frequently, even if you've just done so, and often repeatedly at night
- feeling full even when you've just been.

It can also, not surprisingly, cause sexual problems: according to a MORI poll of 8,000 men, around half said their sex drives had suffered and that they had difficulty in getting an erection and ejaculating.

Medical Treatments

Common medical treatment includes 'watching and waiting' with regular check-ups, as the condition can develop very slowly, hormonal treatment with a group of drugs called alpha-reductase inhibitors, and surgery. Alpha-reductase inhibitors block the production of dihydrotestosterone (DHT), the more potent form of testosterone, which helps shrink the prostate itself but can also have a negative effect on men's sexuality and potency.

Complementary Treatments

204. Natural Remedies

The natural remedy of choice for benign prostatic hyperplasia is **saw palmetto**. It is thought to work against testosterone by preventing DHT from binding on to receptor sites in the prostate, which is how DHT stimulates the gland to grow. In clinical trials, the dosage has been around 160 mg daily of supplements made from whole berry extract. Try Prostex from Nature's Best (90 capsules, £11.95).

Another is extract of **rye pollen**. The product made from it is called **cernilton**, which has been subjected to several proper clinically controlled studies and is approved for medical use in many countries. It is currently unavailable in the UK, however. In the US, you can buy it from a company called Graminex (200 tablets, $25). Take six tablets daily. Having said that, a similar product, Prostabrit, is widely available in the UK in health shops, chemists or via Britannia Health (60 tablets, £19.95) and is taken twice daily.

Looking at an overview of the available trials involving nearly 3,000 men, it seemed that the rye pollen particularly helped with symptoms such as needing to pee in the middle of the night, and men reported all their symptoms had eased somewhat, though when their prostates were measured by ultrasound, they hadn't got any smaller.[2] Saw palmetto did even better, helping with all BPH symptoms including shrinking the enlarged prostate glands.[3]

For all contact details, see under 'Shopping' in the Directory.

See also Men: Prostatitis on page 228.

---

205. Bunged Up

There are many effective and rapid ways to tackle constipation, but a piece of advice especially for men from top UK gastroenterologist Michael Kamm, formerly medical director of St Mark's Hospital for the Colon and Rectum in London, is, don't read on the loo (as many men habitually do), even if it is the one place you get to check the sports pages in peace. It relaxes the rectal muscles, so you can't push stools out so effectively.

See also Fix 37: Constipation.

Black Eye

206. Speed Healing

Try **bromelain**. It is abundantly available in pineapple – and, yes, you could eat loads of that fresh, but unless you want to eat four to six whole pineapples a day for three days, bromelain supplements may be easier to take. This enzyme is anti-inflammatory and great for reducing all sorts of bruising, especially a black eye, a bad bruise anywhere or even a more major injury. Speed healing by taking 500 mg four times daily on an empty stomach for three days. Complementary therapists like naturopaths and nutritionists are now increasingly choosing this one over the more traditional homeopathic remedy, arnica.

Several studies suggest bromelain can reduce swelling, bruising, speed healing time and reduce pain following both injury and surgery.[4] In fact, one official body in Germany, Commission E (similar to the US Food and Drug Administration), has approved the use of bromelain for just these things. Cheaper than putting the traditional bit of raw sirloin steak on it – mind you, you could always up your high-quality protein count by grilling and eating it afterwards.

For bromelain, try Nature's Best (60 x 500 mg capsules, £14.95) or Hollan & Barrett (£8.60). For details, see under 'Shopping'.

See also General: Bruises on page 29 and Fix 313: Bashes and Bruises.

Detoxification

207. The Lazy Way
For men who suspect detoxification is something time-consuming, tedious and girlie that women do at overpriced health spas and which involves drinking gallons of spring water, ingesting unfamiliar (barely edible) macro-biotic foods, with colonic irrigations and scalding Turkish steam baths thrown in, then the foot patch may come as a pleasant surprise.

Feet first
There are several types available, but essentially foot patches are Japanese-style 'sap sheets': big plaster-like affairs, steeped in natural substances that are said to encourage the release of toxic material (from unwanted chemicals like preservatives to heavy metals such as lead) through the acupuncture points on the feet. For instance, one brand, **Revita**, uses bamboo vinegar and wood vinegar essence (from oak, beech and sakura trees).

Detox by sticking plaster? Are you laughing in derision? I might be too if I hadn't tried some recently. Having kept the patches on as instructed overnight, I woke up the next morning to find the material had gone grubby, as if they were facial cleansing pads used to remove a layer of brownish city grime from the face.

Very popular in Japan (they sell £9.5 million of them a month) and catching on in the US and Canada, the detox patches have now found their way to Europe. People wear them for anything from a couple of nights in succession to a few weeks, depending on the level of toxicity they feel they may have in their system.

Results

Some reportedly start feeling better within two to three days, others within a couple of weeks. Usually it would be the lymph system's job to sort this out, but the lymphatic vessels have no pump, unlike the blood circulatory system in the heart, to push the thick spring-cleaning lymph liquid round the body.

Muscular contraction's what does that, and if you also lead a sedentary lifestyle (e.g. drive to work and have an office job), this is another reason why your system may be getting more overloaded with unwanted material taken into the body via food, water and air than it would have done 40 years ago.

If you are interested, try Takara Foot Patches from Body Kind (10 patches, £17.95); in the US, you can buy them direct from Takara (10 patches, $31.95). For contact details, see under 'Shopping' in the Directory.

See also General: Detox on page 46.

208. Driver's Arm

An occupational hazard in summer for anyone, usually men, who spends hours behind the wheel for their job – taxi, bus and lorry drivers, travelling sales executives and, at certain times of the year, farmers – driver's arm refers to those smallish areas that get burnt from having the sun beat down on them for hours through the vehicle window from one side, or even as a result of having rested the right arm on a rolled-down car window frame (during summer city traffic jams and summer-holiday driving).

Small though the area may be (upper surface of forearm usually), it can be very sore even when covered up by a shirt and, being an occupational hazard, risks continual re-exposure to the same sun damage, unless you are a sensible convert to sunblock. Take away the pain and speed healing by immersing in water that's had enough **vinegar** added to it so you can taste it, at two- to three-minute intervals for 60 seconds at a time.

To speed things up, also try **Solaris**, made by Australian Bush Flower Essences, a good remedy for chasing away the sting of burns and sunburn and boosting skin regeneration. You can buy it from Baldwin's (30 ml, £7.95), IFER, Healthlines (30 ml, £7.95) or Australian Bush Flower Essences direct. For contact details, see under 'Shopping' in the Directory.

See also General: Sunburn on page 96.

Exercise

209. Gym Averse but Unfit

Like the car stickers say, 'Green Gym-ers Do It Outside.' For men who dislike the anabolic-steroid-driven ambience, cost or artificial setting of indoor gyms and health clubs, outdoor, green gyms offer a very different way to both de-stress and get fit.

What green gyms involve

Sessions are led by trained facilitators, take place twice a week at varying times of day (weekends too) and involve a warm-up session of gentle exercises, two and a half hours of physical work in a natural fresh-air environment (generally gardening or conservation), a tea break halfway through, then a wind-down session of movement and relaxation at the end.

You could find yourself on a local ecology project such as restoring ancient heath, common or downland, tree-planting, hedge-laying, fostering rare plants or animals, helping build a conservation pond for a primary school, mending old dry-stone walls, weeding an urban allotment or helping out at a city farm. You are also given a variety of different tasks on the same project so that you don't get bored doing the same thing

211

every session but are still able to see the results and continuity of your own work and receive thanks and good feedback from the communities or individuals you've helped.

Green gyms tap into the biophilia hypothesis, which states that a powerful need for contact with nature is an innate part of being human, and if you are deprived of it – perhaps when living in an urban environment and working in a sealed office away from natural air and light for most of the year – your well-being can really suffer. Luckily, taking the nature cure can go a long way towards reversing this for you.

The system is proving especially popular with men of all ages and from all walks of life (though many women are enthusiastic participants too), 70 per cent of whom lead sedentary office-based lives and have never worked either manually or outside. And people seem to really like doing it: the drop-out rate after six months is only 30 per cent, compared with more than 50 per cent for health-club or indoor-gym memberships.

What else is it good for?

Physiologically speaking, green-gyming also:

- supports weight loss and body sculpting – i.e. better abs, gluteals and biceps from all that lifting and digging
- is good exercise – burning up a third more calories than a step aerobics class and improving staying power in all areas
- reduces stress and anxiety levels. In one Brighton-based study in 2002, nearly 50 per cent of those on green-gym programmes reported a marked increase in well-being and more stable moods.
- improves heart rate, bone density, stamina, mobility and helps lift depression (according to two major pieces of research by Oxford Brookes University in 1999 and 2001)
- increases self-esteem – in a review of ten recent studies on green gyms by the UK's Countryside Recreational Network, nine out of ten people said their self-esteem had really improved.

Who's doing it?

There are currently some 50 such projects in the UK alone (Bristol, Manchester, Brighton, Birmingham and Oxford, to name but a few). Men are either taking themselves along to their nearest one or being referred by their GP, usually as an adjunct to, or even instead of, medication when they are suffering from:

- anxiety or depression (according to the mental-health charity MIND, around 15 per cent of men are battling clinical levels of these at any one time)
- burnout – see also Work and Office: Burnout on page 488
- lack of fitness and low stamina
- weight gain that doesn't want to shift
- continuously raised stress levels: surveys suggest 70 per cent of male office workers say these are 'high' most of the time. In one study by the Chartered Institute of Personal Development, over half reported excessive working hours and stress are ruining their sex lives. In fact, there are now 4.5 million workers in the UK alone on a minimum 48-hour week, compared with nearer half that number in 1984.

For further information on your nearest project, get in touch with BTCV. For contact details, see under 'Useful Helplines, Websites and Contacts' in the Directory.

210. Fast-Focus Workouts
The length of lunchtimes for British workers is shrinking, and when last measured (2006), it had diminished to an average of 19 minutes and 42 seconds: barely time to devour a bagel and certainly not long enough to visit the gym. Longer working hours also mean 7 p.m. and 8 p.m. finishes, by which time you may be so exhausted that nothing's further from your mind than 100 ab crunches or 50 lengths.

If you can't find time for a long session, though, you needn't sink under the weight of workout angst and give up on the idea of exercise completely. A new study by the University of New Hampshire has just found that two shorter bouts of just 15 minutes each are *even more effective* than a single 30-minute session.

211. Bigger Biceps
See them bigger and meatier and they will be. In 2001 researchers at the Cleveland Clinic Foundation in Ohio asked volunteers to spend a focused 15 minutes a day just *thinking* about exercising their biceps

. . . and after 12 weeks of mind-over-muscle, their arms were 13 per cent stronger.

This is partly because, as hypnotherapy and Autogenic Training studies consistently show, it is possible to instruct your body to behave in a certain way and have it obey you even under difficult physical circumstances (e.g. to not feel pain, to have more stamina, go to sleep, breathe more freely, slow the body's heartbeat, quicken its metabolic rate or affect the workings of its digestive tract – see 'Mind over matter' on page 205).

It is also because, on an esoteric level, according to one of the major spiritual laws (and also as a corollary to the laws of advanced Einsteinian physics), 'Energy follows thought.' Without getting too New Age about it, this means that if you consistently put energy in the form of thought (willpower, as some call it) into an idea, this can, and often does, manifest in the 'what you see is what you get' three-dimensional world – i.e. it will become solid, a fact, measurably real.

How to think bigger
The first time you ever do this, measure your flexed biceps in millimetres. Write down the measurement somewhere where you can retrieve it after 12 weeks (e.g. your Filofax, computer diary or on a scrap of paper stuck to the wall). Now:

1. Sit or lie down comfortably somewhere where you won't be disturbed. Close your eyes.
2. Take a deep, easy breath in for a count of five, hold it for five and let it out for five.
3. Repeat three times. Feel your body relaxing a bit as you do so.
4. Still with your eyes shut, take your attention to your left bicep. In your mind's eye, see the skin colour beneath your sleeve. Imagine the skin texture, any hair there. Visualise your bicep's curve and shape.
5. 'See' the bicep gently growing bigger, rounder, stronger. Imagine it flexing. Feel pleased with how it's looking now it's larger and stronger. Try and sense how it would feel to flex this much bigger bicep *now*. Hold that feeling in your head for a count of ten.
6. Repeat three times.
7. Do exactly the same thing with the right bicep.

8. When you're done, take three deep, easy, in-for-five, hold-for-five, out-for-five breaths.

9. Now open your eyes. Yawn and stretch a bit.

That's it.

Do this if you can *twice a day, or, at the very least, once*, as like physical bicep training, the more often you do it, the faster and more noticeably it works. Keep tabs on your progress week by week by seeing how much more you can lift. After three months compare the weight you can lift comfortably now with what you could do before and measure the bicep again.

How have you done?

212. Road-Runner Pain

If you're a runner who uses the roads and are finding you're getting a nagging pain, especially in the knees, back or ankles, it could be because you are always running along the same side of the road.

If you are, that may be both the problem and the very easy solution. Most roads slant by 7–9 degrees so that water drains off them when it rains. This sloping surface means that when you run along them one leg is repeatedly hitting the ground higher than the other, points out Martin Haines, who is a physiotherapist and adviser for *Runner's World* magazine. 'Effectively, it's making the leg nearest the middle of the road longer,' says Haines, and the body then compensates by trying to shorten the leg and thus reduce the extra pressure on your back and knee.

The advice? Vary your route – and terrain – as much as you can, and try not to run on a camber all the time. You could find that the pain disappears right away. If it doesn't, see a good sports physio as there may be a bit of damage to correct. For contact details, see under 'Therapies and Therapists' in the Directory.

213. Sports Stiffness

When your calves, thighs, back or shoulders are feeling the effects of a match or workout, try **Microvita Pain Cream**, available from Tranquil Living (125 ml, £8.25); from the Essence Shop, or direct from its makers, Living Essences of Australia (AS$11.90), or as Body Soothe Cream via Victoria Health (£9.99). For contact details, see under 'Shopping' in the Directory.

Having compared its performance with the most popular over-the-counter rub-on pain-relief products like Ibuleve, and even with the very best hospital-standard homeopathic arnica cream, without wishing to sound like an ad, this deceptively gentle cream (also available as a spray) still comes out top and works very quickly. Which is why it's being used in 16 of Australia's state hospital pain clinics, and is catching on in sports clinics worldwide.

See also Fix 473: Endurance Push.

Feet

214. Trainer Taming
Trainers walking about on their own? Clothes cupboard catching the smell so your shirts have that suspect tang of old rubber 'n' sweat about them?

A survey in the *Guardian* on 26 April 2006 found there are 76 times more fungi in the average trainer than in the average toilet.

What to do? You can spend a fiver or so on a pair of Odour Eaters (soft foam insoles impregnated with deodorising chemicals, which seem to last about a maximum of four weeks).

Or you can wash those trainers at least once a month in the washing machine, along with tough items like the bathmat, your grungiest jeans or most ancient gardening sweatshirt. Put on the coolest, gentlest cycle, the one usually used for wool and nylon and no hotter than 30 degrees C, and ideally add five to ten drops of tea-tree essential oil – a champion fungi-fixer – in with the detergent. When they are washed, pack the trainers with loo paper or crumpled newspaper and put upside down on a low-heat radiator to dry. Stretch carefully when partially dry by gently bending back soles.

It has to be said this is not immensely good for the shoes, but it offers a balance between your foot health suffering and your footgear coming in for some additional punishment. Between sessions, reduce mushroom power by loosening the laces, pulling back the shoe tongue a bit and letting them dry out. Ideally, try and have more than one pair.

215. Smelly Feet

If your feet are seriously and persistently smelly, even though you are hot on foot hygiene and washing your trainers, have a word with your GP. You probably have a fungal foot infection, which is extremely common and easily treated with fungicidal cream.

If your feet have been this way for a while, it's a good idea to also take the powerful antifungal agent **Citricidal** for three to six weeks, which is made from grapefruit-seed extract. In the UK, Citricidal is available from Higher Nature (45 ml, £6.90; 100 tablets, £10.50); in the US, it is just called grapefruit-seed extract and is available from NutriTeam (2 fl oz, $6.95). For contact details, see under 'Shopping'.

Persistent fungal infection of the feet is often a sign of a systemic candida infection (a thrush infection in your entire body) and means that though the infection may go for a bit, it'll come back again soon. Systemic thrush isn't a good thing to have anyway as it can affect sperm quality, fertility, energy levels, ability to think clearly and digestion, to name but a few, and it is very common. Citricidal helps eradicate this, too.

Smell-stopper

Try the **lemon** trick. After your morning wash cut two slices of fresh lemon, wipe one over the sole of one foot, then one over the other. Let it dry – it does so quickly – then put on (cotton) socks. The lemon juice deodorises sweat a treat.
Note: this also works for armpits.

See also: Athlete's Foot (Tinea Pedis) on page 25.

Fertility

216. The Essentials

One in five couples has trouble conceiving, and for early confirmed pregnancies (when someone is 8–12 weeks pregnant), the rate of miscarriage is one in eight. If you and your partner want to start trying for a baby, especially if she has experienced miscarriages before, or there have been any birth abnormalities in your existing children, *cutting out booze, cigarettes and any recreational drugs* are the very best things you can do to ensure you conceive soon and that your next pregnancy works out.

Smoking

Fathers who smoke have twice the risk of fathering babies with birth abnormalities. One German study of 8,000 births in 1983 found the most common smoking-related birth defects were harelips, heart defects and urinary-tract deformities.

Herbal Smoke-Stopper

Become like a bear with a sore head when you try and give up tobacco? This can be hell – both for you, and for anyone you live or work with. However, **Nico-Quit,** a herbal mix in a capsule, can help calm the mood swings and depression that nicotine withdrawal can cause. (From www.thinknatural.co.uk, 0845 601 1948, £7.95 for 25 capsules).

Advice on stopping smoking

One of the newest natural ways to stop smoking – and apparently one of the most successful – is using a system called **bio-resonance**, which essentially reads dysfunctional or unhealthy cellular vibrations from your body's cells, changes them round to the correct 'healthy' ones and feeds them straight back for your system to copy. It's also reportedly very quick (one or two hour-long sessions), costs £200–£300 and appears to not only stop the urge to smoke (many therapies from hypnosis to ear acupuncture will do that in the short term) but also claims a 70 per cent permanent success rate.

The therapy has impressed a group of Brighton GPs sufficiently to set up a bio-resonance clinic run by homeopath and healer Meriam Green (who is former manager of the Hale Clinic, London) at their multi-disciplinary surgery in Hove. There is also a dedicated unit in North London, the Healthvibes Clinic, which, thanks to national exposure on *Richard & Judy* in 2005, is very full indeed. For contact details, see under 'Useful Helplines, Websites and Contacts' in the Directory.

I can't find any good study data on bio-resonance for smoking cessation, but it certainly worked for the acute fatigue syndrome I experienced last year following a minor brain haemorrhage and hypothalamus damage, which consultant neurologists had said could take a good 12–18 months to resolve. With just two bio-resonance treatments, it took six months.

If you prefer something more traditional, take a look at www.giving upsmoking.co.uk, which gives details of all the NHS programmes run in the UK from one-on-one counselling to groups; Quit also has a wealth of tips, support and advice to offer. For contact details, see under 'Useful Helplines, Websites and Contacts' in the Directory.

Sniffing black-pepper aromatherapy oil can help curb nicotine cravings. It sounds unlikely, but it is validated by a clinical trial. See Fix 39: Craving Cigarettes.

Booze

A man can wipe out his entire sperm count after a single heavy drinking session, warns andrologist Anthony Hirsh of Whipps Cross Hospital in London.

It doesn't take much

A major blast of alcohol can flatten a man's output of vital sperm-making hormones (follicle-stimulating hormone and luteineising hormone) made by the pituitary and hypothalamus. It takes three months to make a new batch of sperm.

In fact, even as little as a pint of beer a day can produce semen abnormalities, says the Royal Free Hospital's fertility researcher Dr Marsha Morgan. And if a sperm that is less than perfect fertilises an egg, the resulting embryo is likely to either miscarry or develop into a baby that has an abnormality or health problem.

Even if drinking doesn't heppen to affect the sperm you make – and some men's are more sensitive to alcohol than others – alcohol doesn't help the sperm do its job. Those that have had alcohol added to their environment and then been observed under a microscope appear simply too drunk to find their way up a Fallopian tube.

Advice on stopping drinking

All the available resources seem to be aimed at men who either have difficulties with alcohol or are clinically addicted to it – not at the happy social drinker who just wants to stay off it for a while. But, as Foresight, the pioneering preconceptual care organisation, suggests, 'Just stay out of the pub. And drink spring water or alcohol-free wines and lagers at parties. [Take your own, if necessary.] Look, it's only for a few months. It takes just three alcohol-free ones to produce a consignment of good healthy sperm, then wait until your partner falls pregnant, after which you can start drinking again if you wish to.'

Stoned sperm

As with alcohol, smoking marijuana has quite an effect on sperm – they look and behave as if they are, well, extremely stoned (meandering instead of swimming straight, swimming backwards . . . or just sitting there wobbling on the spot, apparently lost in thought). If you are serious about your fertility, any doctor or complementary health worker will say the same – that it is essential you give up *all* and *every* recreational drug *for at least three months* before you and your partner begin trying for a baby in order to create a batch of A-Team Sperm bursting with health and supercharged with major baby-making capacity.

See also Women: Fertility on page 141.

Flatulence

Flatulence is caused by excess gas (flatus) being made in the bowel, and some people just naturally make more of it than others. Passing wind is the only way to get rid of this, since your body can't reabsorb it and your abdomen becomes bloated, uncomfortable – sometimes downright painful – if it remains in the body.

The substance that causes the bad smell is sulphur, which accounts for less than 1 per cent of the gas by volume – the rest is methane, odourless oxygen, CO_2 and nitrogen. However little there is of it, though, it unfortunately carries a big embarrassment factor: other people can detect it in amounts as tiny as one part sulphur to a million of air.

Conventional wisdom suggests that men break wind more than women, so this is more of a male health issue. There are no studies looking at the sex ratio, but it's more likely that, possibly having been raised on locker-room etiquette, many men may be a bit less inhibited about letting their gas go public than women.

On average men pass gas 10–20 times daily; up to 25 is seen as quite normal. But if there is a gastrointestinal problem, this increases. One man counted a record 141 episodes in a single day, 70 of which were over a particularly trying four-hour period.

Causes

Flatulence is usually a symptom of gastrointestinal disturbance and can also indicate that something is perhaps not working too well in your gut. It's a very good idea to check with your GP that your digestive tract is healthy and all is in order. And while you are there, ask about the symptoms of IBS in case this may be at the root of the problem – see also Fix 64: IBS – Have Words With Your Gut. Other common causes include:

- difficulty digesting one particular sort of food or entire food group, such as those made from milk – see also Women: Bloating on page 128 and Young Children: Food Intolerances on page 281. Foods

from the bean and higher-sulphur-content vegetable family (e.g. broccoli and cabbage) are often the culprits too.
- a hefty course of antibiotics, which can wipe out all the useful bacteria in your body, including your gut, as well as those that were causing the infection.

Medical Treatments

Ordinary medical treatments for flatulence not linked to any other condition that requires intervention are drugs, like simethicone, and acti-vated-charcoal biscuits, which you buy over the counter in the chemist's (e.g. WindCheaters). The latter are good old-fashioned gut-gas deodorisers but not that great to eat. Both drugs and biscuits absorb the gas until it has passed out in your bowel motions, which unfortunately leads to smellier stools than usual.

Complementary Treatments

217. Bean Busters

One may wonder why it's worth bothering with beans at all since they are such champion gas-producers. Yet they are so high in fibre, low in fat and highly versatile (not to mention good to eat if cooked correctly) that many people say they would miss them greatly if they couldn't eat them at all. So if you're a bean fan or vegetarian:

- **Soak** any dried beans for four to five hours before use. Afterwards, rinse thoroughly, drain, then cook in fresh water.
- **Rinse** well under running water for two minutes (not less) after cooking. This helps remove some of the indigestible starches on the skins and applies to tinned (pre-cooked) beans as well.
- **Switch** to 'gentler' beans, like split peas, lentils and lima beans. Try anasazi beans too, suggests Bruce Yaffe, a gastroenterologist affili-ated to Lennox Hospital, New York City – they're sweet, mild, versa-tile and available in health food shops.
- **Drink** herbal tea: according to William J. Keller, professor at the North-east Louisiana School of Pharmacy and secretary of the American Society of Pharmacognosy, peppermint (widely available in super-

222

markets), spearmint, anise and caraway (from the health food shop) are the best for digestion.

- **Take** 'good' bacteria in freeze-dried capsule form, to help rebalance a gut unsettled or under-populated with beneficial bacteria thanks to antibiotic treatment, illness or poor diet. However, some probiotic supplements are rather better than others. Try BioCare's, which are good quality, such as Bio Acidophilus (60 capsules, £17.95).

Bravo Beano

Try enzyme power. There's one called **alpha-glactoside**, derived from a food-grade fungus, *Aspergillus niger*, which helps break down indigestible sugars. You can get it in tablet form as **Beano**, which is available in the US from American Lifestyle (120 tablets, $35). It isn't available in the UK, but American Lifestyle will ship to you. Take one per serving of the 'problem' foods each mealtime in warm or cool food – not hot as it kills off the enzymes.

Use eight drops with the first mouthful and 'You could be eating foods you've not been able to have for 20 years,' says Stephen Pray, professor at Southwestern Oklahoma State University Pharmacy, Weatherford.

For all contact details, see under 'Shopping' in the Directory.

See also General: Constipation on page 37.

Penis Enlargement

Most urologists insist that if a man's penis is big enough to reach inside his partner, then it's just fine, but individuals may find they feel a bit differently about that. Which is why in the last 15 years there has been a rise in the number of penile-augmentation operations and a flood of penis-enlarging programmes, pills and patches on the Net.

The old idea that any man with a small- to average-sized penis who is prepared to invest time and money into making it bigger must have psychological problems is also now being challenged, as more men opt to do so. As Dr Hennie Roos of Johannesburg's Millpark Hospital (who's done many hundreds of augmentations) put it, 'These men don't have a small penis, and they don't have psychological problems either. They just want a large penis.'

Just, as many would argue, like women who have perfectly respectable 32B breasts and elect to spend money enlarging them not because they have a deep-seated hang-up but because they would simply prefer to be a 36C and say goodbye to their Wonder-bras.

If you want a bigger penis, you have two options:

- **medical treatment** (i.e. surgery). It has some good proven results. But not all operations either go to plan – or are done by experts (an expert in this case being either a cosmetic surgeon or urologist *who specialises in this area and has done for many years* – not just a general surgeon) so the customer-satisfaction rate can vary.
- **alternative treatments or natural techniques** (like penile-augmentation exercises). There are no reliable medical trials I can find at present, but there are many customer testimonials.

Medical Treatment

Surgery is both expensive and carries the usual risk of any operation – including a not-very-happy client afterwards. Techniques include:

- cutting the penis's suspensory ligament (which runs from its base deep into the pelvis), claimed to add 0.5–5 cm to the length
- exposing the penis down to its root (some 40 per cent of it is internal, to anchor a man's erection firmly so it does not wave about), claimed to add 4–7.5 cm to the length. Erections, having lost their 'guy ropes', might need to be supported or guided by hand afterwards, though.
- injecting fat into the penile shaft to make it thicker, though the effect may sometimes be uneven, or become so over time. Also, this doesn't affect the width of the head itself, so the aesthetic result may be unsatisfactory.

If you would like to explore the option of surgery, it is vital that you first go to a consultant urologist. Unless there are particular medical circumstances such as an injury to the penis, or you are clinically microphallic (born with a very small penis – too small to urinate standing with), you would need to arrange this privately via a GP referral.

Talk it through with the consultant, and if you still want to go ahead and they do not carry out this kind of surgery themselves, they should know a reputable colleague who does. This needs to be a good cosmetic surgeon or urologist with a special interest in penile augmentation. Penile enhancement ads are all over the Net like a rash, but generally speaking, good places – and good surgeons – don't need to advertise as they get more than enough recommendations from other kosher colleagues anyway and the Institute of Urology suggests that most of the ones who do advertise are cowboy clinics likely to do you a less than satisfactory job.

Average erect penis sizes round the world (figures from the International Planned Parenthood Association)

Thai men – around 12.7 cm (5 in.)
White Westerners (UK and US) – 15.3 cm (6 in.)
Black Americans – 17.8 cm (7 in.)

Complementary Treatments

Type 'penis enlargement' into Google and you'll be deluged by information. However, if you want to go the DIY natural methods route rather than the surgical, it is likely that the best results will be obtained from the **Step 1, 2, 3** approach:

Step 1: a penile-enlargement exercise programme
Step 2: a combination nutritional supplement
Step 3: a focused self-hypnosis routine, which motivates, supports and helps you feel 'Yes, I can do this. Yes, it will work for me.'

218. Step 1 – Exercise
Jelqing

A penis-stretching exercise programme usually involves a technique called **jelqing**, said to have been developed by the Arabic civilisation over a thousand years ago and taught to boys there from a young age.

The method, which is claimed to increase both length and girth over time, involves 'milking' your penis by hand. There are also exercises using devices and machines (power-jelqing), but these can be too vigorous and rough, and have been known to cause tissue damage and pain.

Workout time

Daily workouts involve a five-minute warm-up and a 20-minute routine. They should be done on a semi-erect penis (stop if you get a full erection) with a liberal amount of lubricant.

Possible gain over six months is claimed by programme developers to be up to 8.9 cm (3.5 in.), but anecdotal reports suggest that while they do make a difference, it's nearer an average of 4–5 cm (1.5–2 in.). There are several such programmes around, and some are better than others; many 'highly recommend' that you buy their pricey – and reportedly pretty unnecessary – stretching devices as well.

The PC exercise

This is a major part of natural penis-enlargement exercise programmes and involves strengthening the pubococcygeus muscles, located between scrotum and anus, and the area around the prostate gland. Stronger PC muscles help stabilise erections and are important if the penile shaft itself is being lengthened.

One penis-lengthening programme awarded top rating recently by both *Men's Health* and *Men's Fitness* magazines is by **Massive Member**. It costs around $50, offers detailed instructions, 24-hour ongoing email support from the company's trainers, requires no gadgetry and, carries a six-month, no-quibble money-back guarantee. For contact details, see under 'Shopping' in the Directory.

219. Step 2 – Supplements

There is no pill in existence that will make your penis bigger, as such. However, there are nutritional combination tablets marketed as penile-enhancement pills that may help support healthy cell growth, male-hormone output and libido.

Again, there are lots of these around, many of which are no help at all. It may be best to choose one from a well-established company that carries a full money-back guarantee, such as **ProSolution**, which is available in the US (a month's supply, approximately $44). Buyers in the UK can also buy direct from ProSolution. For contact details, see under 'Shopping' in the Directory.

The detailed versions of several different penis pills' ingredient lists all seem to contain certain natural substances that fall into the following categories:

- male sexuality and libido supporters (e.g. muira puama, or 'potency wood' as it's often called)
- male-hormone-output balancers (e.g. saw palmetto)
- traditional herbal sexual tonics, like the Ayurvedic shatavari complex
- blood-vessel dilators (e.g. safflower extract, or circulation-encouragers like ginkgo biloba). These help stimulate blood flow all round the body, including to the penis when a man gets an erection.

220. Step 3 – Self-Hypnosis

Hypnosis has been found to be capable of producing a measurable physiological effect on different areas of the body, including, according to one recent study, enlarging them – see Fix 211: Bigger Biceps. A professional hypnotherapist can teach you a simple self-hypnosis routine for daily use at home.

You do not need to tell your hypnotherapist why you want to do this if you don't want to: simply say you want to use it as a deep relaxation technique. When you've learnt to put yourself into a light trance, you can then devise your own affirmation, or 'instruction', to send to your penis to encourage growth. For contact details, see under 'Training Courses' in the Directory.

221. Prickly Heat

Prickly heat is one of the curses of the summer bare chest, especially for men with hairy ones. It is caused by blocked glands, which prevent sweat from being released, trapping it below the skin's surface so it irritates and itches. Once it starts, it can be difficult to get rid of unless you keep your chest covered by a cotton T-shirt for the rest of the holiday.

But the following can relieve it and sometimes get rid of it altogether:

1. Wash your chest in cold water and pat dry.
2. Add seven drops of Bach's **Crab Apple** to half a cup of cooled water and dab liberally on the affected area. Repeat three times daily.
3. Take three to four drops of the essence in water four times daily too.

Keep your chest covered by a cool cotton shirt for three to four days while using the above remedy.

You can buy Bach's Crab Apple from Healthlines (10 ml, £3.99). For contact details, see under 'Shopping' in the Directory.

See also Fix 234: Anti-Itch Summer Spray – Make Your Own.

Prostatitis

Prostatitis is inflammation of the prostate gland. It is very common in younger men aged 25–45, and one in five men under 40 have had it. This condition can be difficult to diagnose accurately and not easy to treat effectively, especially if it's the chronic, grumbling, non-bacterial kind.

Types

There are two main types of prostatitis:

- acute (i.e. you have developed it recently)
- chronic (you have had it for some time). There are two subgroups under the 'chronic' umbrella: bacterial prostatitis (caused by a bacterial infection) and non-bacterial inflammatory prostatitis (i.e. no infection to be seen, but the gland is clearly inflamed and irritated).
- and a third type of prostatitis, prostatodynia, when no infections or obvious inflammation can be found but you are still experiencing pain and other symptoms, especially during sex.

Medical Treatments

These include antibiotics, anti-inflammatory drugs and painkillers. If some of the symptoms listed here sound familiar, ask your GP to refer you to a consultant urologist or a genitourinary (GU) specialist. Symptoms include needing to pass urine often and burning when you do; chills/fever; lower back pain; pain when you ejaculate; pain in the area between anus and scrotum; inability to urinate.

Self-referral to the experts and how to get it

You can easily refer *yourself* to any local walk-in sexually transmitted disease clinic by just going down there, because while prostatitis isn't a sexually transmitted disease in itself, it can be the result of chlamydia, which is. Ask your hospital's switchboard to be put through to the clinic first and get directions so you can find it easily: they are often tucked away and have discreet but not very revealing names like the James Smith Unit.

Complementary Treatments

222. Natural Help

Extract of **rye pollen** is a successful natural treatment. Trials at the University of Cardiff, the Royal Infirmary of Glasgow and Germany's Georg-August University showed that seven out of every ten men with chronic, hard-to-shift prostatitis did well on **cernilton**, which is produced from rye pollen. However, you need to be persistent as it's three months before the improvements begin to kick in and an average of six months before you are properly better. See Fix 204: Natural Remedies. Zinc and copper supplements and vitamins A, C and E are also helpful.

Keep it coming

Not ejaculating very often may cause fluid to build up in the prostate gland, producing local irritation that can be enough to create the ongoing inflammation that is one of prostatitis's main symptoms. So if you're into Tantric sex, during which the man rarely ejaculates, watch it.

Sports Tip

If you jog, run or play sport, it's a good idea to have a really good pee before each session. Vigorous exercise on even a partially full bladder is one of the risk factors for prostatitis, as the vibration caused by the feet hitting a hard surface as you run and dodge can cause the fluid in the myriad of canals within the prostate gland to shake to and fro. This may trigger irritation in their delicate linings, which could then progress to full-scale inflammation of the entire gland.

See also Men: Benign Prostatic Hyperplasia (BPH) on page 206.

Sex

223. Libido

There are many herbal remedies for enhancing male libido, but if you're looking for consistent results, it's best to stick to the ones that are backed by clinical research.

One of the best

The South American herb **muira puama** is one such remedy. It's used both clinically and traditionally for men and women to increase sex drive. According to GP Dr Sarah Brewer (who has specialised in sexual medicine for 17 years and wrote *Increase Your Sex Drive*), it's 'one of the best herbs for treating erectile dysfunction and lack of libido' that there is.

In one particular trial carried out in Paris with 262 men complaining of lack of sex drive, 62 per cent reported that it was not known as 'potency wood' for nothing as it had had a 'dynamic effect'.[5] A second, smaller study yielded similar results. And as an added bonus, if your memory is starting to play up, it seems it also helps you remember things, according to a Brazilian study in 2004.[6]

Try Rio Muira Puama from Think Natural (90 x 2,500 mg capsules, £19.95).

The most common sexual problem is lack of 'normal' desire or low libido, resulting in 'not having sex often enough'. But how often's enough? A poll by MORI for *Esquire* of several hundred men of all ages found that:

5 per cent never have sex (at present).
13 per cent have sex less than once a month.
19 per cent have sex once a fortnight.
17 per cent have sex once a week.
33 per cent have sex two to three times a week.
11 per cent have sex four times a week.
2 per cent have sex every day, sometimes more.

Which means over half all men have sex once a week or less. Who's normal now?

And . . .
Tribulus is another herb shown to enhance libido, the ability to get an erection and sexual performance.[7] According to the respected medical newsletter the *Townsend Letter for Doctors and Patients*, tribulus boosts male libido, promotes fertility in both sexes and, when used on sports training programmes, can help men reach their peak of physical fitness.[8]

Usually, however, it takes quite a long time to have any effect, but **Libilov** capsules have a far higher level of tribulus's active ingredient, protodioscin, so they work faster. Libilov is made by Nutrica and is available in the UK from Victoria Health (30 tablets, £17.95); in the US, contact Nutrica direct (30 tablets, $29.99) or Food and Vitamins (180 tablets, $22.99).

Not a do-it-now aphrodisiac or instant stimulant, Libilov's effects are steady and cumulative, and ten studies now suggest it is one of the best sexual supplement combinations around for men.

Note: other small studies have additionally found that Libilov can be used to alleviate male infertility, as it improves both sperm quality and their ability to swim fast and straight.

For all contact details, see under 'Shopping' in the Directory.

224. Orgasm Power

If you'd like more earth-shaking orgasms, there is a very simple exercise that can help you get them. Just as pelvic exercises improve strength of orgasm for women, so they can for men. The sensation is partly produced by the contraction of your pelvic muscles, which end deep in the perineal area (that band of thickened muscle between anus and penis base). The harder those muscles contract, the more powerful your climax.

The big Oh!

1. Flex the muscles you'd usually use to stop a stream of urine. Do so ten times, holding each time for a count of eight.
2. Flex the muscles round your anus, the ones you'd usually use to stop yourself emptying your bowels. Do so ten times, holding for a count of eight.
3. Flex the perineal muscles – as if you were trying to pull the whole area further up inside you. Do this ten times for a count of eight.

Start with the exercises once a day for the first week. Work up to twice a day, morning and evening – or even when standing waiting for a drink at the bar as no one can see you doing them – and build up to 20 repetitions each time, then 30. Keep going with those 30 (some men do 50) every day.

See also General: Sex on page 86.

Shyness

Traditionally, men aren't supposed to get shy – they're expected to be confident, up for it and out there at all times. But most men know this is a big fat lie. According to recent social surveys, modern males can be just as sensitive, reactive and insecure as the opposite sex – which is probably one reason why the new generation of men finds it easier to relate to and understand women than the majority of their fathers could ever hope to.

One recent survey of Italian men, who are traditionally seen as sexually upfront and thoroughly opportunistic ('the bottom-pinching princes of Europe'), found two-thirds reported they felt too shy and too insecure about their bodies on the beach to chat up attractive women, and over half said they worried constantly about being given the brush-off. The same survey (in *Riza Psicosmetica* magazine in 2005) also found one in three only went to a beach to sunbathe and would much rather read a book, hide behind their designer shades and listen to their iPod than risk talking to strange girls.

225. Confidence in a Bottle

There are chat-up workshops and confidence gurus galore out there, but an easier and far less expensive option (and even if you decide to go down the behavioural route, it's a very good start) is an essence remedy from the plants of the tough red Australian outback. Called **Confid**, it contains the diluted extracts of six different powerful plants, which work on you at an emotional level. Confid is from the Australian Bush Flower Essences range, available direct, from health shops, Healthlines (30 ml, £7.95) or Neal's Yard (£8.50).

Homeopathically gentle though essences may be, they can be effective all right. So much so that they are starting to be used in hospitals all over the world: in the Texas Cancer Care Center at Fort Worth, the Royal

Perth Hospital in Australia, the University Hospital of Sao Paulo and by the Swiss Green Cross for adolescent victims of Chernobyl, to name but a few.

Another great essence for male sexual confidence – especially if someone has ever experienced distressing rejection from partners in the past – is **Horse Chestnut Leaf Bud** by Light Heart Essences, which can be purchased direct (10 ml, £5.15). The fact that what it's made from looks like a plump, cheerful, alert penis tells you all you need to know about this one.

For all contact details, see under 'Shopping' in the Directory. See also Shyness on page 90 and Fixes 218 and 219 on relationships.

Smoking

226. Giving Up but Edgy
More men die of smoking than women (the ratio's 60:40, according to a report by Action on Smoking and Health in 2001), so if you are trying to give up – and 70 per cent of smokers are at any one time – consider some extra backup from **Nico-Quit**.

It's a natural combination formula that helps soothe the irritability and edginess that goes with nicotine withdrawal. Nico-Quit contains calming ingredients such as passion flower, oat extract, which is used as a mild antidepressant and stress-reducer, St John's wort (extensively researched in clinical trials for mild to moderate depression) and chromium, to help level out the rises and dips in your blood sugar that lead to wobbliness and irritability – caused by fluctuating or dropping levels of nicotine in the bloodstream. It also contains an amino acid called DL-phenylalanine, which the body converts to tyrosine, a precursor for the feel-good neurotransmitters dopamine and norepinephrine. You can buy it in the UK from AuraVita (60 capsules, £13.95). For contact details, see under 'Shopping' in the Directory.

See also Fix 39: Craving Cigarettes and 'Advice on stopping smoking' on page 218.

Weight Loss

227. Fish 'n' Chips Cheats

Are you a sucker for comforting, filling takeaway food you eat on the move or back in your sitting room after being down the pub or playing five-a-side, when you're *starving* but pushed for time or cannot face whipping up a healthy little something? Join the club. So, for fans of (saturated-fat-heavy) fish and chips, there's good news. Shake on the **vinegar** and it'll help keep off the weight.

Why? Being acidic, vinegar can interfere with the digestive enzymes involved in the breakdown of starch, since these need an alkaline environment to activate them. That helps slow down the release of sugar from starchy foods (like chips), as a study published in *Diabetes Care* in 2005 showed. This reduces the body's tendency to make fat cells (pile on the pounds) after a meal.

Tips for Using Vinegar for Weight Control

- Eat a salad that has an oil and vinegar dressing with spag bols, lasagnes and rice-accompanied dishes like curries.
- Dip any bread you eat with your meal (e.g. ciabatta, baguette or pitta) into a mix of olive oil and balsamic vinegar.
- Shake vinegar on to chips.

See also General: Weight Loss on page 105.

Women and Relationships

228. Attracting Women – Top Ten Positive Posing Tips

This fix involves the behavioural science of sex-signalling. So if you've seen a woman you like the look of, here's an expert's ten-point action plan for how to catch her eye favourably and look good while she checks you out. It works.

The following suggestions come from body-language expert and author Judi James, who has her own Channel 5 show, *Naked Celebrity*, several newspaper columns and whose consultancy is much in demand with blue-chip corporates to turbocharge their male executives' body-talk business skills.

1. Stand chatting to other men but casually, not in a tight pack (which can look intimidating and predatory).

2. Look about a bit, but subtly – it shows you are open to meeting women. But don't scan the room too much, as that may give the impression you're desperate to pull and will settle for anyone.

3. If you are listening to someone, including another man, look interested. Women like men who listen.

4. Laugh or (perhaps easier) smile. It's no coincidence that the actors who appeal to women most, like Tom Cruise and Jude Law, have electric smiles that light up their whole face. Practise this in the mirror at home, hone it and it will become one of the best tricks in your repertoire. A really great smile is a deadly weapon.

5. Do the occasional frown. 'It's very effective to do the frown and then throw in a dazzling smile now and again,' says James. 'Get the frown right and you'll look focused and in charge. Again, rehearse at home till you're ready to go public with this one.'

6. Stand tall.

7. If you see someone you like the look of, raise your chin slightly, then drop it back down slowly and soften your eyes a bit.

8. Put your hand in your pocket, as this creates subliminal penis awareness for women. However, only do this if you've practised in the right clothing first. A hand won't fit into tight jeans, and if you do it wrong in baggy ones, it may look dodgy.

9. Hold your drink below chest height: this looks comfortable and confident. If held higher, it can look like a barrier. Use it as a *minor* prop. Enjoy, but don't swig it back too fast or study the bottom as though looking for the meaning of Life, the Universe and Everything.

10. Avoid propping a foot up on the bar rail or standing with your legs too far apart and arms folded. Position your feet at shoulder width, which looks strong and grounded; doing it wider makes someone look like a bouncer, especially if their arms are crossed.

229. Walking for Effect (the 'Drop Dead and Worship Me' Saunter)

This fix is about how to look good as you go over and introduce yourself to someone you fancy.

Even if you're not doing what your father or grandfather probably had to do if they'd spotted a girl they liked (walk from their group of mates across a dancehall to where she was sitting with hers, then back again if rejected), even a few metres can seem like a very long way because you will be subconsciously aware that the way you move is already sending her signals about who you are (and how you are) both in and out of bed.

Going over to a woman you are attracted to for the first time can make the most confident man overly conscious of his arms and legs. He may even start losing his grip on how to walk at all. (If it's any comfort, this can also happen to a woman going past a man she really likes if he's looking at her.)

However, the advice below from body-talk guru Judi James works, especially if you practise it beforehand in the mirror until you're happy with the way you look. Follow her suggestions and the next time you walk over to a woman you won't just be hoping you look OK – you'll *know* you look good.

Try something new

Learning new behaviour can take a bit of courage, since it involves stepping outside your comfort zone and dealing with the fear of (possibly) looking daft. But it is only logical that if you want different results, you'll need to use different methods, and this can be achieved in a matter of weeks. In fact, psychologists suggest that old habits can be changed in just 21 days and new ones learnt even faster.

> 'If you do what you've always done, you'll get what you've always got.' *Judi James*

Style: 'Think Clint Eastwood – laid-back but tough.'

Pace: nice and easy.

Reasons: a good walk can be a serious asset for men. Women won't expect you to walk well, so their eyes will be glued to you when you do. Plus, the way you walk, like the way you dance, advertises your sensuality, personality and sexuality. So you want to make sure it's saying the right things.

How to do it

1. Think about which area of your body you'd like to feature as you walk. A potential lover is going to be most attracted to the face, chest and groin.
2. Consider how you can show this off while you walk. Subtly.
3. Close your eyes and imagine a walk that's easy, fluid and relaxed.
4. Pull yourself right up to your full height by stretching your spine.
5. Take a breath in, then let it out slowly to release any tension. This will give your whole body posture a relaxed but upright look. Slumping or bowed shoulders send out submissive signals that bawl, 'Loser!'
6. Now, focus your energy on your shoulders. Rotate them comfortably in a circle to loosen them, while keeping your arms by your sides. Stop when they are held back and down.
7. Pull in your stomach and tuck in your bottom slightly.
8. Let your fingertips brush lightly against the sides of your legs.
9. Now try walking in front of a mirror. What seems to be the right length of stride for your leg length? Shorter men often overstretch their stride, which can look awkward.
10. Consciously let your fingers relax – ensure they don't curl into fists. Keep your hands slightly cupped with the fingers curved.
11. Keep your body upright without leaning forward.
12. The walking bit: to avoid flat-footing it, put the heel of your foot down first, peel on to the ball of that foot, so the toes propel you smoothly into the next step, and move your hips slightly from the waist as you walk. This gives coordinated movement.

Remember: laid-back, but tough.

If you're interested in finding out more about Judi James's seminars and training programmes, see her website, www.judijames.com.

230. Ranting Partner

Men (and women) often complain their girlfriends (or boyfriends) can harangue them for hours when they are angry or concerned about something – and *will* Keep Going On until all sympathy one originally had has evaporated.

Neuro-linguistic practitioners teach a technique called **timed venting (TV)** for just such an occasion, saying that TV can be invaluable here and has saved many a relationship when one partner claimed their lover wouldn't shut up about a subject, while the other complained they never listened.

It involves saying to your partner, at a time when you are both calm and getting on well, 'About these discussions of ours? You (as I feel) going on – and me (as you feel) not listening? There's a way that you can have your say when you need to and I can listen without interruption so we can sort things out. How about we give it a try?'

1. You can talk to me – or even at me – about whatever is upsetting you for a *mutually agreed length of time*. Say two to five minutes for small issues, up to 15 minutes for bigger things. We agree, before you begin each time, whether we have a small or a big issue here.
2. I listen to you properly, without interrupting, looking around the room or fidgeting, for that length of time.
3. We agree to have a clock or watch or even a buzzing timer around when we talk. And that when time is up, you stop, *whether or not you have finished*.
4. Then either I have my say for the same amount of time *or* that is the end of the session. For today.
5. However, if you have more points you would like to make, we agree to come back together tomorrow, again at a mutually agreed time, for another 5- or 15-minute timed-venting session.
6. We then, if necessary, arrange an opportunity to discuss – together, taking turns – the issues raised.

You would also need to explain, 'I love you and want to listen, but can only do so within my limits. These are what they are. We can work things through if you can help me out here by trying timed venting. If not, I am really sorry but I cannot do this.'

Listening isn't just waiting until the other person's stopped talking.

Timed venting cuts down ranting, going round in circles and repetition. When you both become used to the idea that the window of opportunity is limited, it can help you both to get more into the habit of having shorter problem-solving-orientated *focus discussions* – based on making points as succinctly as possible and then deciding what to do about them.

Young Children

This millennium's children have more incredible opportunities than any generation of kids has ever had before, and they're given more choice, excitement and stimulation in every area of their lives. But the flipside of this is more pressure: pressure to work increasingly long schooldays; pressure to take up all those after-school extras; pressure to consume, look, dress and behave like small adults before their time. This means that on top of the traditional childhood challenges (handling rapid physical growth, emotional development and 'ordinary' childhood problems and illnesses) they're also experiencing increasing psychological stress, which is now nearly as much of an issue for child – and teenage – health as it has long been for adults.

And it's now our job as the grown-ups who love and care for them to offer our children different types of support at different times, helping them handle the challenges they'll face – whether it's dyslexia, anxiety, bullying, lack of confidence, school stress or more 'traditional' health problems, ranging from constipation and chickenpox to glue ear and verrucas.

This section of the book offers as many strategies and suggestions for childhood issues and health problems we can possibly squeeze in, from Buteyko breathing for reducing asthma and broad-spectrum light treatment for ADHD to colour therapy for bringing down fevers; from the quick and easy healing technique for soothing pain to the nutritional supplement that can banish night terrors.

Parents often say they somehow tend to find exactly the right thing to help their children as the need arises, even with hard-to-treat issues that puzzle conventional clinicians. So perhaps a little of this chapter's information may find its way to the right place, at the right time and be of the best possible help to children and parents alike.

After Antibiotics

231. 'Friendly' Bacteria

If your child's had antibiotics, especially if it was for longer than a week or repeated courses, it's an excellent idea to replenish the 'friendly' bacteria in their gut, which the medication can wipe out, predisposing them to food sensitivities, candida overgrowth and irritable bowel syndrome (IBS).

Instead of boring capsules, a far more child-friendly version is a smoothie bio-shake mix in the form of a powdered product called **Strawberry Acidophilus**. This contains both the *Lactobacillus acidophilus* and another beneficial strain called *Bifidobacterium bifidum*, plus freeze-dried strawberry. It's suitable for children *over the age of two*, you can add it to milk, soya milk, rice milk or water; the dosage is half a teaspoon a day for one to two months, and it actually tastes nice. Strawberry Acidophilus Plus is available from BioCare (60 g, £13.75), as is Banana Acidophilus Plus (60 g, £12.90).

Note: if the child is *under two years old*, they'll need a different sort of 'friendly' bacteria supplement. It's called *Bifidobacterium infantis* and is also available from BioCare (60 g, £24.60). It contains the same bacteria as in breast milk, excellent for infant digestion and general paediatric gut health in under-twos.

For contact details, see under 'Shopping' in the Directory.

Anxiety

If a child seems to feel constantly anxious and all other things are equal (e.g. there are no disruptions or divorce at home and no bullying at school), try a gentle two-pronged approach using nutrition and essences.

232. Nutrition
Cut caffeine

While young children may not be coffee-drinkers like their parents, they can get a surprising amount throughout the day from fizzy drinks like colas and from chocolate. This matters, as there is some evidence suggesting small doses of caffeine taken throughout the day can have as much effect on anxiety levels as a single big dose.[1] Other research found even a little bit of caffeine can turn up the volume on someone's response level to 'ordinary stressful events'.[2] So children who tend to be more anxious than most may feel better without any caffeine at all.

Keep blood sugar steady

Low levels of sugar in the blood (hypoglycaemia) can make someone feel edgy and anxious, even downright panicky, as it causes adrenaline to be released in the body. Ensure your child's levels stay fairly steady during the day by avoiding sweet or sugary snacks that will produce a fast blood-sugar high and then cause it to plummet. Bananas, nuts, wholemeal sandwiches and health bars low in refined sugars (see 'Snack attack' on page 514 for which ones taste nicest as some are very disappointing) are all good 'steady-sugar-release' options.

233. Essences

Thini-A (often called 'Thini-Ahh' because of its intensely relaxing effect) is a lovely, peaceful essence from the Brazilian rainforests for someone of any age who finds they feel 'insecure about everything, experience constant fear, anxiety and tension for little reason, is hypersensitive and may have difficulty relaxing'.

It is especially good at evening bathtime. Try three to five drops in the water, depending on the child's age – they may find they are so mellow, they can hardly get out of the water, then sleep like a dormouse all night. It's great for parents who need to relax too.

Thini-A is from Araretama (meaning 'place from which light arises') Rainforest Essences. It is available direct from them or via Healthlines (15 ml, approximately £8).

For worries and fears a child cannot seem to express, consider also **Betony** (*Stachys officinalis*), the plant essence used for helping those with 'unrecognisable, unidentifiable or unconscious fears', from the gentle, yet very down-to-earth Bailey Flower Essences (10 ml, £5.15), which are made in Yorkshire by Dr Arthur Bailey, formerly senior lecturer in electronics and engineering at the University of Bradford.

For all contact details, see under 'Shopping' in the Directory.

See also General: Anxiety on page 11.

---

234. Anti-Itch Summer Spray – Make Your Own

Prickly heat – thought to be caused by blocked sweat glands that become irritated or inflamed – is very common, especially in babies and small children. Research suggests **vitamin-C spray** can reduce the rash and itching. In fact, vitamin C is a histamine-buster in its own right; histamine is the itching chemical released by your body's cells in response to allergy or irritation.

1. Mix two tablespoons of vitamin-C powder with 125 ml aloe vera gel (very soothing).
2. Store in a spray bottle – a small, clean plant-spray one will do fine – and keep in the fridge.
3. Spritz over the rash three times daily.

Vitamin-C powder and aloe vera gel are available from health shops or good chemists. Try Power Health Vitamin C Powder from Goodness Direct (50 g, £3.37) and the Ultimate Aloe Vera Skin Gel from Higher Nature (60 ml, £9.20). For contact details, see under 'Shopping' in the Directory. See also Fix 221: Prickly Heat about topical use of Crab Apple essence.

Asthma

Asthma is a long-term (chronic) breathing disorder in which the airways or breathing tubes have become overly sensitive and narrow temporarily – sometimes very quickly – when the person breathes in substances that upset them. This can be extremely distressing and even life-threatening. As one child put it, 'Not being able to breathe is the most frightening thing in the world.'

Figures and Triggers

Asthma is far more common than most of us think. Britain has one of the highest asthma rates in the world; research shows that in 2001 asthma affected one in 13 adults, one in ten teenagers and one in eight children.[3] That's 5.1 million sufferers, and in 1999 it was 3.4 million, so the problem is rising rapidly. One in four Americans now has asthma or an allergy. In the UK, one in five young children has had asthma-type wheezing attacks by the time they are two; two-thirds will grow out of this by around the age of five, but the remainder go on to develop significant asthma.

This is a condition that doesn't have one single cause but many predisposing and contributing factors, depending on specific triggers. The most common are house dustmites' droppings, house dust, moulds, pet dander, feathers and some foods and drinks – often the ones that also trigger eczema flare-ups (e.g. eggs, milk, certain food additives, and wheat products).

Medical and Complementary Treatments

Fortunately, there is a huge amount that can help a child with asthma. Steroids (both breathed in via inhalers and in tablet form) form the basis of conventional treatment for asthma. Lifestyle adjustments, such as cutting down the amount of salt you eat, can also make a real difference – eating salty food can make an asthmatic's airways constrict, so it is a good idea to avoid adding salt to food when cooking it and not put extra salt on the table. See also Fix 20: Nutritional Anti-Asthma Strategies.

The National Asthma Campaign in the UK can provide lots of information about other treatments; in the US, try the Asthma and Allergy Foundation hotline. For contact details, see under 'Useful Helplines, Websites and Contacts' in the Directory.

Allergy Matters is one of the best places in the UK for useful asthma-combatting 'stuff' like air ionisers (from £25) special vacuum-cleaners (from £300) and anti-dustmite mattress covers (singles from £40). In the US and Canada, contact the Allergy Shop. For contact details, see under 'Shopping' in the Directory.

235. Buteyko Breathing

With something like asthma, there is rarely such a thing as a single fix. However, devotees of the **Buteyko-breathing training method**, which was originally developed in Russia and is now used by over a million people in the former Soviet Union and hundreds of thousands of other people worldwide, reckon it might come close.

Using this breathing method correctly seems to enable asthma to be successfully managed with far lower doses of asthma medicating drugs – and sometimes none at all. For more information about research, see Notes on page 548.

Buteyko breathing is simple, straightforward and has been taught to children as young as three, though usually five is the lower age limit. Basically, it helps avoid the hyperventilation that accompanies, and exacerbates, asthma. The child is taught to:

1. Breathe out fully.
2. Then, try to breathe out just that little bit more until they feel like their tummy may be about to touch their spine.
3. Stay in this 'big-breathe-out' state for as long as is comfortable.
4. Begin to allow air gently back in without gulping.
5. Breathe normally for a little while.
6. When they are ready, begin the technique again by breathing out fully.

To find out more about Buteyko and to locate a class near you, visit the Buteyko Institute of Breathing and Health (BIBH) website, www.buteyko.info.co.uk. For more contact details, see under 'Training Courses' in the Directory.

LifeSource also offers a good self-help package on CD-Rom for children and adults, called *The Breathology Programme* (£29.95). For contact details, see under 'Shopping' in the Directory.

236. Salt Therapy

Inhaling damp, salty air can reduce asthma because it clears and deconstricts the breathing passages. Rock-salt steam inhalation is known as **halotherapy** or **spelotherapy**. And while it has been used for centuries in Russia and Eastern Europe – there are famous curative mines at Wieliczka in Poland and at Praid in Romania, where it has been much researched because salt is so inexpensive compared with drug treatment for asthma – it is not yet well known in the UK or US.

In Russia and Transylvania, halotherapy generally still involves taking patients to the salt-mine chambers for treatment, but now there is a small hand-held device that allows you to have salt steam at home using a porcelain pipe filled with salt crystals. Sucking on the pipe means the moisture of the passing air absorbs tiny particles of salt, which are inhaled down into the lungs, where they cleanse, heal, soothe and help fight infection – the steam is then gently breathed out through the nose to ensure all passages associated with breathing are treated.

How effective is it?

Research suggests regular halotherapy brings an 85 per cent improvement for mild to moderate asthma, and a 75 per cent improvement even for severe asthma, with far fewer episodes of breathing difficulty during the day (74 per cent of patients, compared with 11.5 per cent of those unknowingly using a placebo pipe), less night coughing, and easier expectoration of mucus.

Suck it and see

A standard DIY treatment with a salt pipe lasts approximately 15 minutes and is done two to three times a day, so perhaps an active child could use it in the mornings before going off to school while sitting down to watch a bit of TV, then again just resting peacefully on their bed listening to a story tape when they come back from school and, if they are particularly wheezy that day, have another salt-pipe session in a warm bath with some music on before bed.

In the UK, the BreathEasy salt pipe is available from Tower Health (£29.95). For younger children, there is a model shaped like an elephant – you suck on the trunk – from Cisca (£29.99). In the US, contact Natural Salt Lamps for both children's and adults' pipes (both $89.95).

For contact details, see under 'Shopping' in the Directory.

Note: salt pipes can also be used to alleviate hay fever, bronchitis, croup, whooping cough, colds, snoring and bronchitis.

See also Fix 267: Hay Fever.

Attention Deficit Hyperactivity Disorder (ADHD) and Hyperactivity

Children with ADHD have a short attention span – 90 per cent will underachieve at school because they cannot concentrate on one task for long enough to finish their work or do it properly, and they are often in trouble for disruptive behaviour.

Other characteristics include hyperactivity, being easily distracted, a tendency to distract and interrupt others (which can lead to problems at school, as children with ADHD are often labelled badly behaved), not listening, fidgeting, mood swings, impulsiveness (which often shows itself as not waiting for other people to finish talking), difficulty taking turns and a 'see it, do it', headlong approach to life that often gets them into trouble. Many ADHD children also have disturbed sleep, difficulties with bed-wetting and may find they are frequently thirsty.

Hyperactivity itself is perhaps the main symptom of ADHD and is seldom seen in chronic form on its own. So if your child is hyperactive, they may well have ADHD.

- Worldwide, it is estimated that 1–5 per cent of all children have ADHD.
- In the UK, where the condition's definition is strict, it's thought 1 per cent of children are affected, but in the US, where definitions are far broader, it is estimated to be nearer 10 per cent.
- ADHD is five times more common in boys than girls.

What's in a name?

'New' variants of ADHD are now entering the public consciousness. The terms that come up include oppositional defiant disorder (ODD), conduct disorder (CD) and antisocial personality disorder of childhood (APDC). But are these new disorders, or just new subdefinitions? Genuine, useful clinical distinctions, or spurious new labels invented by drug companies wishing to sell more niche medicines in a profitable, and apparently expanding, market? Perhaps that is up to those parents who hear their children being classified with these new terms.

Help and further information

In the UK, try the Hyperactive Children's Support Group; in the US, try Adders, which is a network of support organisations for parents. For contact details, see under 'Useful Helplines, Websites and Contacts' in the Directory.

Medical Treatments

The medical approach to controlling ADHD involves the use of amphetamine-type drugs; the active ingredient of these, the stimulant methylphenidate (MPH), can paradoxically help an overactive, easily distracted child to focus. These are currently being prescribed for children as young as two.[4] Ritalin is the best known, but there is also Dexedrine, Adderall, Concerta, Cylert, Focalin, Strattera and even a Ritalin patch.

Parents in the US are coming under increasing pressure to use them, and some American schools now insist that all 'disruptive' pupils are given ADHD drugs or they will not be allowed to come in for classes. In many cases when parents have refused, schools have taken them to court – and won.

Medication problems

However, these drugs do not suit around 30 per cent of ADHD children, and in these cases the children become nervous, have even more trouble sleeping than before, experience loss of appetite, dizziness, heart palpitations, headaches, digestive problems, weight loss, itching and skin rashes.[5]

More serious but less common potential side effects include seizures,[6] psychosis (one Canadian neurologist found around 6 per cent of children treated with these drugs became psychotic, developing delusions and paranoia),[7] obsessive-compulsive disorder, which French researchers discovered can develop in as little as ten months,[8] retarded growth,[9] liver toxicity and liver cancer.

Unsurprisingly, though Ritalin is one of the most frequently prescribed children's drugs in the US, it has also attracted more lawsuits than any other medicine – and parents are beginning to look for gentler, drug-free interventions to help their children.

Complementary Treatments

There is a wide range of holistic measures that claim considerable success in moderating ADHD without the use of drugs. The options range from behavioural approaches and supplementation with specific nutrients like zinc, magnesium and essential fatty acids (such as fish oils) to ensuring the child has a really good, healthy, junk-free diet – all non-invasive interventions that are supported by some good-quality clinical research. However, parents usually report that it's not just one single thing in isolation that helps their child, but a considered package of several (together with proper support from their son or daughter's school), which they work out, by trial and error. Try the fixes recommended below.

237. Behavioural Approaches
Providing calm, clarity and a peaceful routine has been found to help. For young and pre-school children:

- Use quiet time and withdrawal to deal with temper tantrums.
- Keep to a steady routine.
- Stay calm yourself and keep the environment peaceful and low-key wherever possible.
- Have very clear rules.
- Explain the programme for the day fully: ADHD children can find the world a very confusing place, so it can help them greatly if you offer clear, accessible information about what is going to happen *each day* (e.g. by using wallcharts) and by avoiding deviating from this without plenty of warning.

- Give lots of notice when something is about to change (e.g. timers and buzzers to give a five-minute warning that it's getting-up time soon, that it's the end of TV time shortly, etc.).
- Praise ADHD children often and within their earshot, as their self-esteem can be low due to frustration and underachievement.
- Play with them as much as you can.

238. A Junk-Free Diet

ADHD children should have a diet that is as additive-free and healthy as possible – low in processed, sugary or instant foods and drinks, high in fresh, unprocessed ones with as much good-quality organic stuff as you can afford.

Studies led by US criminologist Dr Stephen Schoenthaler have repeatedly shown that violent and antisocial behaviour are often linked to poor diet and that supplementing with the right nutrients and improving what the individual eats also improves behaviour. UK research had similar results when working with young male prisoners. For more information, see Fix 297: Nutritional Approach.

And how about the trial with toddlers and drinks high in additives? In 2002 the UK Food Standards Agency carried out a strict double-blind study with a large group of three-year-olds, giving them drinks laced with a cocktail of additives, including tartrazine, sunset yellow and sodium benzoate. Parents noted their children's behaviour worsened almost immediately if they'd had an additive drink but not if they had a placebo one with no additives in it. And these weren't ADHD children, just a group of ordinary pre-schoolers.

Also, when 76 hyperactive children were put on a strict additive-free diet by Great Ormond Street Children's Hospital in London, 80 per cent showed significant improvements – but reintroducing those additives brought the behavioural problems straight back.[10]

239. Helpful Nutrients and Supplements

Interestingly, nutrients and supplements for ADHD include many of the standard ones for mediating other nervous-system-related and emotional disorders (including PMS, depression, anorexia and bulimia).

- **Essential fatty acids (EFAs)** –One Durham-based study of 60 young children aged from 20 months to three years, carried out in 2005 as part of the Child Progress Research Project by Durham Council and three Sure Start children's centres, found EFA capsules had a major positive effect. Not only on behaviour (at the beginning of the study 40 per cent of children's behaviour was rated 'poor' by both parents and teachers, by the end that was down to 4 per cent) but also on learning difficulties, and on hyperactivity levels. Several other centres of research, including Indiana's Purdue University, have also found that a high proportion of hyperactive and ADHD children have all the classic symptoms of EFA shortage (e.g. very thirsty, dry skin and hair, brittle or soft nails) so there seems to be a definite link there.[11] See also 'About EFAs' on page 314.
- **Vitamin B6** – in one small study, vitamin B6 reduced hyperactivity more effectively than Ritalin.[12]
- **Magnesium** – shortage can result in fidgeting, restlessness and contribute to learning difficulties. Polish doctors achieved some dramatic improvements on children's behaviour when they gave them magnesium supplements.[13]

240. Lighting

Using full-spectrum lighting (calming, non-irritant to the nervous system and considered by many natural therapists to be a positive 'nutrient' in its own right) in classrooms rather than the usual fluorescent tubing produces a drop in irritability, headaches, disruptive behaviour, hyperactivity and an increase in concentration, as several American and Canadian schools have found.[14] If the school won't consider this, install them at home, especially in rooms the child spends most time in – e.g. the sitting room, kitchen and their bedroom – so they get a dose of full-spectrum light for at least a few hours a day. This type of lighting is good for the whole family's mood and stress levels too.

For more information and for suggestions on where to buy full-spectrum lights, see Fix 298: Light Therapy.

241. Colour and Décor

A little bit of interior decoration can go a long way. Research published in the prestigious *Journal of the American Academy of Child and*

Adolescent Psychiatry in 1994 found painting classroom walls *soft* pink, decorating the blank white corridors with cheerful murals and putting cheap carpeting on hard floors halved the number of aggressive incidents and outbursts in a school that had had more than its fair share of disruptive children.[15]

See also Fix 437: Clever Colours.

Bed-Wetting (Enuresis)

Almost all children grow out of bed-wetting over time, as the muscles at the neck of their bladder become stronger, their bladder capacity increases, and they begin to sleep a bit less heavily so grow more sensitive to the 'Hey, I'm full' messages the bladder sends to the brain.

Yet bed-wetting is still far more common than most people realise. According to the American Academy of Pediatrics, 20 per cent of five-year-olds wet the bed, 10 per cent of six-year-olds, and 3 per cent of all 12- to 14-year-olds. Children who regularly wet the bed after the age of five are usually offered drug treatment or behavioural retraining therapy.

Help and further information
In the UK, contact Education and Resources for Improving Childhood Continence (ERIC), a very useful and friendly information organisation set up for parents of children of any age who have a continence problem (either wetting or soiling) – including teenagers. In the US, try the National Enuresis Society. For contact details, see under 'Useful Helplines, Websites and Contacts' in the Directory.

Alarms
Alarms: there are many different ones available, but check out the Malem Moisture Alarm, which has a five-star rating from parents themselves. This one does the lot – vibrates, beeps *and* lights up at the first sign of any moisture, waking the child so they have the opportunity to stop the flow. You can buy it in the US via Parentsmart ($89), and it is claimed to take 4–12 weeks to help retrain 'most' children's bladders successfully.

Recommended reading: in the UK, *Seven Steps to Night-Time Dryness* by Renée Mercer (can be ordered from any bookshop though it may take a couple of weeks to deliver) or by mail order more quickly from ERIC itself. Their website is well worth a look as it can give good impartial advice on alarms, books and many other products, and suggests some of the most effective.

In the US, two good books: *Dry All Night* by Allison Mack (see below) and *Getting to Dry: How to Help Your Child Overcome Bedwetting* by Max Maizels, Diane Rosenbaum and Barbara Keating.

Complementary Treatments

According to the Department of Psychological Medicine at the Women's and Children's Hospital in North Adelaide, using simple self-hypnosis and visualisation can work very well indeed for children as young as five.

242. Visualise the Positive
One particular study with a group of 50 children aged 6–16, comparing one of the standard enuresis medications (imipramine) with a special children's programme, *Dry All Night* (a book for parents and children), which uses multi-sensory imagery and storytelling, showed that after nine months nearly seven out of ten were still dry compared with only a quarter of the children on medication.

243. Hypnotherapy
If you would like to try something different but still gentle, according to the University of Michigan, the average time **hypnotherapy** takes to help a child overcome bed-wetting is four to six sessions.[16]

When seeking hypnotherapy treatment for their child, many parents feel reassured if the hypnotherapist is also a medical professional, since while there are several good lay training organisations for hypnotherapists, there are also not-so-good ones. If you'd prefer a medically trained therapist, contact the British Society for Medical and Dental Hypnosis; in the US, contact the American Psychotherapy and Medical Hypnosis Association. For contact details, see under 'Therapies and Therapists' in the Directory.

Is your child constipated? That can be a factor too as the impacted waste matter building up in the bowel may put extra pressure on the bladder. If so, it could simply be a case of offering plenty of plain liquids, fresh fruit and vegetables. You can also add linseed to their food – see Fix 37: Constipation.

See also Young Children: Attention Deficit Hyperactivity Disorder (ADHD) on page 248 and Young Children: Urinary-Tract Infections (UTIs) on page 306.

Breath-Holding

Breath-holding attacks, during which a child can go red, even blue in the face and, in particularly severe circumstances, sometimes actually faint (after which an instinctive reflex almost always starts the breathing off again), can put the fear of God into parents. These episodes seem to be most common in toddlers aged one to two and a half, and often happen when a child is really furious, frustrated or upset. However, though it's often suggested that such incidents are generally 'tantrums' or 'attention-seeking', there is some evidence that iron deficiency may also be a cause.

244. Is It Iron?
In one particular trial in which children who regularly had breath-holding attacks were given **iron** supplements, nearly nine out of ten either had no further attacks or only experienced half their former number.[17]

However, because too much iron can be a health hazard in itself, it is vital your child's iron level is checked before supplementing them with it. This can be done by a blood test at your doctor's. If it turns out to be a bit low, try iron supplementation. However, it is a good idea to see a well-qualified nutritionist to get advice on how much and which *form* of iron would benefit your child. Most conventional doctors have minimal training in nutrition and are not therefore generally the best people to ask, and not all iron supplements are the same. For instance, the most common one – iron sulphate, or ferrous sulphate – isn't actually very well absorbed and can produce constipation and nausea.

Try the British Dietetic Association's practitioner website: their members have three years' training and are approved by the NHS. Also try those who've trained with the Institute of Optimum Nutrition, which again has a three-year course. For contact details, see under 'Therapies and Therapists' in the Directory.

245. Soothing the Shock

A breath-holding attack can be really upsetting for a small child. If yours is shocked or distressed afterwards, offer them a few drops of **Bach Rescue Remedy** or **Emergency Essence**, either as drops under the tongue or drunk in a little water. If they don't want to do this, gently wipe it across the inside of their wrists as there are several blood vessels fairly close to the surface there and some of the liquid remedy can be absorbed that way. Since it's no picnic for parents to stay calm as their child stops breathing (whether deliberately or not), you may want to have some yourself.

You can buy Bach Rescue Remedy from Healthlines (10 ml, £3.99). Emergency Essence is available from Australian Bush Flower Essences, Neal's Yard and Healthlines (30 ml, £7.95). For contact details, see under 'Shopping' in the Directory.

Chickenpox

246. Soothe and Calm – Drip, Dip, Dab

To help calm the often miserable itchiness of chickenpox, drip three drops of **Bach Rescue Remedy** into a palmful of soothing **calamine**, dip in the cotton wool and dab topically on the spots – they enhance each other's anti-itch action and double the soothing power. It is available via Healthlines (10 ml, £3.99) or from most chemists, pharmacies and health shops in the UK.

Another terrific one to use, especially if the child is agitated, restless or in a foul mood because of chickenpox, is the Australian Bush Flower range's **Angelsword**, available direct or from Healthlines in the UK (15 ml, £8.95). Try two drops in the calamine lotion.

For all contact details, see under 'Shopping' in the Directory.

247. The 'Yuck' Factor

If the *look* of so many spots and scabs is distressing them, add two to seven drops of Bach Flower Essences' **Crab Apple** from Healthlines (10 ml, £3.99) to help reduce the 'yuck' factor that can affect some children with chickenpox and other spotty disorders quite strongly.

If they are being especially needy or demanding, give Bach's **Chicory** four times daily in a little water to help them settle. It is available from many chemists and via Healthlines and Healing Herbs (10 ml, £3.20).

For all contact details, see under 'Shopping' in the Directory.

Colds and Flu

248. Immunity

Adults usually tend to get between two and five colds a year; but school-children may catch an average of eight or more, with their immune system getting more tired after each successive bout, until some parents report, 'We just get rid of one, then they go straight back down with another.'

Cold coming on? Nix the sugar immediately – including sweet foods and sweetened drinks. They can halve someone's immunity within two hours.[18]

Some children are also more susceptible than others, possibly partly because their immunity is compromised over time by a not-as-healthy-as-it-might-be diet or too many antibiotics. (One report in 1998 in the *Journal of the American Medical Association* showed nearly half all youngsters going to the GP with an ordinary cold leave with an antibiotic prescription.) Or perhaps they have never really got back on top of things after a particular run of colds or a bad virus.

What helps?

Both **elderberry extract** and **echinacea** are good bets, especially if the latter is combined with a time-release vitamin-C supplement and, if possible, **bee propolis**.

In one particular study in 2004, echinacea extract was found to cut the number of children's colds over three months by half compared with dummy medication.[19] And lab studies carried out at the Hebrew University Hadassah Medical School in Jerusalem in 2005 found that elderberry extract, which contains a hefty antiviral compound called antivirin and bioflavonoids, kills several types of flu – human, swine and, at least in test tubes, even bird flu.

Use the above throughout the winter cold months, or at the *very first* sign of a cold or influenza.

In the UK, for elderberry extract, try Sambucol for Kids, made by Razei Bar Industries and available in the UK from Brunel Healthcare (120 ml, £8.25) or Nature's Way in the US: also available from many indpendent health shops, and health shop chains. Also Echinacea Junior, which are chewable orange-flavoured tablets, from Bioforce (60 tablets, £4.99), and Bee Health's Propolis Liquid (30 ml, £4.45); in the US, see GloryBee's Propolis Extract (10 fl oz, $6.05). For contact details, see under 'Shopping' in the Directory.

249. Colds – Breaking Them
For a 40 kg child, 250–500 mg soluble **vitamin C** every two hours dissolved in water or fruit juice may just head off a cold altogether – and can certainly reduce the number of days it lasts by about a third,[20] suggests UK GP and nutrition expert Dr John Briffa. Be aware that this can also produce looser bowel movements, but this ceases when the treatment stops. Try Redoxan tablets, available from most chemists and pharmacies.

250. Blocked Nose
If it's thick with mucus due to a cold, hay fever or asthma, especially if this is habitually the case, encourage your child to drink as much **water** as they can, perhaps with a little fruit juice in it to make it more interesting (but not milky drinks, as milk encourages mucus production). According to one of the US's top paediatricians Professor William Sears, of the University of South Carolina Medical School, this makes it far easier for a baby or young child to cough up phlegm from their airways.

It's also worth checking for food sensitivities. To find a nutritionist, see under 'Therapies and Therapists' in the Directory.

See also General: Colds and Flu on page 36.

Colic

251. Herbal Help

Generally speaking, hospital consultants are not big fans of herbal medicine, but when it comes to colic, the evidence (both anecdotal from parents and from clinical trials) tells a different story. Dr Dipak Kanabar, consultant paediatrician at Guy's Hospital in London, says offering the colicky baby a little stomach-settling **herbal tea** brings 'significant benefits'.[21]

This is good news for the 10–20 per cent of new babies between one and four months old who have colic – with its tummy pain, wind and exhausting, inconsolable crying, which lasts an average of four and a half hours a day, according to research by the Thomas Coram Institute of Child Health.

British master herbalist Anne McIntyre, a mother of three, says the most effective anti-colic herbal teas are chamomile, dill and fennel. She suggests giving a colicky baby just 30 ml of the herb tea 20–30 minutes before a feed to relax their digestive tract and ease digestion. After the feed, if the baby is still uncomfortable, offer a little more.

Mothers who use this tend to make, say, 500 ml each morning and keep it covered and cool, taking some when they need it. (If it's been in the fridge, warm it slightly before giving it to your baby.) Use half a teaspoon of the fresh herb for every 100 ml freshly boiled water. Cover and let it infuse for ten minutes, then strain and allow it to cool before using.

For very young babies especially, it is best to use organic herbs if you can find them. Try Star Child for dill, fennel seeds and chamomile flowers (100 g, £2.50–£3.23). For contact details, see under 'Shopping' in the Directory.

Commercially prepared herbal baby drinks are also available, but they can contain substantial amounts of sugar.

252. Lactase Drops

Lactase is the enzyme that breaks down the lactose component of dairy foods in the stomach. Some babies are either *lactose intolerant* (i.e. it disagrees with them – *not* the same as a full-blown food allergy) or *lactase deficient* (i.e. they cannot produce enough of the breaking-down enzyme themselves to be able to digest dairy foods). Both conditions can cause colic, and, given that young babies are on an all-milk diet, both are very unfortunate things to have.

If you suspect this may be the problem, the enzyme lactase is available in drop form as a product called **Colief**. You use it by putting some in your baby's milk – whether expressed breast milk or formula – before it is given to them to drink.

It is available direct from Colief (7 ml, £9.99) and from selected major chemists. A 7 ml bottle lasts about a month. For contact details, see under 'Shopping' in the Directory.

253. Natural Healers
Chiropractic
Gentle **chiropractic** treatment may well help too: a Danish study in 1999 showed how useful it could be, but its critics complained the results did not come from a strict placebo-controlled trial (in which a comparative group would be offered 'dummy' treatment). If you'd like to try this option, it's important to find a chiropractor who has a special interest in very young babies and is used to treating them.

In the UK, contact the British Chiropractic Association; in the US, the American Chiropractic Association. For contact details, see 'Therapies and Therapists' in the Directory.

Cranial osteopathy
In a study of 1,250 colicky babies, Dr Viola Fryman, founder of the Osteopathic Center for Children in San Diego, discovered that 80 per cent of them had experienced some form of mechanical trauma during birth and had misalignment around the occiput area (back and base of the skull).

Interestingly, it's the occiput that takes the brunt of labour pushing, and there is a delicate network of nerves sited there that links directly with the gut. If this is disturbed by any displacement of the skull on the neck, osteopaths say this can cause, among other things, colic.

To find a specialist cranial osteopath in the UK, contact the Sutherland Society or try the General Osteopathic Council and ask for local osteopaths who also work cranially and have a special interest in babies. In the US and Canada, again contact the Sutherland Society (it has members worldwide, including throughout Europe) or, for the nearest doctor of osteopathy (DO), contact Osteohome. DOs are fully trained physicians but have an additional 300–500 hours of training in osteopathy; cranial osteopaths have up to a further five years' specialised training on top of that. For contact details, see 'Therapies and Therapists' in the Directory.

Confidence

254. Essences

There are many different essences that can support the development of confidence and self-esteem in younger children. One of the very nicest and most subtle is **Bluebell**. It is helpful for gentle children who may be:

• afraid of being ridiculed
• rather anxious about being noticed *at all*
• shy
• worried that others will judge them
• fear punishment when they've done nothing wrong (e.g. that their teacher will be cross with them).

Bluebell can also gently help children feel good about being just who they are. It is made by Pacific Essences and is available in the UK from Healthlines and IFER (7.5 ml, approximately £6.50); in the US and Canada, buy it direct from Pacific Essences (7.5 ml, CA$11).

If your child likes or connects well with animals, an essence made from animal energies (but without touching a hair on the animal's head) may really suit them. If you think they could do with something more robust than Bluebell, consider **Lion Cub** (for 'fearlessness, confidence, courage, being fully capable and competent') or the delightful **Wolf Pup** (for 'a feeling of belonging, fitting in and knowing that you matter') from Wild Earth Animal Essences' new children's range 'Wild Child', by American ex-wilderness guide, now counsellor and healer, Daniel Mapel. In the UK, Wild Earth Animal Essences are available via

Healthlines (diluted dosage bottle, 30 ml, £7; stock bottle, 30 ml, £8.55); in the US, you can buy them direct from the manufacturer.

For all contact details, see under 'Shopping' in the Directory.

Constipation

Golden Tip

Apart from the usual (i.e. drinking plenty of fluid or very dilute juice, eating fibre-rich foods like vegetables and fruit as much as possible, cutting back on the junk food, and taking regular exercise – from rough n' tumbles on the floor with siblings and parents to playing in the playground, swimming, walking, dancing about, any sports they like . . .) try also:

. . . linseeds. You can buy these tiny, round, golden seeds, e.g. the **Linusit Gold brand,** from any local health shop, including the big Holland & Barrett chain (250 g, £3.95). Tip: the brown variety of linseeds is just as effective as the gold but less expensive.

Soak them in water overnight; drain and mix between a teaspoon and a dessertspoon, depending on your child's size, into their cereal or fruit or vegetable purée the next day. Soaked seeds will keep for 2–3 days in the fridge.

Do this each morning until the constipation eases, as the seeds act like ball bearings on the faeces, easing their transit through, and out of, the digestive tract.

If there is no improvement after two to three days, or if your child's tummy is distended and they are clearly uncomfortable, go to see your GP right away. They can often offer medical treatment, perhaps in the form of a motion-softening suppository or medication that will ease things pretty promptly.

Note: also offer plenty of extra dilute drinks (not milk).

See also General: Indigestion on page 61 and Young Children: Colic on page 259.

Cuts and Grazes

255. Painful Cuts

If a cut is clean, doesn't need stitches and is not infected but still very sore, soothe with the versatile homeopathic **hypericum cream**. Try the St John's wort cream (*Hypericum perforatum*), also known as woundwort, with lavender and chamomile extract from Amphora (60 ml, £3.36).

Or, since **calendula** is also one of the top homeopathic remedies for healing cuts and grazes, bathe the area in a warm solution of one cup (240 ml) pre-boiled cooled water and a teaspoon of calendula tincture. You can buy this in the UK from Baldwin's (50 ml, £2.45); in the US, try Terra Firma Botanicals (1 fl oz, $9).

For a quicker, fuss-free fix, try both calendula and hypericum combined in Nelsons' **Hypercal Cream**, available via the Garden Pharmacy (27 g, £3.95); in the US, it's called **Natural Healing Cream** and is available through Herbal Remedies (1 oz, $5.30).

For all contact details, see under 'Shopping' in the Directory.

256. Grazes

SOS Rescue soothes grazes and cuts (and insect bites), and is gentle enough to use on babies. This is a must for every bathroom cabinet and can be bought from Barefoot Botanicals (75 ml, £9.95).

If, however, a graze is starting to get infected but is also very sore and stingy (meaning even gentle Savlon, and definitely any moderate-strength antiseptic cream like Germolene, would be uncomfortable to put on), use a dribble of runny **manuka honey** with an optional loose gauze dressing that doesn't touch the area.

All honey is anti-infective, but manuka, besides having a great caramel tang and not tasting overly sweet, also has a very high antibacterial action. So high that it has been extensively investigated by New Zealand's University of Waikato Honey Research Unit and is now recommended for clinical use even for serious problems like wounds and bed sores.

All honey contains hydrogen peroxide, which stimulates the growth of new tissues to replace damaged old ones, but again manuka seems to have a higher level than most, and its levels of acidity and sugars are also important factors in the healing process.

Ensure you buy it with a medicinal factor of ten and above from good health shops (100 ml, from £7.50) or via Manuka Honey. For contact details, see under 'Shopping' in the Directory.

For more about the benefits of manuka honey, see also Fix 105: Bee Better and Fix 62: Wound, Ulcer and Sore Healing.

Dyslexia

What Is It?

The term 'dyslexia' comes from the Greek meaning 'difficulty with words'. It is the most common learning disorder among schoolchildren and affects the way the brain processes information. An estimated one in ten children is dyslexic to some degree, causing difficulties with writing, spelling, reading, maths, memory and concentration. There is a lot of variation in how it can affect a child, and it may do so only slightly, moderately or sometimes quite severely. Between 70 and 80 per cent of those with dyslexia are male.

Just to complicate matters, many dyslexics have elements of another learning disorder too, one also caused by information-processing difficulties in the brain, called dyspraxia – see Young Children: Dyspraxia on page 264 and Teenagers: Dyspraxia on page 340. Dyspraxia once upon a time was known rather unimaginatively as 'clumsy child syndrome', though it is far more complex and individualised than that. In addition, an estimated 30–40 per cent of people with dyslexia may also have a degree of attention deficit hyperactivity disorder – see Young Children: Attention Deficit Hyperactivity Disorder (ADHD) on page 248.

Dyslexia often makes life more difficult for the child or teenager at school, producing both frustration and increasingly low self-esteem. Dyslexic children have trouble using and understanding information in the way in which it is normally presented and so they may, very unfairly, be labelled 'careless' and 'lazy' or told, 'You could do better if you just tried harder,' when they *are* doing their best. They may also be referred to by other people who know no better as 'not very bright', even though on average their IQ is just as high – sometimes higher – than that of their friends and classmates. In fact, many dyslexic people are extremely creative, artistic or have special practical skills and abilities. See 'The famous and fabulous' on page 340 for a roll call of talented examples.

Bright stars

Most children and adults with dyslexia will, thanks to the less usual way their minds are wired, excel at the things controlled by the right-hand (imaginative and creative) hemisphere of their brains, including art, photography, architecture, athletics, music, mechanical and engineering skills, creative thought, storytelling, new inventions, new ways of looking at old problems, creative 'big-picture' thinking and intuition (psychology, understanding and empathising with other people). Many are also very good at sports and athletics.

Fortunately, however, dyslexia is now increasingly well recognised and understood in schools and so children are being diagnosed earlier and receiving far more support. (Back in the late 1970s a child would often be labelled 'slow', sat at the front of the class and that was all they got.) There is also a great deal that parents, schools and the children themselves can do to both improve dyslexia and 'manage it' so it is no longer the bar it once was to someone achieving their full potential.

What causes it?
The underlying causes of dyslexia are thought to include:

- 'cerebellar developmental delay' (CDD), whereby the cerebellum, whose job it is to coordinate all incoming sensory information, isn't quite working as it should
- shortage of essential fatty acids in the diet
- possible hereditary element: dyslexia can run in families
- the latest research also suggests that problems with the optic nerve (which transmits information to the brain about what the child sees) may be involved.

Symptoms and Suggestions

No two children with dyslexia are affected in quite the same way. However, there are some common symptoms.

Children up to pre-school age
  A very young child may:

- prefer bottom-shuffling to crawling and may miss out the crawling stage altogether
- have difficulty remembering 'labels' for familiar objects – e.g. names of colours
- begin talking later than expected, and when they do, their speech may be characterised by more stuttering and hesitancy than is usual
- mix up 'm' and 'n', and ' r' and 'l' sounds when talking
- confuse left and right
- use both hands equally (i.e. doesn't become right- or left-handed) until age seven or eight
- like, and be good at, puzzles and constructive toys such as Lego or Connex
- enjoy picture books but not the words that go with them. They may like being read *to* but be slow to try reading for themselves and struggle to master it.
- have an unusual pen- or crayon-grip
- confuse directional words – e.g. may say 'up' for 'down' or 'in' for 'out'
- have difficulty learning nursery rhymes.

One telltale sign of dyslexia is when a child habitually puts their head almost right down on to their desk in an effort to write better.

Children from 5–12 years

An older child may:

- have writing difficulties. Their writing may be slow, laboured and pretty illegible despite their best efforts. They may have an unusual, apparently ham-fisted pen-grip.
- have particular problems with learning to read. The confusion of 'b' and 'd' is a classic, as is reading a word fine on one page, then on the next not recognising it. Substituting similar words for the one they are reading, even if it doesn't fit with the meaning of the sentence, is also common – e.g. 'horse' becomes 'house'.
- continue to confuse left and right
- flub words frequently – e.g. 'bisgetti' instead of 'spaghetti' – something that is common for younger children but not by the time they are seven or eight
- have difficulty remembering 'non-meaningful' information, like the times table
- take longer over their work
- have trouble spelling. Learning lists for tests can be very hard for them and they may have difficulty copying words accurately from the blackboard or from a book. They may also repeatedly misspell words that are used very often, such as 'what', 'because' or 'does'.
- be disorganised at school and at home
- have low self-esteem.

Some things that may help

- **Writing difficulties** – use rubber grips from the Early Learning Centre and many stationers, or even wrap a piece of rough fabric Elastoplast round the pen or pencil where it's held. Specialist teaching support and writing on a laptop or ordinary computer both help. A multi-sensory approach to letter recognition and reading are used increasingly these days – e.g. sounding out the letter while also looking at it held up on a flashcard or board and, at same time, 'drawing' it with a fingertip in a sand tray.
- **Left and right confusion** – write 'L' and 'R' on the back of their hands if young, on their shoes so they know which is which and

also to the right and left of the front door so they are correctly orientated every time they leave the home.

- **Memory problems** – try printing 'non-meaningful' information like the times table on a small piece of paper and encourage your child to carry it around in a maths file or pencil case and use it for reference. Talking 'remember this' pointers into a little Dictaphone can help older children. Boys may like this especially, since it's a small, compact gadget.
- **Taking longer over work** – being taught study skills by the special-needs teacher (i.e. in a way that is relevant to their particular needs as opposed to ordinary subject-based help) can really produce results over time, as can working on a laptop rather than trying to write everything up by hand with much disheartening crossing-out and Tippexing. Try to ensure they do not get overloaded: keep pressure right off them as far as possible.
- **Spelling difficulties** – specialist teaching sessions can support some children. A spell-checker may help when actually writing a story, but not with those school vocabulary tests. Coloured glasses, contact lenses and see-through overlays for book pages can help some dyslexics read easily and accurately.[22] If it's going to work, the effect's immediate (research with 426 children from 12 schools found 50 per cent reported an improvement and easier reading). Contact the Irlen Institute for specialist test centres and supplies of coloured eyewear and overlays (from approximately £7 a sheet), glasses and lenses in the UK, Europe, US and Australia.
- **Disorganisation** – routines, lists, colour-coded charts and timetables, memory aids like colourful Post-It Notes on the front door of what to remember for that day plus ongoing practical support and praise at home and school all help. Resist the temptation to do everything for your child, particularly if they are of school age – aim to help them do it for themselves. As one special-needs teacher of 30 years' experience (she also has a dyspraxic son and dyslexic daughter) put it, 'At this age, do it *with them* – not for them!' For example, help them sort out their room on a regular basis, such as twice a week, so they get used to living in a fairly ordered environment, as opposed to either leaving it in a tip all the time or faithfully tidying it for them every single day.

- **Low self-esteem** – give lots of love, encouragement and support. Boost their confidence in every way you can: praise them for trying at every opportunity and for all the things they do even partially 'right', find out what they really enjoy (you might be surprised) and encourage that as much as possible, rather than trying to give them extra coaching to do everything their peers are doing.

For all suggestions on treatments and support for children with dyslexia, please see Treatments for Dyslexia and Dyspraxia, pp 275–9 (as many of the suggestions are relevant to both conditions). See also Teenagers: Dyslexia: on page 337.

Dyspraxia

What Is It?

Dyspraxia is a neurologically based disorder, the name coming from the Greek word 'praxis', which means 'movement and practice'. It is sometimes referred to as developmental coordination disorder (DCD) and was at one time nicknamed 'clumsy child syndrome' because clumsiness can be one of the main symptoms. An estimated 10–15 per cent of children and adults are affected by dyspraxia, 70 per cent of whom are male, making it one of the most common causes of mild to moderate learning difficulties.

Dyspraxia can also coexist with certain other neurologically based learning disorders (especially dyslexia – see Young Children: Dyslexia on page 264 and Teenagers: Dyslexia on page 337 – and *mild* cerebral palsy) and shows itself in a wide variety of ways. Both those factors can make diagnosis difficult; in fact, some children are not diagnosed until their early teens, and there are young adults who only find out they have it in their early to mid-twenties.

So far as recognition and understanding in schools go, matters are improving (especially in good state primaries and secondaries), but educational psychologists still complain that prompt diagnosis for dyspraxia and subsequent appropriate support provision are currently 'where dyslexia was 20 years ago'.

The good news is that there is plenty the child, professional and parents can do to help a dyspraxic child achieve their potential and make their dreams happen at least as well as their non-dyspraxic schoolmates. Dyspraxic children are just as bright and equally talented as most of their peers (if not, in many cases, with an even higher IQ – see 'The famous and fabulous' on page 340), but they do have to work harder in order to show it.

Symptoms and Suggestions

No two children with dyspraxia have identical symptoms, and there is wide variation in the degree of difficulty they may have. It ranges from children who just have slightly messy handwriting or can't kick a ball quite as straight as their sports teacher expects to those who can only write via a computer, are so uncoordinated that they constantly bump into things and have such difficulty with interpreting ordinary social signals that they find relating to other kids a frustrating mystery. However, the following are some of the most common symptoms.

Children up to pre-school age
A very young child may:

- be unusually irritable and unsettled from birth
- have feeding problems
- be slower than expected to reach developmental milestones – e.g. by eight months they may not be sitting unaided or they may learn toilet-training late
- miss out the crawling stage – i.e. bottom-shuffle, then pull themselves up and walk
- be pretty butter-fingered or 'ham-fisted' and avoid tasks that need good manual dexterity
- have trouble getting dressed and tying shoelaces
- be fidgety
- get stressed or distressed easily. Temper tantrums may persist later than is usual.
- have poor balance and sense of where their body is in space (proprioception), so they may bump into things a lot, lose their

balance frequently, trip and fall easily. They may have trouble learning to ride a trike or bike.
- not have much sense of danger and not seem to learn well from experience – i.e. *will* jump from heights (repeatedly) despite the fact they hurt themselves on landing
- be a messy eater
- avoid construction toys such as jigsaws and building bricks
- have difficulty holding a pencil, cutting with scissors and drawing
- not be into imaginative or role-playing games and not that that fond of creative play either, preferring to be played *with* by carers or have specific games with rules already inherent – e.g. board games and cards
- have trouble socialising with other children and may be rejected or bullied by them for being different, for not picking up on their signals or 'knowing' how to play their games. They may become isolated and prefer the company of older kids or adults.
- dislike lots of noise (especially background noise – e.g. noisy streets, shops and classrooms) and bright lights; rather oversensitive to touch. They may be very ticklish, dislike certain clothing textures and hate their toenails being cut.
- find it hard to concentrate for that long and often leave tasks unfinished.

Some things that may help

- Keep them calm.
- Have a good, predictable routine so they always know what's happening when.
- Ensure the child does not have excessive stimulation and that there are plenty of regular quiet times and pottering times, especially if they have been to nursery or pre-school.
- Liaise with their carers and pre-school teachers regularly. Ask for special-needs help and ensure they get it.
- Check out the room at nursery or pre-school. Look at where they sit (make sure it's not hidden right at the back). Is everything labelled or set out clearly around the room (i.e. work drawers, art cupboard, personal-belongings area, reading or play area) so it is easy for them to find their way around and know where things are?

- Try out small practical strategies – e.g. get extra-chunky cutlery that's easier to use, and grips for their pencils and crayons or paint-brushes from the Early Learning Centre. For contact details, see under 'Shopping' in the Directory. Teach them to fasten their shoelaces using the 'bunny ears' method, with two loops tied together instead of having to wrestle the ends into a bow. Encourage anything that would help with coordination and using their body from an early age, such as swimming, music (especially drumming and percussion) and movement-to-music classes.

Children from 5–12 years

For an older child who has not yet been diagnosed as dyspraxic and received the right support to help deal with it, they will still be having to cope with most of the difficulties they had as younger children and now, in addition, will probably have to manage at least some of the symptoms detailed below. Confusingly, many of them can be fairly typical of young boys (e.g. messy writing, rather uncoordinated, a shortish attention span, a tendency to forget things and be fidgety). However, the Dyspraxia Foundation suggests that you will just know that something isn't quite right, because 'As a parent you will know the difference between a normal child who shows any of these signs and one who is dyspraxic.'

A dyspraxic child from 5–12 years may:

- have social problems. These can really kick in now (e.g. isolation, bullying, difficulty making and keeping friends). They may have trouble withstanding stress (e.g. keeping calm when teased or goaded and losing their temper easily) and can become very upset about this. Your child may also have difficulty knowing 'when to stop' and so may irritate people.
- have difficulties in sports. They may find it hard to kick, catch or hit a ball accurately and might not be well coordinated, so football, rugby, gymnastics, etc., can be hard for them. Team games can be particularly troublesome because they can get confused by lots of rapid sensory input from different sources (i.e. keeping an eye on your team members and on your opposite numbers, listening to the ref, looking out for the ball, seeing where to pass it when you

do have it – 'Over here!' 'No, no! To me, to me!') and also trying to kick it properly when they *have* got it.

- be slow to complete work, which often looks scrappy or messy. They may have immature drawing and copying skills, laboured and not very legible handwriting. They could also have trouble copying from books or the blackboard.
- display difficulty with maths and foreign languages
- have limited concentration and listening skills
- show poor manual dexterity – difficulty with tasks like sewing, making artefacts in design and technology lessons or craft work
- have a poor memory. If asked to do three things in sequence, they may have trouble remembering more than two.

Some things that may help
There are some general suggestions for some of the most common difficulties:

- **Social problems** – drama classes or other activity-based groups and clubs can help, as can playing (supervised, structured) games. Foster one or two particularly easy-going friends. If they come over to your place for a visit, have a fairly short time for the children to hang out at home, then take them out to do something specific (e.g. bowling, the local adventure playground or cinema) and keep the visit to a few hours, rather than all day. This can reduce the potential for any social interaction problems and help ensure it's a 'good' visit that lays the foundations for more in the future. Similarly, if your child is invited over to their friend's place, consider suggesting it's for half a day, not a whole one, and think twice about sleepovers.
- **Short temper and easily stressed** – try role-playing games, mild and good-natured teasing or joking around at home (ensuring they are sometimes the subject of a gentle joke too) in order to help develop their ability to handle 'needling' from other children. Give plenty of quiet time at home to help them recover their equilibrium, which may have been pretty shredded by the average day at school. Facilitate 'grounding and centring' pastimes (if they enjoy them) such as martial arts, children's yoga and swimming at times

when the pool's not packed. If practical, get an affectionate furry pet for them to cuddle (very de-stressing) or, better still, a cheery dog to take out for a walk each day. Dogs are good company, give uncritical affection and provide regular fresh air and exercise combined: very unwinding (unless the weather's really bad!).

• **Difficulty with playing sport** – consider whole-body activities, like swimming or martial arts like karate, as this is very structured for developing coordination and promoting self-esteem, confidence and grounding. Extra private one-to-one tuition in a specific sport can help (so long as sessions are fairly short), especially if they have no option but to play it at school whether they like it or not. However, if that sport is not mandatory and if it just isn't your child's thing, it may work much better to find out what activity they really do enjoy – whether it's badminton or pottery-painting (you may not get the answer you had imagined) – and encourage that as much as possible instead, even doing it with or alongside them at first (if they would welcome this) to support them further until they become confident.

• **Language and maths difficulties** – listening to CDs of the language can help, although many parents choose to let their child opt out of languages even at a fairly early age if they are really struggling, and encourage them to concentrate on the subjects they like better and find easier. Some dyspraxic children who decide not to take, say, French, use one or two of what would have been French lessons to do study skills with the school special-needs teacher instead. Short periods (i.e. no more than half an hour) of gentle private tutoring at home may help with subjects like maths. However, getting help via your child's school from a *specialist learning-support teacher* that is *specific to your child's difficulties*, as opposed to relying on ordinary subject-based tutoring, is *essential*.

• **Difficulties with verbal instructions** – try not to give them several things to remember at once: keep it to three or preferably two. Gently ask your child to repeat them afterwards, again broken down into no more than three small, manageable stages. Encourage them to write down notes on a small jotter pad they carry with them all the time, write bullet points or 'memory-jogger' single words on the back of their hand, etc. Praise them every time they follow instructions correctly.

- **Easily confused** – routines, charts and lists all help here. For school timetables, shading specific subjects in different-coloured blocks (with or without the subject names written over the top) makes them far clearer than an ordinary black-and-white one. Starting a new school or college can be especially muddling. Make sure they know their way around.
- **Spelling difficulties** – as well as specialist teaching help, try working on a laptop with a spell-checker. Using a keyboard can take the stress out of writing, but from a spelling point of view, the child does still have to choose from a selection of correct spellings, so it may initially only be of limited help.
- **Lack of awareness of potentially dangerous situations** – discussion can be very helpful. Talk them through a recent situation in which they put themselves in jeopardy. Use situational games and role-playing, asking questions such as, 'Do you reckon someone would need to be careful of here? Or there?'
- **Low self-esteem** – do anything and everything you can to raise it and keep doing that at every opportunity. Encourage and support any aptitude they have, however minor, and give positive feedback (remember to mention specifics) on everything they do.

For treatments, suggestions and tips on helping children with dyspraxia, please see below: 'Treatments for Dyslexia and Dyspraxia', but also Teenagers: Dyspraxia on page 340.

Treatments for Dyslexia and Dyspraxia

If you suspect your child may be dyslexic or dyspraxic, the first port of call is your family GP. Ensure they arrange for a prompt – i.e. within two to three months at the very most most – appointment to have your child fully assessed by a *professional educational psychologist* to ensure any initial suggested diagnosis of dyslexia, dyspraxia – or elements of both – is definitely correct, and also to asess to the extent to which they are affected (it can often be mildly, but it it may be more severely) and whether there are any accompanying conditions there too, such as ADHD. This is vital, since while it is helpful to be told by your child's school that they think your child may be or 'is' dyslexic or dyspraxic, this is not sufficiently accurate and needs both confirming – and quantifying – by the experts so that you can fully understand your child's individual situation, and so ensure they get *exactly* the help and support they need.

If there seems to be an unacceptably long waiting list to see a suitable professional and you can afford to pay, it is well worth going to a private educational psychologist (approximately £300–£550). Their full report can be invaluable to show to both your child's school and hospital, if they are going to have any help from there, as official backup in writing will help you negotiate the right support for your child.

Through the NHS, your son or daughter could then be offered regular occupational therapy (OC), physiotherapy or both, which can be helpful. NHS OC units in particular often have plenty of useful leaflets – a bonus if your child is dyspraxic and aged 12+, as information on dyspraxia and teenagers is rather thin on the ground. Their school should also provide between one and three one-to-one sessions each week with their special-needs teacher or unit, tailored according to your child's specific needs (not the same as a catch-up subject-based class).

There are also several holistic therapies that can help dyslexic and dyspraxic children. These are often used in conjunction with special tuition at school and either physio or OC. These include:

257. Manipulative Therapies

Manipulative treatments, such as **chiropractic** or **traditional osteopathy**, can help realign the body, encouraging the smooth working of the skeletal and nervous systems. This would probably be offered in an initial run of six to eight weekly appointments to progressively correct the skeletal alignment and posture (and thus the smooth and efficient working of the neurological system), then drop down to monthly or bi-monthly maintenance sessions. Costs are £40–£100 for a first full assessment and treatment (with a chiropractor this usually includes X-rays), then £20–£40 per subsequent appointment.

Cranial osteopathy or its variant, **craniosacral therapy**, can also help calm and settle a slightly jerky or jangled nervous system, and many parents report helpful results for dyspraxic and dyslexic children.

This therapy is calming, soothing and very gentle – so much so that the client tends to fall half-asleep during it. It feels as if all the therapist is doing is gently holding your head; in fact, cranial osteopaths explain that they are subtly encouraging the pulses of cerebrospinal fluid (which bathes the brain and spinal cord) to work smoothly and rhythmically, thereby helping the body's other systems to function harmoniously too. Treatment sessions cost £20–£40, but usually nearer £50–£60 for a first appointment and assessment.

For where to find a qualified practitioner in your area, see under 'Therapies and Therapists' in the Directory. It is also worth asking if they have a special interest in helping children with dyspraxia or dyslexia, and if they don't, ask if they know any good colleagues who do.

258. Brain Re-Patterning

Systems of **neurological retraining** or **re-patterning** can be helpful, such as the **DORE method**, which uses repetitive movements and balancing exercises to stimulate and effectively reprogramme the cerebellum area of the brain over a period of several months. Assessment and tuition are on a private basis, and while not everyone agrees that the technique is useful, academics at the University of Exeter have been monitoring it at a primary school in Solihull and have reported that it produced 'remarkable' improvements – though the children were still behind their non-dyslexic peers – and, just as importantly, the improvements *lasted*.[23] Many thousands of parents have found this treatment well worth the money (£2000+) but there have also been complaints. To find out more about DORE, contact Dyslexia, Dyspraxia and Attention Disorder Treatment (DDAT). For details, see under 'Useful Helplines, Websites and Contacts' in the Directory.

259. Nutrition – EFAs

Essential-fatty-acids (EFAs) can substantially improve dyspraxia, dyslexia and ADHD (see Fix 239: Helpful Nutrients and Supplements) in about a third of cases. There is some good recent research backing this up, and more in the pipeline.[24] One study that caused great excitement was carried out in 2005 with 100 children in normal mainstream schools in County Durham whom teachers suspected were dyspraxic. In many cases, these children were also disruptive.

Half were given fish oils for three months, half placebo pills. Some 40 per cent of the supplement group achieved 'dramatic' improvements in reading and spelling, making nine months' progress in just three months, and half of those who'd been disruptive and thought to have ADHD no longer did so. The programme is now expanding to include more schools – the current study includes 5,000 children in the Durham area.

Good fish-oil supplements to take include Efamol's **Efamarine**, available from Boots, Superdrug, Holland & Barrett and other health shops in the UK (90 capsules, £9.99); in the US, you can buy it from Academy Health (90 capsules, $16.50). Another one is the vegetarian capsules **VegEPA**, available in the UK from Igennus.

Eye Q by Equazen is also good. For a child who is 10–11 years old, they should take six capsules a day with food for 12 weeks, then drop down to a maintenance dose of two. For teenagers, start with six to eight capsules a day, dropping to a maintenance dose of two to three after the first 12 weeks. You can buy it in Boots or via the manufacturer's website (60 x 500 mg capsules, £7.99).

Toddlers and children up to five years old may find it hard to swallow capsules, so try Eye Q Liquid (200 ml, £9.99). Give three teaspoons daily with food for the first 12 weeks, then drop down to a teaspoon daily with food. Or give them Eye Q Chews (60, £8.99). They should take six a day with food spread out through the day's meals, then after 12 weeks drop down to two a day. Again, these are made by Equazen and available from their website.

For all contact details, see under 'Shopping' in the Directory.

See also 'About EFAs' on page 314.

260. Essences

Most essences have not been tested in clinical trials, as fish oils have been, but they are increasingly used by complementary therapists (and even some progressive psychologists) for dyslexia or dyspraxia.

Certain essences are thought to offer gentle, cumulative support – especially **Reunion, Bush Fuchsia** and **Bright Spark** from the remarkable new 'Urban Angels' range, developed by Light Heart Essences in 2006 with the therapists of the pioneering London-based inner-city children's rehabilitation charity, Kids' Company.

Bright Spark is, as its name suggests, used to help children develop their learning skills, especially how to focus, concentrate, organise themselves and their work, and handle the processing of complex information. It is also given to encourage the integration of the right- and left-hand sides of the brain, something that may not be so well developed in people who are dyspraxic or dyslexic.

You can buy Reunion direct from Light Heart Essences (10 ml, £5.15), Bush Fuchsia from Australian Bush Flower Essences (15 ml, £8.95), and Bright Spark can also be bought direct from Light Heart (mouth spritzer, 30 ml, £8.65).

For contact details for all organisations, treatments and products mentioned in this section, please, see under 'Shopping' in the Directory, or under Useful Helplines, Websites and Contacts, and Therapies and Therapists, pp 576.

Ears

261. Earache

Warm a capsule of **garlic oil** in a quarter of a cup of warm (not boiling hot or the capsule will melt) water and remove. With the child lying on their side with the affected ear uppermost, pierce one end of the capsule and carefully drip the warmed garlic oil into their ear until it has trickled into the deepest part. Plug gently with a soft piece of cotton wool. The oil soothes red, inflamed skin, and the garlic is a good anti-infective agent.[25]

Note: if there is no improvement within 24 hours, go and see your GP promptly.

Capsules of garlic oil are cheap and widely available from all chemists, pharmacies and health shops – e.g. Holland & Barrett (100 x 1 g capsules, £2.49). For contact details, see under 'Shopping' in the Directory.

262. Glue Ear

Glue ear is caused by a build-up of fluid inside the ear, which interferes with children's hearing. If they have it chronically when young, they may have trouble learning to speak (as they cannot hear words clearly, they will mispronounce them when trying to imitate them) or have difficulty at school because they simply cannot pick up what is being said by their teachers or classmates.

This fluid can also become infected, causing recurrent, painful otitis media (middle-ear infections), which a GP would usually treat with antibiotics – repeatedly. Another conventional glue-ear treatment is to have slim tubes called grommets surgically inserted into the eardrum (they sometimes later become displaced or fall out), which allow air back into the ear cavity and help drain out the fluid. For persistent cases, surgical removal of the adenoids (glands at the back of the nose) is also used.

However, one German study of 131 children aged from 12 months to 11 years suggests that gentle homeopathic treatment can clear up glue ear faster than antibiotics, takes only four days compared with the standard drug course of seven to ten days and is far better for preventing relapses.[26] The remedies used in the study depended on the children's individual symptoms but included **Apis mellifica**, **Capsulesicum**, **Belladonna**, **Silica** and **Pulsatilla**. See also homeopathic **Mimosa**, a good general ear infection remedy for both children and adults to keep in any home medicine cabinet, pp XX.

In the German study, 71 per cent of the children treated with homeopathy were free of the problem without any relapses for a year, whereas 30 per cent of the other group had up to three relapses during that time.

For best results with glue ear, try and take your child to see a homeopath in person. In the UK, contact the British Homeopathic Association; in the US, check out the National Center for Homeopathy. For contact details, see under 'Therapies and Therapists' in the Directory.

Food-sensitivity link

Glue ear is often linked with food intolerances or sensitivities. These aren't the same as full-blown food allergies: food sensitivity means that though a food won't actually make you ill, bring you up in a rash or cause sudden breathing problems, it still doesn't agree with you. The most common culprits in the food-sensitivity stakes are dairy products.

Suspect a food sensitivity as at least a contributing cause if your child also has:

- a lot of colds
- a frequently blocked nose, even when they don't have a cold

- a love, or craving, for dairy foods, either one in particular (e.g. they are mad for, say, fromage frais or cheese) or all of them.

If so, take them to see a good nutritionist. For contact details, see under 'Therapies and Therapists' in the Directory. If the nutritionist is also a skilled AK practitioner, even better, as they can test quickly and usually accurately to find out precisely what food your child is intolerant or allergic to – and which nutrient(s) they are short of.

Food Intolerances

263. Milk and Dairy Intolerance
There is a sugar in milk called lactose that consists of two other simpler sugars: galactose and glucose. Some children and adults don't have the right enzyme in their gut to break down lactose into its two constituents, so when they eat food with milk in, it causes symptoms including loose motions, wind and bloating. This is called lactose intolerance – i.e. a sensitivity or problem with a particular food, as opposed to an actual allergy (which is a reactive, inflammatory condition).

Three things help here:

1. **Give your child 'friendly', or useful, bacteria,** such as *Lactobacillus acidophilus*. See also Fix 231: 'Friendly' Bacteria.
2. **Give them the enzyme lactase.** You can add it in liquid form to milk 24 hours before your child drinks it or you make a food using milk as one of the ingredients (e.g. ice cream). It is also available in handy tablet form, which can be taken when your child eats the milk products that would usually upset them, like yoghurt or cheese. Alternatively, try Raspberry-Flavoured Lactose Chewits from Milkaid (120, £12.99) or drops from BioCare (15 ml, enough for 36 litres of milk, £9). In the US and Canada, try the Canadian brand Children's Lacteeze (100 tablets, $10).
3. **Use different forms of milk e.g. soya, for cooking and drinking.** Popular alternatives for those who don't like the taste of soya milk, which is available in every major supermarket and health shop, are oat milk – and rice milk, which can be a good one because it's quite sweet so

children tend to like it. Rice milk is available from many health shops, including Holland & Barrett (100 g, £1.49). In the US, try the organic rice milk from Diamond Organics (32 fl oz, $3.59).

For all contact details, see under 'Shopping' in the Directory.

Hair and Heads

264. Itchy Scalp

If the itching is not being caused by the usual (e.g. head lice or candida overgrowth, in which case a six- to eight-week course of probiotics is called for), look to your child's shampoo, suggests top UK nutritionist, applied kinesiology practitioner and osteopath John Taberman-Pichler.

The most common ingredient that causes trouble is the foaming agent laurel sulphate. When my daughter (then aged eight) had an itchy scalp, I spent many months and a lot of money on de-sensitising treatments for a potential allergy until I changed her shampoo to a laurel-sulphate-free brand and found the improvement was immediate.

Try Organic Aloe Vera and Lavender from Green People (200 ml, £7.99), or one from the lovely Urtekram range – try Rose Pure Balance Shampoo from selected health stores or via Love Lula (250 ml, £4.50). For contact details, see under 'Shopping' in the Directory.

265. Painful Hair-Brushing

When you are really trying to be gentle and have a good soft hairbrush yet your young child still yelps, 'Yow, that hurts!' as you brush or comb their hair, the problem is usually a shortage of **vitamin D**, especially if the scalp is tender to touch, says Dr John Briffa, one of the UK's top pioneering natural and nutritional therapists.

Besides ensuring your child gets plenty of D-rich foods, like salmon and mackerel, and enough safe exposure to sunlight, Dr Briffa suggests trying 200 IU daily for four weeks in supplement form followed by a good children's multi-vitamin and mineral supplement that also contains vitamin D, like Dinochews from Higher Nature (30 tablets, £5.30) or Nature's Best Tasty Chews 4–14 Years (100 tablets, £8.95). For contact details, see under 'Shopping' in the Directory.

266. Nits and Lice

Head lice are little insects about 2.5 mm across that fasten on to the scalp and lay eggs – fast. They are also known as nits, but technically that refers to the egg casings, which are dark when they have an occupant preparing to hatch and white when empty. Lice are common in children as soon as they start having mass contact with others – i.e. from playgroup or nursery onwards. And if just one pupil has nits, they can go round a classroom like wildfire.

There are many chemical products for treating lice. However, some parents prefer to avoid these as a) they can sting the scalp, b) the fumes may irritate the eyes, c) they contain organophosphates, which may pose a health risk to children, and d) according to a report in 2005 in the *British Medical Journal*, lice are becoming resistant to some of them.

There are several different natural-ingredient products available commercially, though not all are equally effective. Here's one DIY recipe that certainly is, however: it got rid of lice from my daughter's long, thick hair when she'd had them on and off for a year. (She had a friend who was badly infested and they kept giving them back to each other. The friend got the treatment too, politely promoted as a natural hair-shiner – which it also is.) It was suggested by British aromatherapy pioneer Maggie Tisserand.

The no-more-lice recipe

   12 drops eucalyptus essential aromatherapy oil
   13 drops geranium
   25 drops lavender
   25 drops rosemary
   75 ml light base oil, such as almond or safflower

In a bottle, shake to combine all the oils. This is enough to do one head of long hair or three heads of short hair.

Note: For pre-pubescent boys, leave out the lavender. A small report, based on three case studies, by the US Institute of Environmental Health Services in 2007 found it can, if used repeatedly, affect testosterone balance and encourage slight *temporary* male breast tissue development.

Use this, lose lice

1. Rub gently into the scalp and roots of newly washed, damp hair.
2. Comb back from your child's face, pile on top and clip if it's long. Wind a couple of layers of cling film round their head, with a towel wrapped over the top like in a hairdressing salon.
3. Ensure they keep it on for an hour and a half – many parents bring in a full-length DVD or series of distracting stories or games for this bit – unless the mix starts to irritate them at all, in which case wash off right away in warm water with a gentle shampoo.
4. At the end of the hour and a half take the towel and cling film off and start combing the hair through very carefully with a nit comb. (A white plastic one for 99p from the local chemist's is perfectly effective, but pricier steel or electric ones are also available.) Part the hair in rows at 0.5 cm intervals. Done properly, this will take 30–45 minutes for longer hair, 20 minutes for short hair. *Note:* you need to be a bit obsessive and let the primate grooming impulse take over (satisfying, if time-consuming) or you won't get them all out, and there'll be lots more in there in ten days' time.
5. Wash hair well in gentle shampoo and warm water. It will take two to three rinses to get all the oil out.
6. Repeat seven to ten days later as backup to ensure you get anything you may have missed first time round: there are usually a couple. And since lice mature quickly, what was an egg ten days ago will be laying eggs of its own by now.

Also:

- **Hot-wash all bed linen and towels** the child has used, especially pillowcases, as there may be a live egg or two clinging to them. And that's all it takes to re-colonise a child's head within two weeks.
- **Treat the whole family** (parents and other children) – as lice crawl from person to person (e.g. when you put your heads together for a cuddle, hug or rough 'n' tumble), it's safest to treat everyone alike.

It is best to use organic oils when treating young children: if you can't find any locally, try the ones from Star Child: Eucalyptus Oil (10 ml, £3.50), Geranium Oil (10 ml, £8.75), Lavender Oil (10 ml, £5.95) and Rosemary Oil (10 ml, £4.50).

Ready-made

If your child's class has had an endemic head-lice problem for a while, the quantities of oils listed above will be enough to do an eradication treatment (one initial, one follow-up) plus around 20 monthly preventative treatments. However, if you'd like something natural but ready-mixed, about the best I've so far come across is an eco-friendly shampoo called **Not Nice to Lice** from Naturally Does It (240 ml, £17.99), enough for 24 treatments; in the US, it's sold as **Lice R Gone** from Safe 2 Use ($21.90; nit comb, 55¢).

The shampoo's secret weapon is some protease enzymes that are involved in skin shedding, but it contains no toxic chemicals and so is recommended by homeopaths, hairdressers and GPs alike.[27] Not Nice to Lice stays on for about 15 minutes, and you have to keep massaging it into the scalp at 30-second intervals. Safe for babies, breastfeeding mothers and young children, you can use it weekly to keep the nits at bay during a protracted school outbreak, which may last, on and off, all year.

The 'yuck' factor

If your child is upset by the idea of having lice, Bach's **Crab Apple** can help them get over the disgust. It is available from Healthlines (10 ml, £3.99).

For all contact details, see under 'Shopping' in the Directory.

---

267. Hay Fever

A small but surprisingly useful tip if your child suffers from allergic rhinitis or asthma, suggested by the National Asthma Campaign: put a thin slick of a petroleum gel such as Vaseline round the inside of their nostrils. This helps trap the pollen grains that would otherwise irritate them. Wipe off and replenish as necessary.
See also Fix 55: And for Hay Fever.

Mood-Lifting

268. Grumpiness and Gloom

British aromatherapy queen Maggie Tisserand recommends this simple essential-oil mix either dabbed on the wrists or sprayed around the room if a child is down or grumpy, explaining that it brings 'harmony and light-heartedness'. If my children were inexplicably fed up or had a friend coming round but suddenly weren't in the mood and it was too late to cancel, we used to find it especially good to spray in the playroom. Mix a drop of **geranium aromatherapy oil** with a drop of **orange**, add to 15 ml water (for a spray), or jojoba or almond oil (if it's to be dabbed on the skin).

269. Colour-Breathing

If there is no special reason for being glum and your child is simply feeling a bit negative 'because they are', which happens increasingly as they approach peri-puberty (from ten onwards for girls), or perhaps they've had a disappointment and cannot shake it off, try colour-breathing with them. You can do it with children as young as five.

Colour is a light wavelength and a vibrational rate – different ones for different colours – and has been shown by many studies to have a direct, and sometimes rapid, effect on mood and physical well-being. Imagining a colour – literally 'seeing' it in your mind's eye – can be as powerful as basking under specially tinted light for therapeutic purposes. And children can usually imagine colours especially effectively, as they tend to have stronger imaginations and fewer preconceptions than adults.

The colours for mood-lifting are **blue** and **orange**, says Theo Gimbel, the UK's most experienced colour researcher and practitioner, who founded the Hygeia College of Colour Therapy and the International Association of Colour Therapy. Blue helps bring in peace and relaxation. Orange is for happiness, joy and sheer fun.

For practitioners worldwide, contact the International Association of Colour (IAC). Look for those with 'PMIAC' after their names, as this indicates they are both fully trained and have been in professional practice for at least three years. IAC therapists work worldwide. For contact details, see under 'Therapies and Therapists' in the Directory.

Recommended reading: *Healing With Colour* by Theo Gimbel.

The Happy Colour Breath

Practise the **Happy Colour Breath** yourself first before talking your child through it so you know how it feels.

1. Sit or lie down comfortably somewhere peaceful and close your eyes. Breathe at the rate that is usual and comfortable for you for a minute or two.
2. Now take your mind back to a time or place where you remember feeling *especially* happy: perhaps a special birthday party, playing on a sunny beach or being hugged and swung up into the air by your mother or father if they'd been away for a bit. Enjoy that feeling and stay with it for a little while.
3. Now take a big breath in and, as you do so, imagine a beautiful warm *orange* light growing in your middle, just below the tummy button.
4. As you let out that breath, imagine you're breathing out a beautiful *blue* colour.
5. Keep breathing in and out – with each in-breath seeing that warm orange light spreading all the way through you from the tip of your toes to the top of your head, and with each out-breath imagine breathing out peaceful blue.
6. Continue for a few minutes, or until you feel like you want to stop. Open your eyes, yawn and stretch.

Nappy Rash

270. Dump the Disposables

Repeated nappy rash? If you're changing the nappies often enough and using a good, gentle barrier cream but the soreness persists, try **towelling nappies**. US research suggests babies wearing environmentally sound 'real' nappies get up to five times less nappy rash (and often eczema in the area improves too), so it's not surprising that many parents are switching to Velcro or press-stud towelling nappies and dumping the disposables.

Cushioning care

Other health benefits include proper protection for toddlers learning to walk: US paediatricians are blaming the less-padded disposable for providing insufficient cushioning for bottom falls and therefore being a factor in the rise in spinal injury and hip dysphasia seen in toddlers in the last generation.

Smart nappy choice, smart cost

The disadvantage is that getting real (nappy-wise) can be seriously confusing – there are so many styles, prices, sites, claims and catalogues; but what do you *really* need, and what does it honestly cost? Briefly, the truth is that while disposables will set you back from about £800 a year, real nappies (based on a starter kit of, say, 20, plus linings) will range from £150 for basic towelling squares and plastic pants to around £450 for cute designer all-in-one pull-ons, plus another £35 a year in laundering costs.

Further information

For further information in the UK, contact the UK Nappy Helpline. For contact details, see under 'Useful Helplines, Websites and Contacts' in the Directory.

In the UK, try a company like Kittykins for supplies or So Organic; in the US, see the Born to Love site for practical advice, local and mail-order suppliers, and for diaper services – where they collect dirty nappies from you, launder and return them. For contact details, see under 'Shopping' in the Directory.

If you use real towelling nappies, there's another effective weapon in the anti-nappy-rash arsenal: **vinegar**.

After the washing cycle (at 60 degrees C, using non-biological detergent and a long first rinse cycle), add half a cup of vinegar to a second rinse cycle of the machine. Some of the acetic acid it contains stays in the nappies and helps stop bacteria making the ammonia compounds that irritate nappied bottoms.

Nosebleeds

Nosebleeds happen when the delicate blood vessels lining the nose break open. This can occur if a child blows their nose too hard, picks it over-industriously or has a knock on the area.

271. Immediate Relief
Immediate action to stop a nosebleed involves simply leaning the child forward, pinching the bridge of their nose and asking them to breathe through their mouth.

Homeopaths suggest **arnica 30c** for stopping nosebleeds – give every ten minutes while the bleeding is in progress, then it's suggested following up with the remedy three times daily for five to ten days afterwards.

After about ten minutes any bleeding will usually have stopped. If it hasn't, pinch under the bridge of the nose for a few more minutes.' If it's still not finished after half an hour, seek medical attention.

Arnica tablets are available from most chemists and health shops in the UK, but they may only have the potency 6 (6c) type. If you want to get in some arnica 30c to keep in the medicine cabinet for when it's needed, Helios, the pharmacy supplying patients at the NHS Homeopathic Hospital in Tunbridge Wells, does a 24-hour mail-order service (around £3.75). For contact details, see under 'Shopping' in the Directory.

272. Longer-Term Help
Vitamin C and **bioflavonoids** are good for strengthening the walls of blood vessels and helping them to be less prone to rupturing. Besides ensuring your child eats plenty of fresh fruit and vegetables, consider supplementing with 500 mg vitamin C and 400 mg bioflavonoids (based on a child weighing around 40 kg). Both nutrients are sold countrywide in good health food shops; but if you can't find any locally, try Nature's Best 500 mg Time-Release Vitamin C, which also contains bioflavonoids (100 tablets, £3.50). For contact details, see under 'Shopping' in the Directory.

Should the nosebleeds happen a lot, go and seek your doctor's advice to ensure there is no underlying clinical condition, such as a blood-clotting problem.

Pain

273. Singing It Better

Parents have always known that singing to their young children can often distract them from distress, but now research from the Beth Israel Medical Center in New York with 50 children shows it can also measurably speed their recovery from painful conditions, too.

If you cannot be there giving voice as much as you would like to be, try recording some of the songs your child loves to hear you sing the most (for many it's 'bedtime' and 'cheer-up' ones) on to a tape or CD and encourage them to listen to it via some headphones when you cannot be with them.

274. The Touch that Soothes

There are many different healing techniques, including hands-off spiritual healing as taught by highly respectable healing charities like the National Federation of Spiritual Healers, reiki healing and 'energy healing'. But perhaps one of the simplest for parents to use to comfort their own children when they are ill is **Therapeutic Touch (TT)**.

What is it?

Therapeutic Touch is used by a growing number of nurses and midwives in the UK, is validated by the English National Board of Nursing and backed up by dozens of published clinical trials;[28] in the US, more than a hundred universities both use and teach this therapy. Research suggests that it can soothe pain, calm distress, has a deeply relaxing effect and encourages wounds and injuries to heal more quickly.

It can be especially effective for parents to practise TT with their children, as they love them so much and know them better than anyone else. For this reason, TT is sometimes taught to mothers and fathers who have premature babies in specialist premature-baby units.

Used at home, it can comfort distress of all types, soothe the pain of injury or infection and help a fretful, unwell, wakeful child to sleep. TT can be immensely useful for those really difficult times when they are up – miserable, in pain or both – at 3 a.m. and you've tried everything else. Suitable for all ages from babies to teens (adults and pets too, for that matter), here's how to do a very basic TT:

1. Take six slow, calming breaths. Imagine a golden light settling round you that is dissolving all negativity (tiredness, irritation and worries). It's important to do this or you will 'pass' those emotions and energies through to your child.

2. Sit down by your child. If you've not done TT with them before, explain you're going to try some 'magic no-touch stroking' (as one mother calls it) to help them feel better, and ask them to allow you to try it.

3. If they say OK, ask them to shut their eyes. Look at them kindly, focusing all your attention on them. Now try, as one trained TT nurse put it, to 'send them love with your eyes'. Do this for a few moments, or for as long as feels right.

4. Next, hold one hand about 15–30 cm away from their head and the other, if you can reach, 5–10 cm from their feet. If they are too tall for that, do the head position and hold the other hand above their solar plexus, just below the tummy button. (You need to hold your hand further away from their head than from their feet or solar plexus because this is the area that is the most sensitive to healing energy.)

5. Try to send them love through your palms. You may feel your hands tingling a little or growing warmer.

6. If you would like to do a bit more, try slow 'stroking' along their body from head down to feet or abdomen, still holding your hands away. Do this for as long as feels right to you – for most parents, it's between two and five minutes.

7. To finish, bring your hands back to rest above their original positions (head and feet, or head and abdomen). Let them stay there for a few seconds, then mentally 'sign off' and cease sending your child loving, healing energy for now.

8. Bring your hands down to your sides, rubbing them lightly against your thigh for a moment or two.

9. Take a slow, deep breath in and out, sending the energy down through your body, feet and into the floor to ground yourself. You can also, if you would like to, mentally 'put' a golden ball of protective, healing light round your child. Then quietly withdraw.

Further information

In the UK, contact the Sacred Space Foundation for details of introductory TT courses by teachers accredited by the British Association of Therapeutic Touch, and also for practitioners. To find a TT practitioner locally in the US (where it's called HT, or Healing Touch), contact Healing Touch International. For contact details, see under 'Therapies and Therapists' in the Directory.

Recommended reading: *The Healing Touch* by Suzanne Franzen.

Parties

275. Awkward Social Atmosphere

If there is one of these at a children's party – or even a small social gathering, such as when a couple of your child's friends have come over to play – surreptitiously spray some **Hummingbird** essence around the room.

Make up a spray by adding, say, 21 drops to 200 ml water and spritz away. Hummingbird – made from the energy of the animal but without touching or harming it in any way – tends to produce playfulness, giggles, relaxation and often downright hilarity. It's good for lightening a leaden or tentative atmosphere.

Hummingbird is made by Wild Earth Animal Essences and is available in the UK via IFER (15 ml, approximately £6.50); in the US, you can buy it direct (1 fl oz, $8.99). For contact details, see under 'Shopping' in the Directory.

Premature Babies

276. Kangarooing: Care You Bring Home From Hospital

Eight thousand British babies arrive prematurely (that's 134 a day), and 12 per cent of all American babies are also born too soon.

Parents are often very distressed indeed when their tiny baby is in a special-care baby unit (SCBU) not only because their child is so vulnerable and unwell, but also because it may feel like there is so little they can do to help them. Yet in truth, there is a huge amount.

Kangaroo care

One of the nicest and most medically effective things parents can do, not only to comfort their premature baby – a major thing in itself as the average brightly lit hothouse special-care baby unit is not usually a comfortable place to be – but also to help their little one grow well and strong more quickly, is **kangaroo care**. It involves a mother or father holding the baby tucked inside clothing, so resting against their parent's chest, bare skin to bare skin, like a joey in a kangaroo's pouch.

Most SCBUs are familiar with this method of nurturing premature babies; in fact, some premature-baby nurses also teach it. And so long as the baby is medically stable, kangaroo care can help even some of the very smallest aged 28–30 gestational (in the womb) weeks – they would normally have been born after 40.

How it helps and what it does

Kangarooing premature babies improves their health tremendously, as extensive international research shows.[29] UNICEF and the World Health Organization also highly recommend it, as a kangarooed premature baby:

- sleeps better
- breathes more easily – it's thought that feeling the rise and fall of their parent's breathing helps regulate their own (most premature babies have initial breathing difficulties)
- fidgets less because they are so much more comfortable
- is calmer
- grows faster
- has fewer stop-breathing (apnoea) episodes
- has fewer heartbeat problems
- has a more stable body temperature, thanks to the steady, normal warmth of the parent's body
- breastfeeds more easily. And the skin-to-skin contact helps ensure the mother can make milk for them more readily and for longer (often a problem too).
- gets fewer infections
- can manage without their incubators sooner
- comes home from hospital earlier.

It is also immensely comforting for parents to have skin-to-skin contact with their own baby, helping them give their child love more freely and bond more easily – not an easy thing to do in the unnatural setting of a hi-tech special-care unit when for the initial weeks you may not even have been allowed to cuddle or feed your baby yourself.

Further information
Recommended reading: for demystifying all aspects of SCBUs and *everything* parents can do to help their premature baby (including kangaroo care) both in hospital and in the pre-school years at home, please see *Your Premature Baby 0–5 Years* by myself with Tommy's Campaign, the UK's premature baby research and education charity. For detailed information specifically on kangaroo care, read the booklet by Krisanne Larimer available via www.prematurity.com, or the excellent *Kangaroo Care: the Best You Can Do to Help Your Preterm Infant* by Susan Ludington-Hoe.

Further support and information for parents in the UK is available from the charity Bliss via their website or their helpline; in the US, contact the Pregnancy and Newborn Health and Education Center at the March of Dimes. Log on to their website for email dialogue and advice from one of their specialist health professionals. For contact details, see under 'Useful Helplines, Websites and Contacts' in the Directory.

Relaxation

Children are getting far more stimulation at school, playtime and at home than they were a generation ago. However, more exciting things to do and extra opportunities can also mean less 'downtime', making it harder for a child to switch off and calm down in the evenings. Knock-on effects of this include sleep problems, lack of concentration, mood swings, lower energy levels and a less effective immune system – i.e. they're more tired, crabby, edgy and go down with more winter bugs.

277. Relaxation Techniques
Fortunately, children of all ages respond very well to gentle relaxation techniques – even better than most adults. If you'd like to help your

child wind down more effectively at the end of a busy day but don't want to have to schlep off to junior yoga classes or spend time in the evening between helping with the homework and doing the supper facilitating deep-breathing and visualisation sessions (when even you're not calm, never mind them), there is an easy, effective alternative: relaxation tapes and CDs for kids.

There are many of these around (some of which aren't very good), but one of the best ranges I've come across are by a London-based children's entertainer called Marneta Viegas, who noticed changes in children's behaviour and concentration when she told them stories. She then developed a system of child relaxation for ages two and a half to 13 (works best of all with four- to nine-year-olds) combining well-loved fairy tales with very simple relaxation methods.

The stories are on CD so children listen to them in bed before they go to sleep – setting up a routine of doing so every night works best – and they also tend to return to the stories whenever they are stressed or anxious. A hit on long car journeys too. They are available from Relax Kids (£14.99). You can download audio samples from their website. For contact details, see under 'Shopping' in the Directory.

278. Fever

Besides sponging down with lukewarm (never cold) water, and the colour therapists' favourite – blue or green pillowcases, sheets and duvet covers for the cooling effect of those colours' wavelengths (avoid red and yellow ones) – try the homeopathic **ABC.**

Since children's fevers can peak fast, give every 15 minutes until the fever subsides. It is used for temperature and aches and pains as a natural alternative to Calpol. Helios has an all-in-one combination for feverish children where A is for Aconite, B for Belladonna and C for Chamomilla (30 pillules, £3.50). For contact details, see under 'Shopping' in the Directory.

School and Exams

279. Grades Need a Boost?

If your son or daughter's grades are lower than you feel they should be, you've already spoken at length to their teachers, found nothing untoward and don't want them to be burdened with 'extra learning' at home after the school day when they should be unwinding, there's a gentler holistic option to try: **walking**.

Walking for just half an hour three times a week can improve learning, abstract reasoning and concentration levels, especially for school-age children, and particularly for boys, who have higher-than-average grades at the age of ten if they exercise several times a week.

A senior researcher from the University of Exeter suggests that this may partly be because exercise helps send oxygenated blood briskly to the brain; according to recent American research, walking also puts you into a 'peaceful but alert' mental state, ideal for processing newly acquired information, enhancing memory and de-stressing so a child is in an optimum state to learn.[30]

Further studies suggest walking to school improves fitness levels – no surprises there – and can lower depression, reduce anxiety, enhance body image and raise self-esteem, so exercise can be a useful tool for reducing school stress in general – quite apart from helping ensure they arrive at their first class of the day in a positive, receptive, relaxed frame of mind.[31] No wonder the US custom of taking a **'walking bus'** to school, initiated there in 1993, is catching on in the UK.

Catch a walking bus

To find a walking bus near you, first ask your child's school if they do one and check with your area's Department of Education and libraries, as they will often have details of local schemes. Or, if possible, how about starting one yourself with teachers, other parents or volunteers?

Recommended reading: *The Walking Bus Guide* by Tracy Allatt and Sarah Marshall, which can be purchased through Lollypop Publishing. For contact details, see under 'Shopping' in the Directory.

See also the Walking Bus website (www.thewalkingbusguide.co.uk) and the School Run website (www.school-run.org), which puts parents in touch with others local to them who can not only share lifts but organise walking buses or escorted walks to school, and Safe Kids Walking (www.safekidswalking.org.uk). For more contact details, see under 'Useful Helplines, Websites and Contacts' in the Directory.

280. Better School Test Results

Drink more to score more – **water**, that is. Pupils at Corstorphine School in Merseyside recently found their test results and concentration levels improved after being encouraged to drink water while they did them. They were given sports flasks to stand on their desks, which closed easily and effectively to avoid the chance of spillage, and were asked to just sip when they felt like it as they worked.

Parents, teachers and children were surprised and pleased at the difference such a simple change made, but since the brain is 90 per cent water and efficient neurotransmission requires water too, perhaps it figures.

Despite the proven benefits of water for brains, a fifth of all UK schoolchildren still have no access to a supply of drinking water at school and another 10 per cent are only offered drinking water from washbasins in the loos.

With designer water costing 50–80p for a small bottle, it's worth investing in a big container for home and filling up an acceptably cool-looking flask each day for your child to take in. You could also suggest that the school supplies water-coolers and cups (total cost: around £1 per child per year). Avoid sweet, fizzy drinks: they are all diuretic and just cause more water to be lost from a child's body and brain.

Skin

281. Cradle Cap

This is a form of seborrhoeic eczema (sometimes called seborrhoeic dermatitis) and it is very common, especially in boy babies under a year old. Symptoms are a crusty, greasy, scaly rash that starts on the baby's scalp but may spread to the eyebrows, neck, groin and armpits. In mild cases it looks like dandruff and doesn't need any special treatment.

If it's more marked, try and resist the powerful parental grooming impulse to pick at it, because that can cause infection. Instead, massage a little **cold-pressed olive oil** or **almond oil** into the crusty scales to soften them. Let that soak in for 15 minutes, then shampoo the baby's head – you can do this every day. Try Holland & Barrett's Sweet Almond Base Oil (100 ml, £2.99).

Or you can rub ten drops of **borage (starflower) oil** into the area twice daily for 14 days. You can get the starflower oil by piercing capsules and counting the drops as you squeeze them on to your palm. They can be purchased at Holland & Barrett (50 capsules, £4.11).

In addition to this, if the condition has persisted for some time despite gentle oil treatments, you could also add one drop of tea-tree oil to the starflower, as tea tree is a good antifungal agent and candida (fungal) overgrowth can cause hard-to-shift cradle cap. In the UK, try Neal's Yard Organic Tea Tree Oil (10 ml, £6.05); in the US, try Neal's Yard, Baldwin's or Tisserand (0.34 fl oz, $21). Do also read the note on use of tea-tree oil on page 549.

For all contact details, see under 'Shopping' in the Directory.

282. Eczema

According to a University of Bristol study, paediatric eczema affects a quarter of under-threes, and 10–15 per cent of under-nines. It can be immensely – sometimes destructively – itchy, and difficult to get rid of entirely, but fortunately there's a wide range of strategies (medical, self-help and complementary) that may often help, including **essential fatty acids (EFAs)**.[32]

For children who find it difficult to swallow EFAs in their usual capsule form – choking and saying, 'It won't go down' (indeed, it may not be safe for very young ones to try) – it can be given in liquid form on a teaspoon.

There is a brand called **Linatox**, flavoured with natural strawberry extract, that fits the bill here, and it tastes considerably nicer than the fish oils and evening primrose oil they might otherwise be offered. Get in touch with Cedar Health for stockists.

Also check out Allergenics' special range of skincare products containing extract of soya and liquorice, which can help calm inflammation of the skin, such as their **Steroid-Free Emollient Cream**, available from Wellbeing UK (50 ml, £4.99). Specially designed for people of all ages with eczema, Allergenics' products are used as a natural alternative to steroid-based creams, or at least as a way of reducing their usage.

For all contact details, see under 'Shopping' in the Directory.

283. Impetigo

This is a skin infection caused by the *Staphylococcus aureus* bug, causing red fluid-filled blisters usually around the nose and mouth, which burst and scab over, leaving a golden crust. Very contagious (and itchy at blister stage), it is usually treated with antibiotics.

If you want to treat it naturally, and also boost your child's immune system (see Fix 248: Immunity), use **tea-tree oil**, which can kill the *Staphylococcus aureus* bug. It's pretty strong, so dilute by putting five drops in half a cup of water and dabbing it on to the sores with cotton wool two to three times a day; this may sting a bit even when watered down so much. See also the note on use of tea-tree oil on page 549.

Hot-wash all clothing, bedding, towels and flannels that have been in contact with those blisters too. Ensure your child washes their hands well with hot water and soap; also keep them from close contact with family and other children until the infection is gone – a case of 'hug from behind'.

Note: if it is not improving after three to four days, go and see your GP as it can spread quickly.

See also Young Children: Nappy Rash on page 287 and Fix 264: Itchy Scalp.

Sleep

284. Gentle Bedroom Atmosphere

Jacquie Wilton, an experienced gem therapist and senior healer trainer with the UK's National Federation of Spiritual Healers, suggests using a **pink rose quartz** (the 'love stone') in a young child's bedroom to promote a soft atmosphere and peaceful sleep.

First, cleanse and 'programme' the stone with love and peaceful thoughts (see Appendix 1: Cleansing and Programming Crystals and Gems on page 536), then place it near the child's bed – first checking it's too big to be swallowed. You can get rose-quartz pieces, say, 7–10 cm across, from gift, New Age and gem shops (£6–£8).

Choosing a stone

Finding the right one for your child is easy. If you're looking at several pieces, first see which one attracts you when you look at it. Pick it up and hold it for a few moments while you think of your child and see how you feel about it then. If it still seems like the right one, buy it.

Extra peace

For an extra feeling of sheer peace, bliss and protection for children in their room at night, especially if they are a bit nervous of being left alone, spray a little of the combination essence **Calling All Angels** in a circle round their bed and around the periphery of the bedroom. One mother describes the spray as feeling 'like someone just put loving arms round you'.

It is made by Alaskan Essences and can be bought in the UK from Healthlines (150 ml, £17.50, or £11.95 for 60ml); in the US and Canada, you can buy it direct. For contact details, see under 'Shopping' in the Directory.

Further information

Recommended reading: on the subject of angels, for a bit of background if you are interested, see *A Little Light on Angels* by Diana Cooper, a lovely but very sensible, practical and straightforward book about angels – and the availability of angelic protection to everyone who asks for it.

See also Houses and Gardens: Atmosphere on page 435.

285. Night Terrors

Night terrors are a distressing medical sleep disorder, also known as sleep terrors, sleep terror disorder or pavor nocturnes. They can affect anyone of any age but seem to be most common in young children aged three to five. Canadian and American research suggests night terrors are produced by increased activity in the brain during what is usually the deep phase of sleep (Sleep Stage 4) and tend to happen 15 minutes to an hour after going to sleep. Night terrors are *not* the same as nightmares, as anyone who's seen someone having one, or had one themselves, will tell you. Characteristics include:

- sudden awakening, or sometimes the child can be very difficult to wake while in the throes of the night terror, which can last 5–20 minutes
- sweating and confusion
- extreme fright or terror that is very difficult to soothe
- inability to explain what the matter is or what just happened
- may have no memory of the episode the following day
- may feel they are seeing alarming things in the room (the most common reports are snakes, spiders and non-specific dark figures), which, despite the fact this is so common and well documented by sleep scientists, has led some people to worry the cause may even be a sinister spiritual one.

Sleep terrors, like other sleep problems, tend to have a hereditary aspect and, again like other sleep disorders, can be triggered or made worse by stress, tiredness or over-tiredness, worry, even a heavy meal and certain medications.

Tips for Parents

Anti-sleep-terror measures for young children that parents report they found helpful include:

- five to ten drops of organic lavender oil in the evening bath
  Note: See Nits and Lice on page 283 for advice on use with boys.
- homeopathic Chamomilla 6c
- rests in the afternoon with a cosy blanket and perhaps a taped story to prevent over-tiredness, promote relaxation and reduce any stress build-up.

Something to take

Researchers in Rome have also found that a form of **tryptophan** called **5-HTP**, which is the forerunner of feel-good brain chemical serotonin, helps. They gave it at bedtime in doses of 2 mg per kg of bodyweight to a group of children aged three to ten years. After a month over 90 per cent had at least improved, and by the end of the six-month trial period 84 per cent were completely free of night terrors. In comparison, the study's control group of children (who were given no 5-HTP) got no better over that six-month trial period.[33] For details of supplies of 5-HTP, see Fix 304: Mood Enhancement.

Anti-night-terror essences

Essences can be a gentle way of supporting other night-terror-reducing measures. The powerfully protective remedies **Angelsword** and **Fringed Violet** mixed together would be indicated if you felt there might be a possibility of a spiritual element in the night terrors for a particular individual.

Both are from the Australian Bush Flower range, available direct or from Healthlines (15 ml, £8.95 each). For around £7, the staff there can also mix a remedy bottle up for you – less than half the cost of buying the essences separately yourself. Explain the combination is for a toddler or young child and the Healthlines staff (a cooperative of essence practitioners, teachers, healers and homeopaths) will adjust it accordingly. The mix needs to be taken as dilute drops under the tongue morning and bedtime.

Still on the same subject, Alaskan Essences' sacred-space spray **Guardian** can be very helpful for those who are either a bit more vulnerable than most or very sensitive to their surroundings. It has a lovely, delicate, but refreshing scent. Spray sparingly around the perimeter of the room and the child's bed each evening before they turn in, or they can help you as part of a reassuring going-to-bed ritual.

In the UK, Guardian spray is available via Healthlines (60 ml, £11.95); in the US and Canada, buy it direct from Alaskan Essences (2 fl oz, $11).

For all contact details, see under 'Shopping' in the Directory.

See also General: Sleep on page 92.

Teeth and Teething

286. Tooth Knocked Out

If a tooth is actually knocked clean out of your child's mouth (not uncommon in toddlers unsteady on their feet and active kids who are still learning to control their bodies and balance – one in 12 damages a tooth before the age of five) head straight for the dentist.

If one's not available, go to the nearest A & E. However, *don't* rinse that tooth off under water or put it in an envelope for safekeeping during the trip. Instead, place it in a covered container in some milk. This will help preserve the nerve fibres and any tiny blood vessels inside, thus maximising the chances of a dentist being able to re-implant it success-fully.[34]

287. Teething Babies : Top Quick-Tip

Buy some plastic ice-lolly sticks from the supermarket, dip them in water and place on a small tray in the freezer. The water forms an ice coating, and teething babies find chewing on these cooling, satisfying and soothing. When my children were teething, I used to pour warm water on a soft pillule of **Chamomilla 6c** homeopathic remedy and add that to the lolly-stick water dip as an extra teething-soother.

Chamomilla 6c is available from Boots, health shops and most pharmacies or via Ainsworths. For contact details, see under 'Shopping' in the Directory.

See also Teething Toddlers on page 305.

288. Fluoride – Fearful?

Most ordinary toothpastes contain fluoride, intended to help fight tooth decay. However, not all parents are happy for their children to have it, either in tap water or in toothpaste (lots of pre-schoolers tend to swallow some toothpaste when brushing), as many hundreds of pieces of research have linked it with health problems ranging from mottled or pitted teeth to birth defects, brain damage, bone cancer and osteoporosis.[35]

Fluoride has also been found to cause hyperactivity in rats, but may not have the same effect on children – no one has yet studied it properly to check. The US now has fluoride warnings on toothpaste labels, but the UK doesn't.

'Natural' toothpaste

However, just to make life difficult, there are also some potentially harmful chemicals in 'natural' toothpastes, such as propylene glycol, sodium lauryl sulphate (SLS) and triclosan. Propylene glycol inhibits bacteria growth but is also a neurotoxin and carcinogen; SLS, the ingredient that makes toothpaste (and shampoo for that matter) foam up so becomingly, can strip off the skin's protective oily layer, producing irritation and erosion (which is why it's used in car-wash soaps and de-greasing products for garage floors); and triclosan is an antibacterial agent sometimes added to counteract the irritating effect of SLS, but it can mix with it to create an even more irritating combination – definitely to be avoided if someone's got ulcers or bleeding gums.

Some alternatives

So what's a parent supposed to do? Perhaps see if your child likes one of the following children's fluoride-free natural toothpastes (they also have no artificial sweeteners, colours or preservatives):

- **Children's Tooth Gel**, from Weleda (£1.95), is made from extract of calendula.
- **Children's Mandarin Toothpaste**, from Green People (£2.99), contains organic orange and mandarin essential oils and vitamin C (all of which are natural preservatives).
- **Salvadora Toothpaste**, made by Sarakan, contains extract of *Salvadora persica* – the 'toothbrush tree' – which research has shown to inhibit plaque. [36] Try Goodness Direct (50 g, £1.84).

You can buy these products direct from the companies named above or in selected health shops, via mail order or the Net. Prices will vary. For contact details, see under 'Shopping' in the Directory.

Another alternative is to make your own . . .

Teething Toddlers

Has your toddler got a bright-red teething cheek? Add two drops of chamomile Roman essential oil (which has soothing and anti-inflammatory properties) to a palmful of sweet olive oil, suggests Dr Vivian Lunny, medical aromatherapist and former head of scientific research for the Aromatherapy Organisations Council. Rub the mixture gently on the outside of the affected part of the face. You can buy chamomile Roman from Baldwin's (5 ml, £7.85). For contact details, see under 'Shopping' in the Directory.

See also Fix 287: Teething Babies.

289. DIY Toothpaste

If you've offered your kids a few 'natural' commercial ones and they don't like them ('Ee-*yew*, Mum!'), try this quick and easy DIY recipe:

1 cup baking soda (a gently abrasive, decent tooth-whitener and antibacterial agent)
1/3 cup sea salt
3 teaspoons glycerine (available at pharmacies and major supermarkets)
organic mandarin essential oil

Mix the baking soda, salt and glycerine together. Add a little water to make a good thick paste, plus a few drops of the organic mandarin essential oil to make it taste nicer. And go brush.

Always use organic essential oils for children if you can. Try Star Child's range: Mandarin Oil (10 ml, £5.95). For contact details, see under 'Shopping' in the Directory.

Note: the toothpaste can be kept in an airtight jar, somewhere cool, for a week at a time.

For a version of this for adults, see Fix 117: Tooth Powder – DIY and Fluoride-Free.

Travel Sickness

290. Ginger

The misery of travelling to family holiday destinations may become a thing of the past if you give your child **ginger**. It comes powdered in convenient capsule form, but if these prove awkward for small children to swallow, try ginger tincture, taken as a few drops in water half an hour before setting off, then every three hours or so throughout the journey.

It is well researched for seasickness by the British Navy, and Chinese sailors used to keep a slice of fresh ginger between cheek and gum for the same reason. Ginger can also be really helpful for morning sickness – see Fix 183: Morning Sickness (No. 1) – and the nausea produced by chemotherapy, as well as all types of motion sickness. My own children, who used to be carsick the second we hit any kind of asphalt, would report that they felt 'Not brilliant, but OK' after the tincture or capsules, which was a serious improvement.

If you want to give the capsules a go, try Nature's Best Ginger (90 capsules, £7.95); in the US, try Nutrivea USA (100 x 500 mg capsules, $29.45). For the tincture, go for Organic Ginger Tincture from Napiers (100 ml, £5.15); in the US, try Ginger Root Tincture from Wilderness Family Naturals (1 fl oz, $13.99). For contact details, see under 'Shopping' in the Directory.

See also Teenagers: Travel on page 384.

Urinary-Tract Infections (UTIs)

Infections of the internal plumbing system may involve the bladder, urethra, ureters (tubes bringing urine from the kidneys to the bladder), the kidneys or all of these. Bladder infection, also called cystitis, is the most common type.

Symptoms include painful urination ('stingy wee', as my daughter called it) and stronger or bad-smelling urine, which may also be a bit cloudy, the repeated urge to pass water but only being able to do a little each time and an ache in the lower abdomen when walking or running. Back pain, fever and bed-wetting may be present, and very young children may also feel tired, irritable or have vomiting and diarrhoea. The usual cause is a very common bacteria called E. coli, which is present in waste matter from the back passage, finding its way up the urethra (urine passage) and into the bladder.

If your child is already suffering, encourage them to drink plenty of plain water – glasses and glasses of it – to dilute the sting of the urine and help flush out the bacteria.

To help prevent cystitis and other UTIs in your child:

- **Keep encouraging the water-drinking habit** – though it doesn't have to be the large amount used for the first-flush effect.
- If they are going to the loo rather than using nappies, **teach girls (and boys) to always wipe from front to back,** to discourage the migration of E. coli from the rectal passage to the urinary passage, whether it's recessed in the vulva or emerging at the tip of the penis.

291. Natural Treatments
Cranberry extract
It contains substances called proanthocyanidins, which help stop the E. coli sticking on to the bladder wall. For children, try 200–400 mg a day, depending on their age and weight. Cranberry in packaged juice form is often promoted for cystitis, but this isn't a great option if it contains sugar or artificial sweeteners (and almost all brands do). For **cranberry-extract capsules**, see Higher Nature's Super-Strength Cranberry Extract (30 x 500 mg capsules, £8.90) – for a young child of 40 kg, take half a capsule a day; in the US and Canada, try the Canada Drug Superstore. For contact details, see under 'Shopping' in the Directory.

Cat's claw
Anti-infective and anti-inflammatory, the herb **cat's claw** is sometimes used for UTIs as a second-line treatment for low-level, grumbling infections if the usual measures, either holistic or medical (usually antibiotics), cannot quite get rid of it, says top UK nutritionist and osteopath John Taberman-Pichler. A good infection-fighting complex containing

cat's claw, the immune-system-booster echinacea and goldenseal is available from Solgar in the UK, or, in the US, via Healthy4You (30 capsules, $11.55). For contact details, see under 'Shopping' in the Directory.

Note: check with your nutritionist to see if cat's claw would be suitable in your child's case and to refine exact dosage. For details of organisations that can put you in touch with a nutritionist, see 'Therapies and Therapists' in the Directory.

> ### Warning
>
> UTIs can accelerate fast, becoming extremely uncomfortable and, if they reach the kidneys, may damage them. Should there be *no improvement within 24 hours*, if your child is getting worse instead of better, if there are any traces of blood in their urine or if they have a temperature, see your GP right away.

See also Young Children: Bed-Wetting (Enuresis) on page 253. For more general advice on UTIs, see General: Cystitis on page 41.

Verrucas and Warts

A verruca is a wart that is growing on the sole of the foot, and warts and verrucas of all types are caused by the tenacious little human papilloma virus (HPV). A GP would freeze them off with liquid nitrogen (cryotherapy). However, if you don't much like the sound of this, there are some low-tech natural remedies that have been compared with this conventional medical treatment and come out on top.

292. Getting Warts Taped

One is plain, ordinary **duct tape**. One study compared up to six cryotherapy treatments given two to three times a week with duct tape stuck over the warts. When that tape was changed every six days, the wart was also soaked in warm water and sanded down with a pumice stone, a routine that lasted for two months. At the end of the trial period, 60 per cent of the cryotherapy group were cured, but 85 per cent of the tape group were wart-free.[37]

You can also dab a little tincture of **greater celandine** (*Chelidonium majus*), a traditional anti-wart remedy (ask a herbalist to make it up for you), on the warts each time you change the duct tape to enhance the effect. Preliminary research in China and Russia suggests this is effective, and another study in Sweden found the same.[38]

To find a professionally qualified herbalist near you, contact the National Institute of Medical Herbalists. For contact details, see under 'Therapies and Therapists' in the Directory.

Banana-skin remedy

You can do the same with banana skin, following an old folk remedy for verrucas and warts. Put a small piece of the peel on the affected area, with its soft white inside against the wart, and keep it in place with, yes, a piece of duct tape. Change peel once or twice a day and keep doing so for three weeks, or until the wart has gone.

Worms

There are several natural substances to treat threadworms, sometimes called pinworms, which are thin white things measuring 1–1.5 cm in length. They're very common in children : up to 20 per cent are estimated to be affected at any one time, though they may not realise it.

The problem begins if a child inadvertently swallows a worm egg, which can be passed on via bedding, under the fingernails or in food. They take up residence in the intestine, and the females migrate to the host's anus at night to lay yet more eggs. That tends to cause a very red and itchy anal area; scratching puts yet more eggs under the nails and so the cycle goes on.

Anti-worm DIY

- Wash hands thoroughly on waking each morning, every evening and after every loo-break.
- Nail-brush (you can use an old toothbrush) under the nails to remove any eggs.
- Keep nails short.
- Add a few drops of tea-tree oil to the water you're washing in to help kill the eggs. (See note on page 259 about use of tea-tree oil.)

293. Natural Anti-Parasitics to Take

- **Grapefruit-seed extract** – UK holistic physician Dr John Briffa suggests giving five to ten drops in diluted fruit juice three times daily for seven days. Try Citricidal from Higher Nature (45 ml, £6.90; 100 tablets, £10.50); in the US, it's called just grapefruit-seed extract and is available from NutriTeam (2 fl oz, $6.95).
- **Garlic** – try giving 1 g garlic-extract capsules (odourless, unlike the oil capsules) once or twice daily for 7–14 days. You can buy garlic extract from Healthy Direct (60 x 1 g odourless capsules, £2.95).

For all contact details, see under 'Shopping' in the Directory.

Note: if the worm problem hasn't resolved within 14 days of using natural remedies and prevention measures, you'll need some extra help in the form of medication from your GP, who will probably suggest treating the entire family.

Teenagers

Teenagers aren't just younger versions of adults, whatever advertising and marketing agencies may say, though they may look (and act) like them sometimes. Halfway between childhood and maturity with many sensitivities, problems, issues and challenges that are totally unique to the six years between 13 and 19, teens are a very special species unto themselves.

This section looks at all sorts of things that teenagers may find helpful, from which natural hangover cures actually do work (one particular homeopathic remedy packs a remarkable punch here) and the gentle holistic acne treatment that's as effective as conventional drugs but without their side effects, to the essences that help heal a broken heart, the aromatherapy oils that ensure teenagers revise better and the specific nutrients that reduce aggression. Whether it's body odour or eating disorders, you might just find the very thing you need – just when you need it – in the following pages . . .

Acne and Spots

294. Acne

You can make an excellent natural anti-acne cream by adding five to seven drops of pure organic **tea-tree aromatherapy essential oil** to 50 ml base cream or oil; a bland one containing vitamin E for healing any acne scarring is ideal. Shake well to mix.

Tea tree is antibacterial, as confirmed in 2000 by a review of four strict randomised controlled clinical trials (the sort respected by doctors and scientists as gold-standard research).[1] In fact, another clinical trial found a 5 per cent tea-tree cream performs just as well as conventional spot-zapping cream containing the standard 5 per cent of the chemical benzoyl peroxide (BZ) – and caused considerably *less* of the 'scaliness, redness and itching' often seen with conventional BZ-containing anti-acne products from the chemist's.

Products containing tea tree are available from most health shops, including branches of Neal's Yard, Holland & Barrett and the Body Shop – e.g. the Body Shop's antiseptic Tea-Tree-Oil Facial Wash (250 ml, £5.50/$10). In the US, there's a stronger ready-mixed product available called Skin Energizer Cream (available direct from Skin Energizer). For contact details, see under 'Shopping' in the Directory.

Note: do not use on inflamed acne. As tea tree can also cause skin irritation and an allergic reaction, keep a close eye on how your teenager's skin reacts. It is not suitable during pregnancy.

295. Spots – Beat the 'Yuck' Factor

If your teenager has spots and is distressed by them in the sense that he or she thinks these are yucky, gross or that they themselves are 'ugh' or 'unclean', soothe this feeling with **Crab Apple** (*Malus pumila*) essence by Bach Flower Essences, from Healing Herbs or Healthlines (10 ml, £3.99). For contact details, see under 'Shopping' in the Directory.

This one's the 'feeling clean all through' remedy from Dr Bach's original collection, made from plants in his gentle Oxfordshire country garden. Take four drops under the tongue or in a glass of water three to four times a day. They can also add ten drops to a warm, relaxing, evening bath until they feel better about themselves

308. Spot-Zapper

Get some of that old-fashioned **magnesium-sulphate paste** from the chemist's and dab it on overnight. It draws out spots nicely, especially the red, angry ones that need to come to a head fast so you can get rid of them.

Belonging – a sense of

Being a teenager can be hard, and living with one who is finding life difficult isn't easy either. The Native American Indians call this period when you are journeying into adulthood 'the thundering years'regarding this as the time for the boy or girl to listen to intense feelings, dreams, desires and goals, and to be outrageous, even downright difficult, *because they need to be*. They acknowledge adolescence as an exciting, energy-powered time full of potential and creative energy – but also one which can be painful, seething with turmoil and riddled with self-doubt.

296. The Essence that Helps You Feel Part of Things

There is a lovely essence called **Wolf** that can help see teens through their thundering years as and when they need it, developed by an ex-wilderness guide, therapist and spiritual counsellor called Daniel Mapel, which he recommended especially for this section in the book. He has a remarkable range of 88 essences based on different animal energies from both the US plains and forests and the African savannahs (all made without touching a hair on any animal's head).

'Wolf is primarily used for helping people feel socially connected with others – a big part of the teenage years, especially for boys, is feeling isolated in one's own experiences, not having a language or community to talk with and make sense of what is going on,' says Mapel. 'Wolf helps with all that, nurturing a feeling of kinship and connection with others, breaking down that sense of isolation.'

Wolf is made by Wild Earth Animal Essences. In the UK, you can buy it from Healthlines (30 ml, £8.95); in the US, buy it direct from Wild Earth Animal Essences. For contact details, see under 'Shopping' in the Directory.

Aggression and Disruptive Behaviour

Excessive aggression is multi-causal, so there are no quick fixes, but different strategies work for different individuals, depending on their own particular mix of contributing factors and triggers. And it tends to be a considered package of separate techniques, all complementing and backing each other up, that helps the most – with parents and teenagers working together to discover, often by a spot of trial and error, what suits best.

However, recent clinical studies show that **a nutritional approach**, one using both supplements, and healthy food, improves things to some extent for the greatest number of teenagers (and adults too for that matter) so this one's a very sensible first-base measure, especially if the person's diet is not too terrific.

297. Nutritional Approach

1. **Dump the junk.** Remove all junk, fast and processed foods and drinks from the teenager's diet and feed them as healthily as possible. See also Fix 238: A Junk-Free Diet.
2. **Up EFAs.** Give essential fatty acids (the omega-3 and omega-6 varieties), plus certain key minerals and vitamins. These include magnesium, zinc and B6, all well known for their beneficial calming and balancing effect on the neurological system. See also Fix 239: Helpful Nutrients and Supplements.
3. Take **a good quality one a day multi vitamin and mineral supplement**: VM-75 (Solgar, 60 capsules, £17.50) or Multiguard (Lambert's, £17.50 for 90) are both good – see Shopping. Keep this up for three months, as this is how long it takes for a decent concentration of the minerals and vitamins you are short of or lacking altogether, to build up in your intercellular fluid (which is what needs to happen before they can start making a real difference). It is possible, though, that you may notice improvements starting after just 4 – 6 weeks.

About EFAs

- Essential fatty acids are called that because they are essential to us.
- We can't synthesise them for ourselves – we need to get them from our food or from supplements.
- Pro-EFA foods include *oily* fish (e.g. salmon, mackerel and tuna), **nuts, seeds** and **green leafy vegetables**.
- Modern food-processing techniques tend to strip many of the EFAs from our food before it even reaches our mouth.

- Nutrition experts believe this may be one of the reasons why aggression and behavioural or learning disorders are now more common than they were 50 years ago.

Research studies led by US criminologist Dr Stephen Schoenthaler have shown that antisocial and violent behaviour are often linked with substandard nutrition and that supplementing with EFAs improves matters.[2]

A recent UK trial by the University of Oxford has shown supplementation with EFAs plus additional minerals and vitamins can even calm down young adult prisoners. The investigators saw a reduction of 35 per cent in just two weeks in violent incidents and 'antisocial behaviour' among the inmates who were given supplements, whereas those who received dummy pills carried on as before.[3]

In one study when chemical additives, sugar and refined-flour products were taken out of the diets of 8,000 youngsters in youth detention centres in the US, their levels of difficult or disruptive behaviour dropped by almost half. Another piece of research involving 500 young offenders is now under way in Holland; French prison services have also expressed an interest.

Once someone's nutrition is improved and they have enough EFAs in their system, they are likely to be more stable neurologically and so more willing to try out any other treatments or initiatives which could help to help combat their aggression (whether these are behavioural techniques and counselling, or defensive martial art training and regular outdoor exercise). Those interventions are more likely to work for them now, too.

Better brain food for teens
It is probably no coincidence that most antisocial behaviour is down to teenage males. This is partly fuelled by rising testosterone levels, but it also happens when their fast-growing bodies start competing fiercely with their brains for vital neurological nutrients (the sort that junk food doesn't provide much of). 'Around puberty is a really crucial time – it's the second biggest burst of brain development after foetal

development,' says John Stein, professor of neuroscience at the University of Oxford.

The brain is a metabolic powerhouse. While it only makes up 2 per cent of our body mass, it takes up 20 per cent of available energy from food. Brains are also 60 per cent fat, and the insulation around nerves ensuring smooth conduction of signals up and down them is also fatty, two more reasons why EFAs are so valuable for the nervous system.

Where to get EFAs

Try brands like Efamol's **Efamarine**, which was used in the UK prison trial, available from Boots, Superdrug, Holland & Barrett and other health shops in the UK (90 capsules, £9.99); in the US, you can buy it from Academy Health (90 capsules, $16.50).

Also see **Eye Q** by Equazen, which contains fish oil and evening primrose oil. For teenagers, it's usually recommended that they should take around six to eight capsules a day with food for the first three months, then drop down to a maintenance dose of approximately two to three capsules daily, unless otherwise directed by their physician or nutritionist. You can buy it in Boots or via the manufacturer's website (60 x 500 mg capsules, £7.99).

Another option is **VegEPA**, which is suitable for vegetarians and available in the UK from Igennus.

For all contact details, see under 'Shopping' in the Directory.

298. Light Therapy

> What's natural, non-invasive and encourages good behaviour? Daylight.

Light – that is, real outdoor full-spectrum (FS) daylight unmediated by tinted glasses or contact lenses, windscreens and windows – plays a powerful part in our health and affects many aspects of it, from our blood pressure and rate of dental decay to hormonal output, fitness levels, sporting stamina and weight loss.

Natural light is a vital nutrient in the form of pure raw energy – one that is both free and limitless. It has long been used to treat neonatal jaundice, psoriasis and herpes infections; it also has a powerfully positive effect on behaviour, mood and learning ability. There are many good studies with adults, animals and children (both primary-school age and teenagers) that support this.[4]

Most of us – including teenagers – spend the majority of our time in surroundings that have the wrong kind of artificial lighting: at school, college and most work environments, especially if they involve computer screens and harsh fluorescent strip lighting. Added to that, we spend less and less time out of doors. Yet photobiologists – the scientists who specialise in the study of light's effect on living creatures, working, for instance, in the American Society of Photobiology – plus doctors, psychiatrists and natural therapists who use FS light treatment for their patients, all agree you can use *both natural and artificial FS light* to:

- reduce behavioural problems
- improve learning difficulties.

And, as extensive research in Russian schools and the Center for the Improvement of Undergraduate Education at Cornell University both found, FS lighting also:

- cuts study fatigue
- helps students concentrate better.

Experience in US schools backs this up too. After full-spectrum lights were installed in five classrooms in Sarasota, Florida, in 1973, a group of extremely hyperactive, learning-disabled children calmed down significantly and learnt to read. Absenteeism dropped. However, children in four classrooms with ordinary lights continued to act up – they were being tracked by concealed motion-detecting cameras – and their learning disabilities and numbers of days off school remained the same.[5]

Similar results were reported from schools in California, Colville in Washington and Alberta, Canada.[6] A classroom comparison in Vermont accidentally found full-spectrum lighting strengthened the students' immunity. And Texas's Fort Worth Education District, which was one of the first in the US to bring in sodium lighting (which isn't full spectrum) when it was initially fashionable, was also one of the first to take it back out again because so many pupils and teachers complained of headaches, eye strain, difficulty concentrating and other problems. The list goes on. You get the idea.

FS light therapy for teens at home

To help strengthen your teenager's concentration and promote calmer behaviour (perhaps especially for boys at a time when these qualities may traditionally start to slip a bit):

1. Ensure they get at least half an hour outside in full-spectrum light every day. How about suggesting an extra outdoor sport after school in longer daytime hours, biking or walking part of the way to college or an after-school paper round, which also boosts their spending money?
2. Up their FS hours at home. Install full-spectrum lighting (ceiling, or maybe a bedside or desk lamp) in the room or rooms where your teenager spends the most time: perhaps the kitchen, if that's somewhere your family tends to congregate to talk and eat, the TV den or rumpus room, or your teenager's bedroom.
3. Lobby their school or college to change classroom lighting to full spectrum, if they've not already done so.

Further information

Recommended reading: for further information to use as informed ammunition, see the excellent *Light, Radiation and You* and *Health and Light: the Effect of Natural and Artificial Light on Man and Other Living Things*. Both titles are by the pioneering photobiologist Dr John Ott, who's been researching and working in this area for 50 years. Dr Ott is also director of the Environmental Health and Light Research Institute in Sarasota, Florida. See also Michael Holick MD's *The UV Advantage*. Holick is a world authority on the effect of light on health and was head of department at Boston University before, it is alleged, being asked to step down because of his radical views.

Product possibilities

There's a flood of full-spectrum light products currently on the market, and some are rather better than others.

In the UK, the following are flagged up in a special report by *What Doctors Don't Tell You* magazine (prices 2005): the Lumie Bodyclock Advanced (an alarm clock and light that you can set to create FS gradual sunrise and sunset – teenagers like this one as it's gadgety but has a cool design and another practical function apart from being a 'health lamp'), available from Allergy Matters (£97); the Sunshine Simulator (flicker-free desktop light) from Natural Collection (£169); Solux True Daylight lamps from Outside In, such as the Single-Arm Task Lamp (61 cm high, £99.95 including UK delivery); and Daylight Bulbs from the Natural Approach (from £3.50 each).

In the US, OttLights' Chromalux lamps fit into existing fixtures and simulate natural daylight. Although initially more expensive than ordinary lights, they use lower wattage and last ten times longer. You can buy them direct from OttLight Systems.

For all contact details, see under 'Shopping' in the Directory.

For more product information, see General: Seasonal Affective Disorder (SAD) on page 85 and Fix 72: Bright Light. For information about the difference between full-spectrum and broad-spectrum light, see Notes on page 548.

See also General: Anger and Aggression on page 9.

299. Bashes and Bruises

If your sporty teenager responds to offers to 'put something soothing' on a bash or bruise with, 'Leave *off*, I'm fine,' they're unlikely to accept a nice rub with arnica cream three times daily. A **stick-on arnica patch** may be a different matter, however. Just stick one on-site for sore areas. You can leave them there for up to 24 hours, useful for relaxing stiff muscles, especially shoulders, and for relieving bruising and sprains, as they help reduce local inflammation from soft-tissue damage. If the area's large, you can use several of them.

You can get Naturopatch in the UK from Victoria Health (10 patches, £7.99); in the US and Canada, you can buy them direct from Naturopatch of Vermont (10 patches, $15). For contact details, see under 'Shopping' in the Directory.

See also General: Bruises on page 29 and Men: Black Eye on page 208.

Alcohol

It's a fact – underage teenagers are drinking more than ever in both the UK and the US, with British teens taking more drugs and drinking more alcohol than in any other European country, despite having the most restrictive laws. In fact, one study by Belfast's Royal Victoria Hospital found 40 per cent of 15- to 16-year-olds had been binge-drinking or drunk in the past month and 50 per cent drank regularly.

And the latest research (2006) by New York's Columbia University stated, 'America has an epidemic of underage drinking which germinates in the *elementary* – and middle – schools,' adding that they estimated a quarter of all alcohol sold was consumed by underage drinkers. Focus Adolescent Services estimates that the average age for US boys to begin drinking is 11, for girls it's 13, and the average age for teens to be doing so regularly is from around 16.

Parents can help their children out here by talking with them about how to drink safely, so they don't end up doing something they would not normally have wanted to and put their health or personal security in jeopardy.

300. Hangover Prevention

A decent stomach-lining snack before going out partying, clubbing or pubbing is key to being able to drink enough to get happy but reduce the risk of drunkenness and hangover.

A glass of **full-fat milk** (as opposed to skimmed or semi) is good. Not because, as traditionally thought, it 'lines the stomach' – any food will do that – but because its high fat content makes the body produce a substance that slows the stomach-emptying process, meaning any alcohol someone then drinks will go through their system more gradually, reducing the risk of major drunk-making alcohol-absorption peaks.

301. Hangover Cure

This simple, tried and tested natural hangover cure deals with both the dehydration and the low blood sugar (hypoglycaemia) that excess drinking causes. Dr Andrew Irving (author of *How to Cure a Hangover*) suggests a little **porridge** sweetened with **honey, sugar** or **maple syrup**. The carbohydrates in the oats have a low glycaemic index (GI) so they are absorbed slowly, thus steadily raising and maintaining higher blood sugar ratings, while the sweet topping works fast to boost blood sugar levels right away.

302. Concerned?

Although alcohol and getting drunk may often be seen as a rite of passage for teens, if parents do find they are becoming concerned about the amount they believe their teenager is consuming, help and information is available in the UK from Alcohol Concern, which provides free fact sheets on teenagers and alcohol, and has a helpline. You can also talk to ParentLine Plus, a charity running a free helpline for parents needing support and information about a range of issues, including teenage drinking. In the US, for treatment referrals try National Drugs and Alcohol Treatment Referral Routing. For contact details, see under 'Useful Helplines, Websites and Contacts' in the Directory.

Anorexia

Figures and Triggers

Anorexia is an illness involving severe, deliberate restriction of food intake and an obsession that you are fat. It can develop when someone is having difficulty coping with the problems, worries or feelings they have and begins to use food reduction as a means of trying to regain some control over their life or of expressing profound distress, anger or resentment that they don't feel they can communicate in any other way.

The number of people suffering from anorexia has more than doubled in the West since 1970,[7] and the number of people affected to some degree at some point in their lives is between one in 50 and one in

100 of those aged 15–30 in both the UK and the US – that's half a million in Britain, and some two million in the USA.

Teenagers most at risk include those training to be or working as dancers, actors, athletes and models. There is also evidence that high-achieving girls who set themselves (or are set) demandingly high standards can be especially vulnerable because of the pressures and expectations that are often placed upon them by their schools or colleges, their parents or both. Being bombarded with media images of size-zero girls like Keira Knightley, Victoria Beckham and Amy Winehouse really doesn't help either.

Around 10 per cent of school-age teenagers affected by anorexia are boys who have become obsessed with exercise and physical training.

A survey in 2005 of more than 2,000 girls by the British teen magazine *Bliss* found that 92 per cent were unhappy with the way their bodies look and *one in four* had some form of eating disorder (anorexia, bulimia and binge-eating)

Symptoms

Symptoms include severe weight loss, absence of periods, obsession over calories and weight, excessive exercise, difficulty concentrating, dizziness and a distorted self-image (dysmorphia – i.e. looking in a mirror and genuinely perceiving the reflection to be much fatter than the person truly is). Anorexia may also coexist with other eating disorders, such as bulimia, and with self-harming.

Medical Treatments

The conventional medical help available includes helping the person to learn to eat normally again and to gain weight. However, that often isn't enough on its own to prevent relapse, because the underlying issues and causes need to be addressed as well, and many enlightened psychologists now take the approach that anorexia is as much a symptom as a disorder.

It is something that won't go away on its own unless its form is mild and transitory – and, if left unchecked, can be fatal. A teenager with anorexia will usually need:

- expert help
- a good support system in the medium to long term.

This may include specialist counselling from a health professional, backup from a self-help support group, behavioural therapy and group or family therapy. It is important that your teenager not only feels comfortable with their health professional but that the person has solid experience of, or a special interest in, the disorder (which rules out the average GP and many psychologists).

Antidepressants or being an in-patient for a while at a specialist unit may sometimes be suggested. And though the majority of people with anorexia do get well over time, this may take anything from several months to several years, and during that period they will need lots of love and support at home.

The Eating Disorders Association is a good first port of call for teenagers affected by anorexia (or any other eating disorder) and for parents who would like to understand the condition better and find out where to get help. They have a Youthline number for under-18s, and if you email or text a support worker there, they will reply to you via the same route. For contact details, see under 'Useful Helplines, Websites and Contacts' in the Directory.

Complementary Treatments

A two-pronged approach has been found to help with anorexia: this includes normalising and improving self-image and stabilising mood. Nutrition can be helpful – not just from from the 'eating more' point of view, but also taking some very particular minerals, vitamins and other nutrients that seem to speed recovery and redress biochemical imbalance. Zinc is one, tryptophan another.

303. Self-Image – Zinc Supplements
Which and why
Zinc has a lot of different roles in the body, but one of them is the

normalisation of brain function and perception. In one study published in *The Lancet*, it was found that anorexics and bulimics have, biologically, a lower uptake of zinc and that their eating patterns and digestive behaviour (such as making themselves vomit regularly after eating and using laxatives excessively) further reduce the amount of zinc they absorb, making the problem worse.[8] But work in 1992 by Dr Rita Bakan and her colleagues at the British Columbia Institute of Technology found that taking extra zinc can help stabilise someone with anorexia and encourage faster weight gain.[9]

The best and most easily absorbed type of zinc is **zinc picolinate** – in fact, it's so well absorbed that you may need only half the dose you'd take of ordinary chelated zinc.

Try Holland & Barrett's Zinc Picolinate (100 x 25 mg tablets, £6.99). For contact details, see under 'Shopping' in the Directory.

Note: if you suspect zinc deficiency, also check what sort of fillings your teenager has in their teeth, if any.

Visit a mercury-free dentist

'Silver' dental amalgam fillings containing mercury may well be linked to zinc deficiency, says pioneering British holistic dentist Jack Levenson. Amalgam mercury leaches progressively into the body as the filling material ages. (You can tell this is happening if a silvery one's gone grey or, worse still, black.) Mercury, besides being highly poisonous, blocks zinc absorption, and as we have seen, zinc deficiency can be a significant factor in anorexia.

Levenson says he has seen many young girls diagnosed with eating disorders recover after their amalgam fillings were removed and harmless white ones put in their place. For where to find a holistic dentist in both the UK and the US who does not use amalgam and can remove old mercury fillings *safely*, see under 'Therapies and Therapists' in the Directory.

See also Fix 119: Mercury Amalgam Fillings and Fix 116: Addressing Mercury Toxicity.

Note: do not, whatever you do, ask an 'ordinary' dentist to remove old mercury amalgam fillings – you risk ingesting a massive dose of mercury when they are drilled out.

304. Mood Enhancement – Tryptophan

Nutritionist Maryon Stewart, and clinical nutritionist (a doctor with specialist nutritional training) Dr Alan Stewart, the pioneering team behind the nutritional approach to beating PMS and menopause and founders of the UK's excellent Women's Nutritional Advisory Service (which has now become part of the Natural Health Advisory Service) suggest trying **tryptophan** supplements.

This is because even moderate dieting lowers levels of tryptophan and of the mood-moderating hormone serotonin – both of which affect your eating behaviour and the way you feel about food. Research suggests that serotonin levels in anorexics are lower than normal and remain that way even when they've put weight back on.[10] If you would like your teenager to try this, look for a 5-HTP supplement (5-HTP is tryptophan's precursor) like Higher Nature's Serotone 5-HTP (30 x 30 mg capsules, £8.10). Or, some nutritionists say better still, look for pure tryptophan itself but do not use it with antidepressants.

Note: pure tryptophan is banned in the UK and US, but not in mainland Europe or Canada, and is widely available in Japan. You can therefore buy it in the UK and the US through the Internet from Physician Formulas (60 x 500 mg capsules, $33.95). 5-HTP can be bought freely both over the counter and via the Net in the UK and the US. It does not work quite so well, but it is easier to get hold of.

Add to this a **good-quality one-a-day multivitamin and mineral supplement**, as after restricting food intake so drastically, someone with anorexia will be short of just about everything, but particularly vital are iron, calcium, the B vitamins, folic acid and vitamin C. Good ones to take include Solgar's Formula VM75 from Green's (60 capsules, £17.50) and Multi-Guard for Young Adults from Nature's Best.

For all contact details, please see under 'Shopping' in the Directory.

305. Essences for Anorexia

These are increasingly used in conjunction with other natural therapies for anorexia to help normalise a person's perception of themselves and their appearance and to raise their self-esteem.

Three of the most helpful are **Loquat, Salvia** – and the **My Body** combination, one of the new Urban Angels range developed specially to support teenagers facing major challenges to both their emotional and physical health (see pp 379). Salvia was developed by master herbalist and aromatherapist Dr Judy Griffin, who also works with the Baylor Medical Center in Dallas and the Texas Cancer Care Center in Fort Worth. The essences are taken as drops under the tongue or in a glass of water two to four times daily. They can also be added to a gentle, healing bath every night.

Loquat is available direct from South African Essences (15 ml, approximately £7), and Salvia is available in the UK via IFER (3.8 ml, £7.50) and the Nutri Centre; in the US, try Petite Fleur Essences ($18). My Body is available direct from Light Heart Essences, or via Victoria Health. For contact details, see under 'Shopping' in the Directory.

306. Aromatherapy for Anorexia

The one every therapist I have ever spoken to recommends is **rose absolu**. This the most nurturing, beautiful and female of aromatherapy oils. It can be added to a bath (just a couple of drops, since it's pretty powerful and is also quite expensive, though worth it).

The effect of this queen of essential oils has been described as 'feeling like someone just put a loving mother's arms round you' (which is why it is also often used for post-natal depression). Also a mood-enhancer, this rich form of rose helps users feel good about their femaleness too – something that many anorexics do not.

For suppliers in the UK and the US, try Neal's Yard's Rose Absolute Oil (2.5 ml, £15.40); or if you want some special good-quality organic rose oil, try Star Child (trial bottle, 1 ml, £7.95). For contact details, see under 'Shopping' in the Directory.

307. The Forgiveness Process

This is a great deal more important and effective than it may at first sound. There is nothing weak or wet about forgiveness. Done in the right frame of mind and the right way, you are not surrendering your power, nor are you saying that it no longer matters that someone has wronged you.

Forgiveness is a powerful emotional and spiritual choice whereby you acknowledge that, yes, this person *has* hurt you and that, yes, it does matter – perhaps it matters a great deal – but that you now choose to let this go in order to be free from the person who harmed you. And perhaps even more importantly, you are making a conscious and deliberate choice to set aside the burden of energy-consuming resentment, distress and anger against them that you have probably been carrying for some time. This may be especially relevant for someone who has developed anorexia, because there is frequently great resentment (and other major issues) involving parents in the equation somewhere. For a girl, the issues are often to do with her relationship with her mother.

Yet bad as things may have been, forgiveness can actually set you free of them for ever and let you get on with your life without anything holding you back. Not for nothing do healers say that forgiveness, if it's freely and unconditionally given when a person is good and ready, is – next to unconditional love – the most powerful healing force there is.

For a way to go about the **Forgiveness Process** so that it brings maximum relief, freedom and benefit to both you and others, see Appendix 2: The Forgiveness Process on page 541.

If, as a teenager, you feel you might like some support with this (and proper back up can help greatly here), either a good trained counsellor or a professional healer could, with your parents' permission, support and guide you. In the UK, try the National Federation of Spiritual Healers and the British Association for Counselling and Psychotherapy; in the US, try the American Association of Healers and the American Counseling Association. For contact details, see under 'Therapies and Therapists' in the Directory.

See also Teenagers: Body Image on page 330.

Anxiety

308. Nervous and Worried

There's a quick, easy, 'keep calm' trick to teach a teenager – for those times when deep breathing and the mantra 'I will not panic' just don't cut it. Suggested by Angela Parker, a former NHS nurse in the special care unit of the Royal Sussex County Hospital, now a clinical reflexologist and aromatherapist with two teenage daughters and a busy practice based in Sussex.

Use the tip or nail edge of your index finger to feel around halfway down the ball of your thumb of the same hand, just in the centre. If you're anxious or hyped this usually feels tender. Rotate your fingertip there gently but firmly for two minutes. Release, then repeat every five minutes until calm descends.

One of the best things about this one, apart from the fact it works, is that no one can tell you are doing anything. Results are not sudden or dramatic, but you gradually realise that you are feeling better than you were.

309. Presentation or Interview Nerves

When your child reaches 15, this is the time they have to start being more proactive academically – doing stand-up presentations of their own work, oral exams for languages and interviews for sixth-form colleges and then universities – all of which can be pretty daunting for most until they get used to it, and a source of real stress for some.

Help soothe their nerves and boost their confidence quietly with a great anti-worry essence called **Crowea**, made from the rather regal little five-petalled *Crowea saligna* flower, which grows on tough metre-high shrubs along the sandstone ridges of coastal New South Wales.

Seven drops under the tongue the night before the presentation or interview, again in the morning and, if required, another discreet seven just before they go in soothes worry and stress, bringing balance, calm and promoting that wonderful '*I can do this*' feeling.

Crowea is an Australian Bush Flower remedy. It is available direct or from Healthlines (15 ml, £8.95). For contact details, see under 'Shopping' in the Directory.

Bedrooms

310. Their Room – a Fetid Teenage Pit?

Apart from opening the window (and tidying up if permitted), what will freshen up a fetid pit of a room that your teenager has been lurking in with the door firmly shut for days?

Try the **Silver-Violet Flame**. This is a fast, powerful technique that can be very effective at removing atmospheric dross and stale vibes, yet takes only seconds.

It is based on the first law of physics – and one of the first laws of esoterics as well – which states that 'Energy can neither be created nor destroyed, merely changed from one form into another.' For all practical purposes, this means that it is possible to change or 'transmute' negative (oppressive, gungy and unpleasant) energy into positive (fresh, bright and light) energy, which is far nicer to live with.

How to do it

1. Open the door and window. Let fresh air blow through.
2. Tidy up minimally if you're allowed to. If not, proceed to Step 3.
3. Say clearly and firmly, either in your head or out loud:

> Dear Silver-Violet Flame of Transmutation and Grace,
> which was given to this planet by the mighty Archangel Zadkiel
> to increase the level of positivity here, in love and respect in the
> name of Light, I ask you to come to this room.
> Blaze all the way through it, from its very lowest point to its
> very highest point, under every object, and in every corner –
> transmuting everything and anything that is of a negative
> nature within or upon this room to 100 per cent positive
> vibration and burn away all the dross.
> Please – do this – NOW

As you speak the word 'now', imagine a bright silver flame tinged with violet appearing in the centre of the room – or on the bed – as if someone has just lit a firework.

See that silver-violet light grow and become blindingly bright, until it fills the entire room.

'Send' it under the bed, into the corners, blast into the cupboards, sweep it along shelves and across all surfaces like a flame-thrower and especially aim it at piles of discarded clothes – unless you can take them all away and wash them – and the bed.

When you've finished, give the entire room one last huge blast of silver-violet fire.

Repeat three times if you feel the space was pretty bad. One of the other major laws of the universe is that if you ask with positive intent for something to be done (so long as it's for the best) three times, it will be.

Say thank you and mean it. Leave the room (preferably still with the window open). Put your head back round the door five minutes later. There. How does it feel now?

Body Image

311. Getting Real
If your teenage daughter is unhealthily obsessed with her 'chunky thighs', thinks her hips or waist is too big, that she's fatter than everyone else, cannot be talked out of it and it's making her unhappy – that way dysmorphia and eating disorders lie. So try offering some real facts and statistics (the reality-check treatment). Positive, accurate information is an empowering holistic healing approach to dysfunctional self-perception. She may be slightly reassured to hear about what's genuinely normal in the sense that 'Everyone else is like this too.'

In a March 2006 survey, *Heat* magazine reported that in fact:

The average waist in the UK is 84cm (33in); in the US, it's 90cm (35.5in)

The average set of British hips is 104cm (41in); in the US, it's 109cm (43in)

The average weight for a 16- to 24-year-old British girl is 64.5kg (10 st. 2lb).

Oh, and stunning Liv Tyler's a size 14, actress Kate Winslet's hips were 99 cm (39 in), which suited her lush *Titanic* costumes to a T, and Beyoncé and Charlotte Church are also curvy and proud.

Bulimia

Bulimia nervosa is a psychological disorder that disrupts a person's ability to keep to a normal eating pattern. Not just an eating disease, as it has been labelled in the past, this is, says the UK's Royal College of Psychiatrists (RCP), a serious mental health problem. People with bulimia tend to binge (over-eat frantically), then panic and get rid of what they just had as soon as possible by self-induced vomiting, laxatives, diuretics, or a combination of the three.

Figures and Triggers

Bulimia has many of the same causes and triggers as anorexia and shares some of its characteristics – i.e. it's a condition that starts gradually, often almost accidentally, but can quickly become a destructive, compulsive coping strategy; and it also tends to begin around puberty.

It's thought that a quarter of all women will, at some time in their lives, suffer from a degree of bulimia, especially if they were overweight as children or young teenagers.

Bulimia may start in the early teens, but, unlike anorexia, it often stays hidden for many years before becoming apparent in someone's later teenage years or early twenties. The disorder affects an estimated one in 30 of all teenage girls, and while young men also experience it, it is ten times less common for them.

Bulimia is a complex and secretive illness. And because there is often no drastic weight loss as with anorexia, it tends to remain unnoticed for longer, though a person may leave small deliberate clues in the hope these will be found, and that they will either be heard or offered the support they would like to have.

Bulimic?
Consider the possibility of bulimia if two or more of the following sound at all familiar. Your teenager:

- is spending long, inexplicable periods in the bathroom with the door locked

- has become really obsessive about calories or exercise
- is becoming secretive about eating and shopping
- has regularly started having what they explain as tummy upsets
- has bought laxatives or dietetics
- has left occasional signs of vomiting, perhaps not totally erased, in the bathroom or loo
- has a puffier face and fingers than usual.

Other symptoms may include:

- poor sleep
- persistent tiredness
- depression
- constipation
- irregular periods
- tooth decay
- increased hair growth on the face or body
- difficulty concentrating
- decreasing interest in life or other people.

Medical Treatments

Bulimia is not easy to overcome, but over half all those who have it recover completely, with perhaps only the very occasional lapse in stressful times. Because it is a serious mental disorder and not deliberately disruptive behaviour, it is important not to become angry or blame the person for something they are unable to stop doing, but instead to show them you love them, be there for them without judgement and persuade them to allow you to help them get the right professional support as soon as possible.

Professional help for bulimia comes in two forms. One is antidepressants (like Prozac), which, though often useful in the short term, are of no real value long term and can have unwanted side effects. The other is talking therapy. Two types of the latter are used for bulimia: interpersonal therapy (looking at the person's relationships with others) and, the most successful one, cognitive behavioural therapy, which looks more at the individual's own feelings and fears and then encourages them to develop different behaviour patterns.

Complementary Treatments

See the essential aromatherapy oils, gems and essences under Teenagers: Anorexia on page 321 for boosting self-esteem, helping someone feel loved and enhancing a positive body image, as they will support people with bulimia too. The following nutritional approach can also be of considerable help to bulimic teenagers:

312. Nutritional Method

Stabilising blood sugar
Bulimia is thought to be essentially a psychological disorder, but there is evidence that there can be underlying nutritional factors at play too. One is blood sugar balance.

When blood sugar fluctuates or drops, this can trigger food cravings and mood swings in *everyone* (e.g. the 4 p.m. energy dip at work that makes the most sensible eater want – or actually go buy and eat – a large, squashy Danish pastry). In one study, a group of bulimic women were put on a diet designed to keep their blood sugar levels steady. Every single one of them stopped bingeing while they ate this way and, continuing the regime, were still binge-free two and a half years later, which is impressive, given that the standard recovery rate using psychotherapy and/or medication is around 50 per cent.[11]

For a try-it-and-see DIY approach, try the **glycaemic index (GI) diet** (an eating plan that keeps blood sugar rock steady) – see Fix 181: Eat the GI Way. Also see Snack Attack on page 514.

Tryptophan and vitamin B6
Tryptophan is an amino acid that the body makes into the feel-good chemical serotonin. Serotonin affects eating patterns and appetite. In one study, researchers, suspecting bulimia might be connected with lower-than-normal levels of serotonin, gave women who binge-ate 3 g tryptophan, plus 45 mg **vitamin B6** (which is thought to help with the conversion of tryptophan into serotonin) a day for four weeks. They gave

a control group a dummy placebo treatment. The group taking trypto-phan and B6 felt happier, and their eating patterns and feelings about food in general were more stable.[12]

Top British nutritionist and author of *Natural Health for Kids* Dr John Briffa suggests that teenagers over 16 might benefit from 50 mg 5-HTP two to three times daily. For more information and sources, see Fix 304: Mood Enhancement – Tryptophan.

Note: do not use pure tryptophan with antidepressants.

To find professional nutritional help, contact the Natural Health Advisory Service (incorporating the Women's Nutritional Advisory Service) or the Institute of Optimum Nutrition. For contact details, see under 'Therapies and Therapists' in the Directory.

See also Teenagers: Body Image on page 330 and Fix 307: The Forgiveness Process.

Colds

313. Student Sore Throat

Teenagers burning the candle at both ends, refusing anything but a cute little short jacket (girls) or a T-shirt (boys) in freezing temperatures and being in a hothouse of other students' germs all winter are prime candi-dates for the student sore throat (also known as the winter throat that just won't quit). It can last weeks and weeks, and result in repeated time off.

Manuka honey is great for getting rid of these. It can be taken on bread if they can swallow, off a teaspoon if they like the taste, dissolved in hot milk or in hot water with a spritz of lemon juice 4–5 times daily. For more information about manuka honey, see Fix 105: Bee Better and Fix 62: Wound, Ulcer and Sore Healing.

Night-waking

For those who wake in the night when the soreness is at its worst (my son describes it as 'like red-hot carpet fluff and grit down my throat'), use the tried and tested homeopathic favourite – a gargle with five drops of **hypericum** and five of **calendula** mother tincture in 300 ml cooled boiled water. Make some up at night and keep it in the fridge, perhaps leaving some in a covered glass by their bed so it's right there if they need it at 3 a.m.

You can buy the tinctures in the UK from Helios via mail order, which will arrive within 24 hours. Helios also supplies many individual US customers. In the US, you can buy calendula mother tincture from Homeopathic Educational Services (½ fl oz, $8.99). At the time of writing, I can't locate a reputable US supplier of hypericum; however, Neal's Yard in the UK do supply individual customers in the US and sell hypericum (15 ml, £4.65), and may also be able to point you towards a local stockist. For contact details, see under 'Shopping' in the Directory.

See also General: Colds and Flu, on page 36.

314. Cramp-Buster

Cramp's quite common for teens who are going through a growth spurt or not, for the moment, eating a very balanced diet.

If the attack's a persistent, painful one and none of the usual soothing techniques (massage and kneading, hot water bottles, walking about) is working, try adding two to three drops of **Angelsword** to a blob of good-quality arnica cream or Body Soothe Cream – enough to fit into your cupped palm – and massage with that. This was the only acute-attack cramp-buster that used to work for my teenage daughter, who used to get vicious calf-muscle pain in the middle of the night.

Angelsword is by Australian Bush Flower Essences and is available direct, via Healthlines (15 ml, £8.95), IFER and Flower Sense. Body Soothe Cream is made by Living Essences of Australia and is available in the UK from Victoria Health (125 ml, £9.99). For contact details, see under 'Shopping' in the Directory.

315. **Crisis Point**

If your teenager is in such a state that they have literally locked themselves in their room and can't bring themselves to come out in order to deal with an issue – perhaps they are hysterical, feeling hopeless, depressed or are really flipping out and feeling like doing damage to themselves or others – you need to do something fast. Something which will not be seen as intrusive, as that may tip them over the edge altogether, but something effective. This is where the right essence can stop a drama or developing crisis gently, but effectively, in its very tracks.

What helps?

There are a couple of really good ones here, both developed especially for teenagers who have reached the end of their tether. One is called **The Works**. Try offering them a small glass of water, if they'll take it, with a few drops of this one

The Works gem essence is part of a range especially for children and teenagers called 'First-Aid for Feelings'. It was developed by Ann Callahan, former director of the Irish School of Homeopathy, and her remarkable nephews, Ben and Mica, who were 11 and 10 at the time. It's a gentle but surprisingly effective remedy for acute situations that is catching on all over Europe as a young people's alternative to Emergency Essence or Rescue Remedy. (It can be bought from Healthlines(15 ml, £8.95) or direct via www.indigoessences.com (00) 353 – 1 – 201 8029. For more contact details, see under 'Shopping' in the Directory.)

Another good one is from the Urban Angels range, made by Light Heart Essences in conjunction with the therapist team (including psychologists and complementary therapists) who work with the teenagers at the London-based children's rehabilitation and support charity Kids' Co. It's called, very appropriately, **Don't Give Up.** Taken longer term it can help a despairing teenager find new ways of looking at old, previously seemingly insurmountable problems, empowering them not to give up on their goals, dreams or tasks. In the short term, i.e. taken as an acute crisis remedy, it can help address 'desperation, confusion and hoplesssness or even suicidal feelings'. (Available from both Victoria Health; or Light Heart direct, see Shopping, £7.50, for 30ml mouth spritzer.)

Either The Works or Don't Give Up can work quickly to calm and balance, so that you and your son or daughter are at least able to talk something through. Then together you can perhaps agree on, and arrange for, some extra appropriate help and support if needed.

Dyslexia

For a general introduction to the condition, see page 264.

Symptoms and Suggestions

Teenagers

A teenager with dyslexia may:

- have continued trouble writing and spelling
- dislike reading at all, find it hard and not 'enjoy words' as a result
- have real trouble learning foreign languages and maths
- display growing disorganisation and forgetfulness at school or college (e.g. games kits and handing in pieces of work) and home as the amount of things they are expected to manage, and take responsibility for, grows. They may often run late for appointments and classes, and have difficulty sorting out their work – i.e. planning essays, coursework and revision schedules, which can lead to anxiety, panic, going into outright denial and a teenage reluctance to either face or discuss the problem, which seems increasingly insoluble as work and tasks pile up. Their files may be a mess; they may lose pieces of work easily and drop behind with deadlines.
- have trouble getting abstract ideas and logical arguments out of their head and on to paper in the way they want
- consistently get lower marks than their intelligence would suggest they can reach, despite considerable effort
- confuse verbal instructions, especially if given a long string of them
- muddle up phone numbers and email addresses
- show signs of dropping self-esteem and growing frustration.

Some things that may help

- **Spelling and writing difficulties** – get help from your child's school from a *specialist learning-support teacher* that is specific to your teenager's difficulties as opposed to general extra subject-based tutoring – this is crucial. Your teenager could try working on a laptop with a spell-checker (which at least flags up incorrect spellings and suggests correct options). For words with transposed letters (which many dyslexics do a lot – 'becasue' instead of 'because' is a classic), a spell-checker will often only offer one correct option, which does make life easier.
- **Reading inaccurately, laboriously or without understanding** – transparent coloured overlays developed by the Irlen Institute to put over the page may help.[13] For contact details, see under 'Shopping' in the Directory. Another way of using this therapy is through reading glasses with coloured lenses. Blue often does the trick, say researchers at the University of Oxford, because that colour wavelength calms down the functioning of the magnocellular pathway in the brain. This is the route via which the brain perceives and registers both motion and 'where things are' (like letters in a word or words on a page).
- **Lack of 'enjoyment' of words** – encourage listening to stories and plays on tape or CD, or discussions, plays and other programmes on the radio, to help foster an enjoyment of words in a different way.
- **Trouble learning foreign languages and maths** – listening to CDs of the language can help, although many parents suggest their teenager drop languages if they are struggling and encourage them to concentrate on the subjects they like more and find easier. Again, for both languages and maths, ask for help from a specialist learning-support teacher.
- **Trouble managing their workload** – it can help to set aside time to help them devise a work or revision schedule broken down into small 'chunks' with a logical progression; writing lists and routine both help. Ensure they have a personal mentor or tutor at school whom they like and whom they meet with regularly and often. Get any support at school that your teenager is happy to have: from

extra mentor meetings to specialist learning support sessions to help teach them work skills in a way that is specific to their needs. The skills taught that are likely to help the most across the board are general literacy, study skills, memory, essay planning and organisation. For essays, offer more assistance at home and feed-back on drafts.

- **Working more slowly than their peers** – lots of things help here, from writing on a laptop instead of by hand to encouragement and practical support both at home and from a school special-needs teacher. Also consider suggesting doing slightly fewer subjects when exams come round – e.g. seven or eight GCSEs instead of the now more usual 9–11, or three AS levels instead of the usual four. Ask their teachers to ensure they are given more time for exams: any child who has been diagnosed as dyslexic is legally entitled to 25 per cent more time if they want to take it. Many parents ask for this on an 'in case' basis, so their children can use it if they need it.

- **Trouble with verbal instructions** – try not to give them several things to remember at once: keep it to three or preferably two. Politely ask your teenager to repeat them afterwards, again broken down into no more than three small, manageable stages. Encourage them to write down notes on a small jotter pad they carry with them all the time or write bullet points or 'memory-jogger' single words on the back of their hand. Praise them every time they follow instructions correctly.

- **Muddling up phone numbers** – suggest they put them immediately into their mobile, checking the number back slowly with whoever gave it to them right there and then. If taking messages over the home line, have a notepad by the phone and encourage them to read any numbers back to the giver before putting the handset down.

- **Low self-esteem** – do anything and everything you can to raise it and keep doing so at every opportunity. Encourage and support any aptitude they have, however minor, and give positive feedback (remember to mention specifics) on everything they do. See also Teenagers: Self-Esteem and Confidence on page 373.

For complementary therapies for dyslexia, see 'Treatments for Dyslexia and Dyspraxia' on page 275. See also 'The famous and fabulous' below.

316. Beat Body Odour

A burst of adolescent hormones can trigger stronger underarm odour for a while. If ordinary deodorants just aren't doing much, this is a holistic freshness fix used in Brazil. Cut a fresh slice of **lemon** and wipe well under your arms. Kathy Phillips, former health and beauty director of British *Vogue*, now beauty director for Condé Nast Asia and director of the excellent aromatherapy-based products company This Works, says lemon's acidity nixes odour, the juice works cumulatively so after a while you won't need to use it every day, and it won't stain your clothes. She's right on all counts.

Dyspraxia

For a general introduction to this, see page 269.

The famous and fabulous

Dyslexic and dyspraxic people are just as smart and talented as any other group – often more so. For instance, all the following were, are or have shown signs of dyslexia or dyspraxia:

- **Smart?** Not half: inventors Leonardo da Vinci, Thomas Edison and Albert Einstein, plus entrepreneurs like Henry Ford of Ford Motors and Virgin's Richard Branson.
- **Famous writers:** F. Scott Fitzgerald, Agatha Christie, Irish poet W. B. Yates and Hans Christian Anderson.
- **Artistic?** You bet: Andy Warhol, Picasso and the sculptor Rodin, photographer David Bailey and designer Tommy Hilfiger, to name but a few.

- **Actors and singers with stage and screen presence to burn:** Tom Cruise, Jodie Kidd, Orlando Bloom, Robbie Williams, Cher, Noel Gallagher and Robin Williams.
- **Charisma:** world leaders including Winston Churchill, General Patton, Thomas Jefferson, John F. Kennedy and George Washington.

Symptoms and Suggestions

Teenagers

If a dyspraxic teenager has not yet been diagnosed, or received the right support, they will still be having to cope with most of the difficulties they had as younger children (see 'Symptoms' on page 270) and now, in addition, will probably also have to deal with at least some of those listed below.

Confusingly, many of these are not unheard of in non-dyspraxic teenagers either (boys in particular). Careless appearance, being a bit awkward and monosyllabic, messy writing, getting heavily into MSN and computer games, trouble organising their work, of uncertain teenage temper – isn't that all pretty normal at their age? Yet mothers and fathers usually know intuitively if something is making life harder for their child than it needs to be, no matter how many times their recurring concerns may have been dismissed by teachers and health professionals.

Because dyspraxia is such a complex and variable condition, and often masked for years if the child is bright, many dyspraxics are not diagnosed until they are 11 or older, despite their parents' repeated enquiries. My own son wasn't until he was 13.

Social
With regard to symptoms, a dyspraxic teenager may:

- be less mature than their peers and find it difficult to socialise. They could be one or two years behind their classmates, so perhaps prefer the company of older or younger friends. They may have increasing difficulty decoding social signals and responding appropriately. Unless they have had the right support, dyspraxic teenagers can find their peers hard to keep up with, as teenagers' language and chat is fast, idiosyncratic, increasingly witty and has started to play with sarcasm, irony, verbal manipulation and charm.

- may not feel ready to form a sexual or emotional relationship until one to three years after their contemporaries have started going out with each other, then find it harder to do so when they do want to. Chatting up someone they fancy may be more difficult for a dyspraxic teenager. They may have subsequent trouble forming normal positive girlfriend-boyfriend relationships and will have to deal with the distress, puzzlement, loneliness and frustration this causes. They might, as a result, retreat into pastimes that don't require skill with face-to-face interaction – e.g. playing more computer games and becoming overly dependent on Net-based communication like MSN and MySpace.
- still have difficulty knowing 'when to stop' and so may annoy others unintentionally
- find conversation awkward, especially starting one up and disengaging at the end
- have difficulty with grooming skills (e.g. shaving, doing hair and make-up) and working out what clothes go together or are appropriate for a particular occasion. Dyspraxic teenagers often appear to notice less about their appearance than most others their age.
- have difficulty understanding what's cool and what isn't. This doesn't just apply to personal appearance (as above), but to things like music, pastimes, films, books, the way they decorate their room, the design of their MySpace site, so it can be hard to favourably impress – or even fit in with – peers who are becoming increasingly hip and wise to every aspect of popular culture and consumerism. Your teenager may be seen as weird or not plugged in, and so be labelled geeky or daggy. This can make them feel, and be, isolated.

Below are some things that may help with social skills:

- **Socially less mature than peers** – being reassured that everyone's got their own personal internal timetable that means they do things at their own pace and in their own time (not other people's) can help. So can joining a loosely supervised social group where they will mix in with the opposite sex in a mediated, activity-based way, whether it's a local community youth club with a youth worker on hand, a drama course, a church group or even youth volunteer services. Try Millennium Volunteers for 16–24s. For contact details, see under 'Useful Helplines, Websites and Contacts' in the Directory. Anything that has instructors showing you how and encouraging you on is good. All of these are better options than just hanging out and eyeing each other up, which can be intimidating as they offer a dyspraxic teenager, who misses many subtle cues anyway, few pointers as to how to behave.

- **Tendency to withdraw** – role-playing games, mediated social activities and anything to boost their confidence are just some of the things that could help here.
- **Knowing 'when to stop'** – again, try illustrating acceptable limits through role-playing and example.
- **Conversation** – offer some short, general 'entry' and 'exit' scripts that they can use and adapt as necessary. Practise these with them in role-play and put this on a tape or burn on to a CD so they can listen at their leisure if they want to.
- **Grooming skills and appearance** – strategies could include complimenting them with specifics when they *do* look good (e.g. 'That top really suits you: the colour turns your eyes much bluer'); helping them choose clothes in *short* shopping trips if they'll let you; for girls, a professional make-up lesson or two, having briefed the (preferably young, friendly) beautician first; for boys and girls, a step-by-step session with an amiable hairdresser, having first spoken to them yourself, at a time when the salon is mostly empty and quiet; for boys who are beginning to need to shave, electric rather than manual razors can be easier to use.
- **Cultural perception and knowing what's cool** – this can be a difficult one, but perhaps strong visual, cultural images from mainstream films, MTV and reading style or music magazines can give a few clues, as may encouraging them to chat with you about who was wearing what, how it looked, what they thought of them and whether they would like that sort of look themselves.

Physical

Your teenager may:

- get tired and drained by others more easily than their peers and may miss out socially because of this. It doesn't help that teenagers' sleep patterns are changing anyway because their brains are temporarily becoming more reactive to light (see Teenagers: Sleep on page 380), so though they start staying up much later, they actually need more rest, not less. This can cause ongoing fatigue, which can make any existing difficulties with things like poor memory or being disorganised worse.
- have poor coordination in sport, a tentative sense of rhythm and poor posture when dancing
- have difficulty learning to drive and it may take them longer to learn than non-dyspraxic teenagers.

There are lots of things that can help physical symptoms in a dyspraxic teenager:

- **Stamina** – encourage plenty of rest, suggest afternoon kips or chill-outs if a party is coming up that night. Offer lifts back at, say, midnight, if you sense they are worried about how they are going to manage to stay the course: they can always invent a face-saving excuse for why they have to leave a bit early – e.g. they have to be up early the next morning as they are going somewhere or have friends coming over early. Try to discourage them from taking on too much and encourage them to pace themselves and get early nights when they have the chance. Also ensure their diet is good. Suggest taking at least one full day off at the weekend (i.e. no Saturday job or homework on that day) and consider supplementation with energy-boosting nutrients like co-enzyme Q and good-quality ginseng – see Teenagers: Energy on page 351.
- **Poor coordination** – some dyspraxic teenagers may find whole-body sporting activities, such as swimming and skiing, or equipment-moderated pastimes, like sailing, mountain-biking or canoeing, easier than traditional team sports like football or rugby. Martial arts, teen yoga and Pilates, as they are slow and controlled, can all be useful

because they not only develop coordination and confidence in movement but are calming and grounding. Pilates and yoga may, however, be rated as girlie and so shunned by boys.

- **Learning to drive**: suggest trying a driving simulator a couple of times before they begin – some bigger driving schools have them – until they feel confident enough to get in a vehicle for the first time. Offer lots of low-key practice opportunities, keep the pressure off and let them know they can take as much time as they want, with no expectation of them passing their test quickly. Offer praise for even slight progress. If they're finding the difference between right and left especially confusing, try putting L and R stickers on the relevant sides of the wheel. For later when they have passed their test and are needing to find their way about, if their sense of direction is not good, try a talking GPS.

Emotional
Emotionally, your teenager may:

- be more easily confused than others and find new territory particularly hard to get used to. If they go to a new school or to sixth-form college at 16, it can take them a long time to familiarise themselves with the new layout (for non-dyspraxic teens, it's a month on average), to remember teachers' names and become confident with finding their way around. They may get lost more than most, arrive late for classes, even miss some altogether for many weeks because they simply cannot find them in time. Changes of rooms and venues for lessons can really throw them.
- tend to worry (e.g. 'travel anxiety', exams and interview panic)
- feel more pressured than their classmates by deadlines for work and homework. They may become anxious and feel harassed by academic demands and requirements that their peers take in their stride. The jump in academic expectations and work standards that happens at the beginning of Year 9 (at the start of GCSEs) and beginning of Year 12 (or their first year at sixth-form college) comes as a shock to most teenagers until they get used to the higher standards required and heavier workload. This may be especially discouraging for dyspraxic teens – so discouraging in fact

that it may lead to them dropping subjects, going part-time at college or even eventually dropping out of higher education altogether.
- have increasingly low self-esteem
- be the target of bullying. Dyspraxic children are more likely to be bullied, especially around the ages of 13 or 14.

Fortunately, there's lots that can be done to help:

- **Easily confused** – routines, charts and lists all help here. When going to a new school or college, 'walk the course' before they join (more than once if need be). Encourage the teenager to visit the new premises before the start of the new academic year with you, a teacher or an older student on a quiet day (as trying to check the premises out on an open day or evening can merely be confusing as they're usually packed). Check out other main areas they'll need to use, like the library, loos and changing rooms, and have a drink or snack in the dining room or coffee bar: anything to help them get the feel of the place before they officially start. They could carry a map of the new school, with the rooms they use for their own lessons marked up in fluorescent pen or coloured in. Timetables coloured in by subject are easier to follow. Suggest they keep this in their bag in a protective plastic folder at all times.
- **Worrying** – leave plenty of time, make lists, tick off items on a checklist, break things down into small tasks and rehearse or 'walk through' the forthcoming event.
- **Feeling pressurised by schoolwork** – lots of support and praise, a regular routine put together with their agreement and a quiet place for doing their homework with help on hand if need be can all help greatly. Take some of the pressure off where you can (e.g. consider suggesting they take fewer subjects at GCSE and AS level), so they can concentrate on them and feel less overwhelmed.
- **Low self-esteem** – do anything and everything you possibly can to boost your teenager's self-esteem and keep doing it. Praise any talent or aptitude they may have, and always congratulate them on anything they have done well, even small things, with specifics – e.g. 'This bit in your essay about George Bush is interesting: never

knew he'd said that' or 'Your hair looks good today. It suits you spiky in front' or 'You handled that call to the cinema well: got all the times you need *and* some alternative film ideas.' Encourage them to join activity-based groups, especially drama and martial arts, or anything they show even a small aptitude for. Animals can help too: get a responsive, tactile pet of their choice if they don't already have one that is solely theirs – a cat or a dog if they like these animals are ideal, as they offer unconditional love, uncritical company and, if they are calm-natured, can be very soothing and grounding. A cute or characterful dog is a great conversation-facilitator for someone who is shy or not great at starting up conversations. The exercise they ensure you get is stress-reducing, plus in halfway decent weather, it produces that feel-good factor. See also Teenagers: Self-Esteem and Confidence on page 373.

Academic
Your teenager may:

- work more slowly than others. Homework and essays seem to take a long time and the results do not reflect the amount of time and effort they may have poured into them. They may tend not to finish tasks properly, so this combined with 'scrappy' work may result in lower grades being awarded than they otherwise might have got.
- have trouble managing, organising and planning their workload, whether for coursework, ongoing homework or revision. Their files are often in a mess, and they may lose pieces of work easily. Your teenager may often be overwhelmed by their homework, which has piled up and is frequently handed in late.
- have trouble learning foreign languages and maths
- find it hard to express ideas clearly or take in what is being said to them, despite being quick-thinking. They may find there is a frustrating gap between what they know, or feel, and what they can put across in the written or spoken word.
- have difficulty writing legibly or quickly
- have spelling difficulties
- dislike reading, find it hard and not enjoy words as a result

- feel more anxious about exams than their peers and withstand this sort of pressure less easily

Some strategies which can help a dyspraxic teenager academically:

- **'Slow worker'** – regular help at school from a *specialist learning-support teacher* as opposed to ordinary subject-based support like extra maths or English coaching, especially general literacy and study skills, can help considerably. By law, a child who has been officially diagnosed as dyspraxic is allowed between one and three periods a week *instead of* other lessons, not on top of them.
- **Organising workload and planning** – give ongoing extra support and encouragement with homework, coursework, revision and organisation. Post-It Notes, breaking down tasks into small 'chunks', writing lists and routine all help. Set aside time to help them devise a work or revision schedule with a logical progression. Ensure they have a personal mentor at school whom they like and whom they meet with regularly. Get any support at school that your teenager is happy to have.
- **Learning languages and maths** – listening to CDs of the language can help, although many parents would encourage a dyspraxic teenager to drop languages if they are struggling and encourage them to concentrate on the subjects they prefer. Again, get help from your school from a specialist learning-support teacher. Extra tuition at home can help too, but remember that tutors do not teach in the same way as a trained special-needs teacher and that they charge by the hour (£15–£30) even though half an hour's concentrated one-to-one in a subject they find really hard may be more than enough for a dyspraxic teen (possibly too much) after a long day at school. If you feel a conventional tutor might suit their particular needs, consider seeing if a tutor would do half-hour sessions – you may still have to pay the full hourly rate – say, on a Saturday or Sunday when there are no school lessons.
- **Expressing ideas** – talk your teenager's ideas through with them whenever they want to. Encourage, listen with interest and give feedback, but try not to hurry them or put words in their mouth 'to help them along', even when things are progressing rather slowly.

Paraphrase what they've said at the end and offer it back to them for consideration if something's been a struggle to say – e.g. 'So when you miss the bus in the morning and there's not another for 20 minutes, you reckon going to the pub stop is best as lots of different ones go past there? Yes, sounds very sensible.'

- **Writing** – try a laptop. If they can learn to think straight on to the keyboard, without the mental 'interruption' of trying to form letters with a pen while simultaneously struggling to spell correctly, a dyspraxic child (or adult) will usually find they can express themselves in writing far more easily.

- **Spelling** – as well as working on the laptop, your teenager could make use of the spell-checker. However, this may be of limited help to some, as while it flags up misspelt words, it usually offers several options, which the user then has to choose between. Your teenager may still need to get out the dictionary when they are going through a draft.

- **Reading** – encourage listening to stories, plays, discussions and other programmes to help foster an enjoyment of words.

- **Exam stress** – don't push them to do the 'higher' exams, as easier ones actually passed can be better for their confidence and far less stressful. Keep exam periods calm and quiet for them at home. Help keep unnecessary pressure off by encouraging them to drop any 'extras' – e.g. ask them to put any Saturday or after-school jobs on hold for a couple of months – and don't expect them to do all their usual jobs (if they do any) at home during this time. Ensure their diet is good and they get plenty of early nights; all the ordinary, sensible support non-dyspraxic teenagers need here will be doubly necessary for your child. Ask their teachers to ensure they are given more time for exams: any child who has been diagnosed as dyspraxic is legally entitled to 25 per cent more time if they want to take it. Many parents ask for this 'just in case'.

Life skills
Your teenager may:

- find serial verbal instructions confusing, especially if given a long string of them

- muddle up phone numbers
- have a tendency to forget time and be unaware of how much has passed
- struggle to retain information ('in one ear and out the other'). Remembering more than two instructions in sequence may still be difficult, which becomes more of a problem now they are a teenager as many of the instructions given are more complex.

Here are some useful tips:

- **Serial instructions** – try not to give them several things to remember at once: keep it to three or less. Politely ask your teenager to repeat them afterwards. Encourage them to write down notes on a small jotter pad they carry with them all the time, write bullet points or 'memory-jogger' single words on the back of their hand. Offer praise whenever they follow instructions correctly.
- **Phone numbers** – suggest they put them immediately into their mobile and check the number back slowly with whoever gave it to them. If taking messages, keep a pad by the phone.
- **Time-keeping** – suggest they use the beeper on their watch and put easy-to-read clocks in main rooms, including theirs.
- **Memory** – if you possibly can, avoid the temptation to do it all for them (e.g. 'Here's your games, kit, lunch money, mobile all newly charged up for you, spare pair of socks'). Look instead at techniques that will support them in remembering and praise them when they do. Try strategies such as Post-It Notes on the front door, pinning up a tick-list of things to take to school in their room and writing things down and asking them to repeat instructions back to you.

For fixes for dyspraxia, see 'Treatments for Dyslexia and Dyspraxia' on page 275.

Further information
Recommended reading: there's almost nothing written about dyspraxic teens (most of the material is for parents whose children are younger), but there is some good advice in *Dyspraxia, the Hidden Handicap* by Dr Amanda Kirby.

Other resources: contact the Dyspraxia Connection, a small Nottingham-based charity offering much-needed services for teens and parents – social groups, adventure holidays, social-skills courses, clubs and outings. Teenagers may like www.matts.hideout.co.uk, which is written by a dyspraxic teenaged boy, or the teen website at www.dyspraxiafoundation.org.uk. For help and advice for parents, get in touch with the Dyspraxia Foundation. For details, see under 'Useful Helplines, Websites and Contacts' in the Directory.

Energy

317. Exhaustion

Teenagers' energy levels can nose-dive quite suddenly and just keep on dropping. This may be triggered by a virus they cannot quite shake or a tough period of studying, stress or worry, then become endemic, exacerbated by a teen's tendency towards going to bed later yet needing more sleep (see Teenagers: Sleep on page 380) and their burgeoning social lives.

If you are already encouraging healthy meals, early nights and rest yet your son or daughter simply cannot seem to get back on top of things, first take them to the GP for a thorough check-up to exclude anything like low-level glandular fever or anaemia.

If all else is equal, a simple energy supplement could be just what's needed – but which one? There are literally hundreds of nutritional and herbal products on the market, but some are better than others and not all are suitable for teenagers. British biochemist Shabir Day, founder of Victoria Health, who has formulated many of his company's cutting-edge supplement products, suggests a combination of **co-enzyme Q** and good-quality **ginseng**. The former helps our cells' tiny powerhouses (the mitochondria) release the maximum amount of energy from food; the latter is an adaptogen and energy-enhancer, which, encouragingly as teens like quick results, tends to start making a difference in just five days.

Try Health Aid Strong Sibergin 2,500 mg Ginseng from AuraVita (30 capsules, £13.49), available as small, sleek, teen-friendly black-and-red-striped capsules – 'go-faster capsules', as my 18-year-old son calls them.

Take one a day. In the US, try SMARTbomb (30 capsules, $23.99). Co-enzyme Q is available from many different retail outlets. If you can't find any, try Health Direct's 30 mg ones. Take one a day. For contact details, see under 'Shopping' in the Directory.

Exercise

318. Ugh?

If that's the response the word exercise gets from your teenage daughter, why not try something fun, cool-looking and relaxing that doesn't feel or look like ordinary exercise – but will flatten a puppy-fat tummy and trim a wodgy waist a treat? Try **hooping**.

> Q. When is a hula hoop not a hula hoop?
> A. When it's a hooper.

What is it?

Hooping is a hot new workout option for a teenage girls who loathe traditional enforced school exercises like netball, tennis, hockey and jogging, find frenetic street-dance classes too much and will only put on any kind of swimwear if they're sunbathing. It is also enormous fun and, because of the gentle, rhythmic, circling pelvic motions, is grounding, calming and centring too.

This is the latest exercise craze to come up via the festivals route and start seeping into the mainstream. Savvy girls and women realise how relaxing it is, how sexy it looks and how terrific at toning up stomachs, waists, arms and hips it is, so hooping classes and parties are springing up all over the UK and parts of the US.

The new way to do it is to music like a modern dance class – acid, ambient chill, reggae, hardcore dance, Celtic, jazz-funk, you name it, you can hoop to it, as you loop that lazily spinning ring from waist to neck, to arm, wrist and back again. People get the hang of this one fast and can look graceful from their very first session, because the hoopers are weighted (often with sand inside) so beginners don't have to throw themselves all over the place to make them stay up.

In the UK, see Gaiam Direct for the Betty Hoop starter kit of weighted hoop (unclips and folds up for easy carrying) and exercise DVD (£27.98); in the US, you can buy it from Betty Hoops direct (hoop and DVD, $39.98). For contact details, see under 'Shopping' in the Directory.

For parties, school classes and community events in the UK, contact local hooping instructors – often trained dance teachers too – like Sharna Rose, who also makes her own brightly coloured metal-weighted hoops. For contact details, see under 'Training Courses' in the Directory.

Hair

319. For Reluctant Male Hair-Washers

Until they discover girls, most teenage boys seem pretty reluctant to bother much with personal presentation and hygiene. For some families, the weekly confrontation about greasy hair, filthy nails, etc., and subsequent nagging or arguments can become a real source of conflict. Luckily, the **60-Second No-Water Clean-Up** is a hit with both boys and parents alike as it:

- is effective
- gives the hair body as well as removing grease
- takes less than a minute
- does not involve hot water or removing clothing.

The 60-Second No-Water Clean-Up

1. Shake a fine layer of calendula talcum powder (soothing on the scalp but doesn't smell 'scented') on to the head. Massage it briskly into the roots of the hair. Try the aluminium-free one by Bay House (220 g, £2.89). For contact details, see under 'Shopping' in the Directory.
2. Hang head down and, using a brush with good-quality natural bristles (not hard plastic ones), brush hair briskly from root to end until all the powder's gone.

That's it.

Obviously girls can also use this one. Because of temporary loss of slipperiness, if they are styling or putting longer hair up afterwards, the hair will be far easier to manipulate into place.

> **Tip**
> If bristles are a bit clogged afterwards, just flick the base of the brush along a shelf edge, then brush it with another brush to get rid of any residual powder.

Headaches

320. Computer-Game-Induced Headache

This fix, the **Anti-Headache Tug**, can be done in three minutes or, if your teenager needs a very quick fix, just 20 seconds.

The Anti-Headache Tug – three-minute version

1. Switch off the screen and close your eyes.
2. Place your hands flat against your temples, then slide them upwards and backwards towards your crown.
3. As you reach your crown, close your fingers so they are grasping the very base of the hair where it emerges from the scalp.
4. Clench your fingers so you can feel the scalp lifting and becoming taut. Hold this for a count of five.
5. Release slightly and clench five times.
6. Move further back round the sides of your head (see diagram) and repeat.
7. Move to the back of your head and repeat.
8. Repeat all round the hairline, starting in front in line with your nose and working round to the back, but just doing two clenches in each place.
9. Finally, rub your head firmly, rapidly but lightly all over, mussing your hair, as when a hairdresser shampoos you.
10. Lay your hands gently but firmly on your head, fingers on your crown, palms resting on the sides of your head, heel of hand touching top of the ears, and leave for a count of five before taking them away gradually. This helps 'settle' the nerve endings in your head. Mmmm.

You can do this for your teenager, but unlike most massage techniques, self-administered is better as the recipient can judge the degree of traction and pull more accurately.

The Anti-Headache Tug – 20-second version
A simplified version is simply to tug handfuls of hair right at the roots (if you do it further away down the hair shaft, it pulls and hurts) and progress round the crown area in a circle, holding each tug for a controlled four seconds.

See also General: Headaches on page 57 and Migraines on page 64.

321. Leaving Home
Below are some invaluable remedies for teenagers who've gone away to their first year at university or are living away from home for the first time, suggested especially for this book by the senior homeopath at Helios, the specialist pharmacy supplying patients with prescriptions for the British NHS Homeopathic Hospital in Tunbridge Wells:

- **homesickness** – Ignatia
- **exam stress** – *Argentum nitricum*
- **confusion** (it's all so new, or the campus seems huge and complex) – Belladonna, *Carbo vegetabilis*. If it's making the teenager feel a bit panicky – *Argentum nitricum*.

You can buy all of these remedies in the UK from Helios and Ainsworths (£3.30–£4.50); in the US, try the National Center for Homeopathy. For contact details, see under 'Shopping' in the Directory.

Mobile Phones

322. Protection

Almost every teenager has one (more than 94 per cent of high-schoolers) and uses it regularly, but controversy about the precise nature of the health risks mobiles present continues to ebb and flow with every new report.

Some of the most interesting reports are coming out of Russia – the only country conducting trials on mobile safety not to have a home-grown mobile-phone manufacturer on its soil and, some might suggest, therefore rather freer of vested interests than the research coming from certain other countries including the UK and the US. Findings include the suggestion that a mere two-minute call can disrupt the biochemistry of a teenager's brain and the recommendation that children, teens, pregnant women and drivers with pacemakers should avoid making mobile calls where possible.[14]

> **Mobile Tip**
>
> Hold your mobile well away from your head (e.g. a couple of feet) while it's searching for a connection after you've dialled a number, since that is when the power surge happens, and this is therefore thought to be the most damaging time to have it close to your head. Place by your ear only after it has started ringing.

If you, like most parents, reckon the safety benefit of your teen being able to reach you in emergencies outweighs the potential health hazards, mobile-smart advice includes:

• Choose a phone with radiation emissions that are as low as possible and certainly, suggests the European Union, well below 2 SAR (Specific Absorption Rate), but variation is tremendous: one Nokia model weighs in at 0.68, whereas a Sony Ericsson Z600 is a quarter of that. Shop around. See www.mmfai.org to check the SAR rating before you buy.

- Go for a cheap plan with the fewest inclusive minutes possible.
- Encourage texting, instead of calling, except in emergencies.
- A hands-free system like Bluetooth is claimed to reduce radiation to the head by 50–90 per cent. Unfortunately, radiation can still travel up the wire and reach the brain, so Professor Challis, vice-chairman of the National Radiological Protection Board and chairman of the Mobile Telecommunications and Health Research Programme, has suggested attaching a small **ferrite bead** to the wire and recommends that all companies adopt this. They've not in fact done so, but such a bead is cheap, simple and unobtrusive, so you can get one yourself if you like. There is some evidence to suggest it works best when placed below the hands-free kit's microphone. Ferrite beads are available from electrical suppliers like Maplin Electronics (they call them ferrite clamps). Check out their range of clip-on ones on their website – type in the code 'N89AB'. For contact details, see under 'Shopping' in the Directory. *Note:* most hands-free systems have wires less than 4 mm in diameter, so ensure you know the size before you buy.

See also Fix 158: Protective Earrings for Mobile Users.

Night Cramps

Night cramps seem to hit teenagers (especially younger ones) and children in the evenings more than at any other time. The cramps may only last a few moments, but, as used to be the case with my 14-year-old daughter, may persist for many painful hours – defying treatment with hot-water bottles, massage, movement and painkillers alike. The problem is often related to a shortage of **calcium, magnesium, potassium** or **B vitamins**.

323. Nutrients and Supplements
One approach is to encourage the teenager to eat plenty of sesame seeds or tahini paste and tinned fish (for extra calcium), nuts, seafood, green leafy vegetables and bananas (for extra magnesium). If that doesn't help, consider supplementation.

A teaspoon of Marmite a day – on toast or off a spoon – can help prevent cramps (if the problem is lack of B vitamins). Having it on toast for breakfast every morning is a good and easy way to remember to take it regularly.

Giving additional magnesium in pill or capsule form can work within anything from a few days to a few weeks, says one of the UK's top holistic doctors, Dr John Briffa. He suggests giving 300–350 mg daily for a teenager. One particular study found magnesium cuts cramps by more than 70 per cent.

If the cramps persist, seek advice from a professional nutritionist or your GP. For organisations that can put you in touch with a nutritionist, see under 'Therapies and Therapists' in the Directory.

Periods

324. Starting Periods

If you're a woman and you're reading this, do you remember what happened the day you had your first period? A party? A treat? Anything special *at all*? Probably not: all most of us get is a packet of sanitary towels plus a hug and/or a lecture from our mother. Periods, in Western society, are seen as slightly inconvenient or a bit messy, rather than a reason to celebrate.

Yet traditional societies usually celebrate them, for they see this as a joyous day – like a birthday, but better – when someone is making the honourable and exciting transition from being a little girl to a young woman, capable of bearing children of her own.

Native American Indians regard the beginning of a young girl's menstruation as a special gift and tell their daughters, 'All you now touch is blessed by your womanhood.'

Some societies still hold terrific women-only parties to mark a young girl's first period (first blood, new moon or menarche celebrations) in which everyone dresses in their best and there's great food, drink, dancing, singing, presents, candles and a beautiful new outfit for the girl concerned.

According to Anke Mai, a specialist youth counsellor in Wales who works with teenage girls on all sorts of issues including rites of passage, 'The way you mark your first menstruation, and how people around you relate to you during this special time, will stay with you for ever.' She adds this also has an important influence on how you feel and react to the other 'big times' in your life.

Ideas

Apart from inviting over your daughter's friends and those of yours she really likes, plus favourite older female relatives from sisters and aunts to grannies, ideas to make a first-period party special include:

- **Red rose petals** – lay out a path of flower petals for her to walk on as she comes downstairs, all dressed up to meet her guests. Give some of these to guests so they can shower her with them like confetti. Put some to float on the surface of a scented bath for her to have before she gets ready. Star Child sells dried red rose petals if fresh ones are in short supply. For contact details, see under 'Shopping' in the Directory.
- **Pretty red beads** – each one can be given to her by a different girl or woman during the party with good wishes and love, then strung together into a special necklace for her to keep for ever.
- **Small red candles** (can be the tea-light variety) – give one to each and every girl at the party who has not yet begun her period. Suggest they may like to light this for their own celebration, when their time comes. Ask them to pass this light on to younger girls too.

Further information

Recommended reading: for suggestions about creating a first-period party for a daughter, see *Rites of Passage* by Christine Hall.

Ceremonies and parties: 'The Maiden's Voyage' ceremony from 5 Rhythm dance teacher and young shaman Kate Shela, who also works extensively with teenage girls.

The Dolphin Connection offers holidays and weekends away with specialist facilitators for teenage girls to honour their transition into womanhood – and one's a week-long wild-dolphin adventure in the Azores.

For all contact details, see under 'Training Courses' in the Directory.

Tampon Tip
For younger teenagers who are just beginning to try tampons for the first time: if it's uncomfortable or won't slide in right, coat the end and the first centimetre or two of its length with Vaseline, or do the same to its applicator tube if it has one.

See also Teenagers: Rites of Passage on page 364.

325. Premenstrual Syndrome (PMS)
PMS can be mild, non-existent or raging during teenage years. For some, it may be especially troublesome in the first 12 months or so when a girl's menstrual cycle is settling down, and also around the age of 15–16, when GCSE exam pressures are starting to put the boot in and raise stress levels, as stress hormones interfere with the output of, and balance between, oestrogen and progesterone.

Three-hourly eating
According to the Natural Health Advisory Service (incorporating the Women's Nutritional Advisory Service), which originally pioneered the nutrition and sensible-eating route to combat PMS, one of the very best – and easiest – things you can do to help your daughter if she is experiencing PMS is to encourage her to *eat every three hours, taking healthy snacks in between meals if necessary.*

Healthy snacking means foods low in refined sugar and high in complex carbohydrates, *not* chocolate, sweets or pastries. Good anti-PMS between-meals fillers include:

• a health bar low in refined sugars (for some of the ones that taste nicest, see 'Snack attack' on page 514)

- a banana
- a *small* wholemeal bap, filled pitta, tortilla wrap or sandwich
- a bag of unsalted nuts
- oat biscuits.

Suggest she carries whichever of these she likes best around with her in her pocket, schoolbag or backpack so she can stick to the three-hour rule like glue.

326. Period Cramps
Menstrual (period) pain is, statistically, the most common gynaecological complaint there is. Between 60 and 93 per cent of adolescent girls suffer from it, especially on the day before their period begins and on day one.

Pain at school
The trouble is that if the pain strikes while they are at school, the child-protection laws are now so stringent that there may be little the staff are allowed to offer as help beyond a lie-down. In the UK, parents must pre-sign a permission form or send in a letter even for paracetamol to be given to their child at school – and permitted dosage of that is not high, so it may not be enough to dispel some types of vicious period cramp.

A child is not allowed to carry their own supply of analgesics in their schoolbag either: they have to be handed in to school officials, again with an accompanying note from parents. Then to obtain them, the child has to present themselves to the school sickbay.

For a far less complex alternative that's just as effective as two to three painkillers (possibly more so), suggest simple 'press-here' **acupressure**. A study in 2003 of 50 healthy teenagers with period pain compared the following technique, which the girls were taught to do themselves, with traditional bed rest. The acupressure came out by far the best.[15]

How to do it
The researchers used a point called **spleen 6**, which is on the inside of the ankle, three fingers-width above the anklebone. Press this for six seconds, release for two seconds and repeat using two five-minute cycles on each ankle.

The fast, easy version
That is all very well, but a girl may become a bit self-conscious if she has to keep reaching down to her ankle and holding it for five minutes in the middle of class.

A far simpler and very discreet DIY technique using a different acupressure point called the **shousanli** seems just as effective as spleen 6 and was suggested to me by top London acupuncturist, naturopath, osteopath and senior lecturer at the British School of Osteopathy, Phil Beech. For details of how to do this, see Fix 180: Period Pains – Immediate Relief.

327. Period Blahs
If your daughter comes home from school crabby, stressed and with gnawing period pains, run her a hot **lavender** bath (with eight to ten drops of organic lavender essential oil) and suggest she soak in there for a good 20 minutes.

A British medical trial in 1995 showed lavender really reduced distress levels and increased the well-being of 122 patients in the hothouse and stressful conditions of an intensive-care unit, which is quite a challenge.[16] And the essential oil is so effective at relieving the abdominal cramps caused by womb contractions (responsible for both period discomfort and labour pain) that when used for a high proportion of the 8,000 mothers in an eight-year study on aromatherapy as pain relief for childbirth by Oxford Brookes University, the women's use of hefty opiate painkilling drugs plummeted from 30 per cent to 0.4 per cent.

See also Women: Periods on page 165.

That 'periods are gucky' feeling . . .
Crab Apple essence (Bach Flower remedies, £3.75, 15ml, from most major chemists and health shops) can really help girls who feel distaste for menstruation (especially if they have started their periods recently), encouraging them to see these as natural, healthy renewal and cleansing processes, rather than messy or unpleasant. Add seven drops to a bath and soak on period days as a there-and-then sorter; or for longer term help, take 4 drops under the tongue or in a little water 3-4 times daily for 2-4 weeks.

Relationships and Dating

328. Heartbreak

Listening, nurturing and treats, confidence-boosting, keeping busy, lots of unconditional love from family and the support of good friends are all vital to help heal a broken heart – something that can temporarily destroy even the most confident of teenagers. Essence therapy can also be invaluable here.

For a shattered heart

Wild Horse carries a strong, brave, loving energy with it that is a favourite to help heal a shattered heart as it also helps encourage a feeling of 'a loving belonging to others'. It is available through Wild Earth Animal Essences in the US and through IFER in the UK (15 ml, approximately £7).

For 'hurt-givers'

Mauve Meleleuca helps boost self-confidence and heal the sadness or hurt if someone is a 'hurt-giver' – i.e. feels they have given out a great deal but received very little love back from a person in return. It is available worldwide from Living Essences of Australia (15 ml, approximately £7).

For rejection

Red Deadnettle is a gentle but subtly powerful essence that seems especially helpful for girls and women. It is used to take away the sting of rejection if someone has been turned down or passed over for another and is feeling bitter, angry or lonely yet still longing to feel loved. You can buy it direct from Light Heart Essences (10 ml, £5.15).

For nostalgia and obsessing

Boronia (for pining and obsession) mixed with **Bottlebrush** (for brushing away the past and making positive new beginnings) can both be very helpful if someone cannot or will not let it go and move on, are stuck in nostalgia ('I just want it to be like it used to') or are holding on to a worn-out relationship despite the fact it is no longer making them happy.

Both Boronia and Bottlebrush are Australian Bush Flower remedies. You can buy them direct or from Healthlines (15 ml, £8.95 each). Health-lines will also do a special personal mix of the two (approximately £7). In the US, you can get most of the essences mentioned in this book, including these two, from Flower Vision Research ($13.50 each).

For all contact details, see under 'Shopping' in the Directory.

329. 'Love-Stone' Therapy

Place a cleansed and programmed (see Appendix 1: Cleansing and Programming Crystals and Gems on page 536) piece of **rose-quartz crystal**, also known as the 'love stone', in their room. Ensure it's neither too tiny nor too overwhelmingly large: 7–10 cm across seems to be a good size.

Rose quartz sends out a gentle, soft, loving energy that can help comfort a battered heart (since the age of four my daughter has called hers the 'there, there' stone). By the bed (or on the bedhead if it's the right design) are optimum places to put this crystal, as the feelings of sadness are often worst when you're trying to get to sleep and immediately on waking.

Rites of Passage

Traditional societies have always had rites of passage for their teenagers: specific ceremonies and challenges that mark their becoming young adults and ensure their society respects and honours them for it after-wards. But what do we have? We have 18th- or 21st-birthday parties if the young adult's luck is in and their parents are happy to foot the bill – dancing, lots to drink but rarely any 'What does it mean?' or 'Why's this special?' bits.

Apart from that, it may be easier to say what we haven't got. We don't have the answers to questions like, What does it mean to be an adult – not just legally, but emotionally and spiritually? How does a girl or boy teenager manage to come of age these days in our fast-paced, materialistic and highly technical Western culture? How do they know when they've come of age at all? Just how can adults help boys to become men – and girls to become women – who are sure of their own identity, happy in their own skin and unafraid of life? All things most parents hope for very much for their children.

330. Rite-of-Passage Camps
Why a rite of passage?

Israel Helford is a specialist counsellor for men and boys, has been a rite-of-passage leader in Vermont for more than 20 years and also runs courses for fathers and sons, adult men and business corporations. He suggests that teenagers who aren't offered some skilled mentoring and positive guidance 'throughout this life-defining time tend to remain stuck in adolescence – adult-sized children . . . with all childhood's self-absorption and, often, aggression'. He's not the only one. Several different organisations (including some Christian ones) specialising in offering adolescents this sort of support and arranging positive teenage rites of passage to mark their transition to young adulthood have sprung up in the UK, Canada and the US over the past decade.

What they involve

On some courses, the teenagers participate with their parent of the same sex (fathers with sons, mothers with daughters); others are run under the guidance of trained facilitators and involve a wide range of activities from wilderness survival skills, physical (and often intellectual) challenges, dance and drumming to discussion, sharing experiences and counselling, all ending in congratulations and celebration.

How a teenager may feel afterwards

Both boys and girls who have attended the rite-of-passage camps (which last for between three and ten days) usually report a major sense of achievement, excitement, increased self-confidence and a real understanding of who they are; but having said that, the idea of a traditional ritual coming of age don't suit everyone. Get as much information as possible about any rite-of-passage events in your area, then discuss them fully with your son or daughter – they will know whether it's likely to be for them.

Finding out more

There are some terrific courses out there, but they're not all of equal quality, so shopping around, safety checks and personal recommendations are important.

As a start, in the UK, try Circle of Life, which offers three-day summer courses for groups of up to 14 teenagers from 14 to 16 years old (£160); in the US, check out Soul Awakening (Helford's organisation in Vermont) and the Youth Vision Quest course in Santa Rosa, California, which lasts eight to nine days ($350). For contact details, see under 'Training Courses' in the Directory.

Note: wilderness courses, like Trackways in the UK, are not the same thing as rite-of-passage ceremonies – though they too can be great confidence-builders.

331. Transition-Soothing Stone

Amethysts are said to purify and to help transmute negative energy to positive, helpful in both bringing a person in turmoil back into balance and in clearing a room that has become rather negative thanks to a build-up of brooding teenage vibes. (See also Teenagers: Bedrooms on page 328 and Appendix 1: Cleansing and Programming Crystals and Gems on page 536.)

For teenagers in transition to another phase of their development – whether it's a growth spurt, an academic jump, an emotional change or a sexual shift – top Canadian crystal therapist Karen Ryan, who practises in Ontario, suggests that, with your child's permission, you place an **amethyst crystal** near their bed (not right on top of it or on their bedhead: they can be pretty powerful).

Safety

332. Late Back?

It's night-time, they are late back and you are waiting up and worried. However, you are not helpless here – there is something you can do. Help them stay safe by quite deliberately *sending them protection and positivity* rather than worry – because worry is a negative emotion and as such can attract yet more negativity (i.e. trouble) to the recipient. Two of the most important laws of the universe are that Like Attracts Like and Energy Follows Thought. This means that on a spiritual or emotional level, if you think hard about someone, your thought flows in the form of mental energy from you to them and it will be coloured by the emotions you are feeling. If it's a worried or angry thought, your 'sending' will be tainted by worry and anger; if it's loving and calm, the energy you are sending that person will be loving and calm. For instance, for a son:

Negative sendings
Thinking, '*I just know something's happened to him:* he's in a bad part of town and I don't trust those friends he's with . . ." will send negative energy to him, as will imagining him hurt or in trouble.

Positive sendings
However, thinking something along the lines of, 'He is fine – he's probably just getting on the night bus now. He's sensible even if he is a bit late. His friends are a good bunch; they'll all be looking after each other,' and 'seeing' him as clearly as you can in your mind's eye arriving home at the front door safe and sound will send out positive energy to him and thus help him attract more of the same, so maximising his chances of staying safe.

You can take this one stage further by 'sending' him, again in your mind's eye, a big ball of protective golden light, 'seeing' him enclosed in it and quietly asking the Angels of Light to keep him safe.

As a belt and braces approach, next visualise wrapping him in a dark-blue **Cloak of Invisibility**, zipping it all the way up the front from feet to neck and draping its hood over his head. You can use this mind-spirit technique on yourself but also to project on to others who may need it. This helps ensure he's less likely to attract unwelcome attention. For how to do it, see Fix 188: Threatening Situations.

333. Protection – the Silver Roller Blind
If your teenager is aware that someone is staring at them in a hostile, lecherous or otherwise unwelcome way, or perhaps whispering about them while sending them unfriendly looks, this is an instant mind technique that can be used to block them out completely.

The Silver Roller Blind

1. Without even looking at the person, imagine reaching up and tugging hard on a sash cord, which whips a shining silver roller blind down swiftly between you and that other person – bang!

2. See this silver blind deflecting everything the other person is sending at you, as if you're holding up a mirror. Know your silver blind is *impenetrable and indestructible.*

3. As you let each breath out, 'breathe' power and energy into your silver barrier to make it stronger and stronger. Then, when you don't need it any more, just mentally flip the blind back up again.

334. Staying Safe

Are there ever times when your teenager feels threatened when he or she is out and about and wishes not to be noticed in order to pass by safely? Perhaps a disruptive group of boys has just boarded the bus where he or she is sitting quietly minding their own business upstairs; or they are walking down the street and a gang of boys or girls who've had a few drinks too many are coming down their side of the road.

There is a very fast, simple spiritual technique that takes only seconds, but can help screen someone from hostile notice. It is known as the **Cloak of Invisibility**, and involves imagining you are flinging a concealing dark-blue hooded cloak over yourself, pulling the hood down over your face *Star Wars*-style and quickly zipping it closed from feet to chin up the front. For how to do it, see Fix 188: Threatening Situations.

Longer term, street awareness and non-confrontational ways of dealing with potential trouble can be invaluable. Schools and community youth workers may know of a reputable group in your area. They use many techniques drawn from numerous different disciplines, including non-verbal communication, body language, martial arts and role-playing.

See also classes at places like Dorset's award-winning **StreetWise Safety Centre**, the courses for teenagers run by **Kidscape** and, in the US, an organisation like **Kidspower**, which runs courses for children, teenagers and college students (Teenpower and Fullpower International). For contact details, see under 'Training Courses' in the Directory.

Scars

There are many different reasons why a teenager may develop a scar. The most common causes include a sports injury, accident or fight and fast weight gain or loss, because of a rapid change in body shape –

e.g. if a girl's breasts grow large very quickly, she may develop some stretch marks. Scars can also be the result of self-harm – see Teenagers: Self-Harm and Cutting on page 375.

335. Scar Reduction

However, once any mechanical tissue damage has healed over, if the teenager would like to help heal and diminish their scarring – sometimes if the wounds were self-administered deliberately, they might not wish to yet, for a variety of reasons – rubbing in a little high-quality, pure, natural (not synthetic) **vitamin-E oil** daily can reduce the appearance of scarring and speed up healing.

Try Health Aid Pure Vitamin-E Oil, which can be bought in the UK from AuraVita (50 ml, £7.72); in the US, buy it from Worldwide Shopping Mall, a company based in Yorkshire that also supplies to the US.

Pure vitamin-E oil has long been used by natural health practitioners, especially masseurs and aromatherapists, to encourage scar reduction of all types. It has to be said that there is little hard clinical evidence that it works, but plenty of the anecdotal variety.

The only slight drawback is that you have to rub Health Aid's oil in very thoroughly as it's so rich, thick and sticky. Oil obtained from piercing a natural vitamin-E capsule and squeezing it on to your palm may be easier for many. Or try **rosehip oil** – not so sticky.

> **Rosehip oil** also has a good folk reputation for encouraging scar healing as it contains scar-erasing trans-retinoic acid. A small American study using rosehip for the severe scarring of ten mastectomy patients was reported to help the marks fade considerably over a four-month period, though it did not erase them altogether.
>
> Try Rose Mosqueta Oil (£9.99 for 20ml from Rio Trading).

For all contact details, see under 'Shopping' in the Directory.
See also General: Scars on page 83.

School, Homework and Exams

336. Peak Performance – Mental

Kick the sugary breakfast snacks and go for **beans on wholemeal toast** for teenagers who would like to boost their school or college performance without any additional effort whatsoever.

Research by the University of Ulster published in 2003 found children breakfasting on fizzy drinks and sugary snacks got the scores of the average 70-year-old in tests for memory and attention, yet good old beans on wholemeal proved to be a winner for brainpower. Beans are a good source of both protein and fibre, and other research has shown a link between a high-fibre diet and improved reasoning ability.

> How to be smart – eat breakfast.

And if they aren't keen on the idea of cooked food that early in the morning – as many teenagers seem not to be – *New Scientist* suggests **Marmite on wholemeal toast** instead, as Marmite is packed with the B vitamins shown to have brain-boosting abilities in many other studies and wholemeal bread has plenty of cognition-boosting fibre.[17]

337. Brain Boost Through Sleep
The night before an exam

An old-fashioned early night is one of the best brain-boosts a teenager (or indeed anyone else) can get before an exam, important presentation or performance. Even one makes a difference.

If someone has been up late many times in a row, the effect on their reasoning and mental performance is similar to that of someone who's legally drunk, says researcher Sean Drummond of the University of California, San Diego.

However, the University of Loughborough's Sleep Laboratory suggests this can usually be reversed (unless it's really chronic) with as few as two early nights – though you may need as many as five consecutive ones, depending on how long you've been short of sleep for.

So if someone's got a maths exam or a college interview tomorrow, turn off MSN, MTV, the cable showing of *Sin City*, or whatever they are glued to that doesn't finish till midnight, and send them off early with, for girls (see page 283) a relaxing hot bath plus 10–12 drops of lavender oil on their pillow. For boys, 7–10 drops of Thinni-A essence in a bath may be best.

See also 'Early bed, better grades' on page 381.

Immediately after learning a new subject

Einstein's law of relativity tying your teen in knots? Quadratic equations flooring them? Advice from education researcher Carlyle Smith of Trent University in Peterborough, Ontario, could help all teens wrestling to process, and understand, information – read it through, then *sleep on it.*

When you sleep, your brain is processing new facts or memories and practising new skills you've just been trying to teach it. It reactivates the neurological circuits you were using for what you just learnt to do – say a type of maths calculation – 'rehearses' them, then shuttles those new memories down into the long-term storage area, from where you can retrieve (remember) them when you need them next.

This works for other skills too – like playing a musical instrument, mastering a new complex video game, and driving – and scientists like Smith believe it also works for memorising facts and figures. He adds that even taking a short nap after a learning session (if you can switch off sufficiently) will help, which is why participants at corporate training seminars are increasingly encouraged to have 'quiet time' after sessions and even get their heads down for ten minutes' kip.

Teens might not be up for a post-learning nap (the Instant-Energy Breath – for how to do this, see Fix 156: Feeling Drained – and a few minutes' subsequent switch-off time might find favour as it's so quick), but it could work for them to do any theoretically hefty homework in the early evening, rather than mid-afternoon, then sleep to facilitate the brain-sorting and downloading process.

338. Homework

Many teenagers say they work best with an iPod in their ears and their favourite downloads on full blast. Parents generally don't see how this can be so, but recent research published in *New Scientist* in 2005 confirms that a person always concentrates best if the music's familiar.

Apparently, it is this familiarity that matters far more than what sort of music it is. If someone doesn't know a tune, this breaks their concentration no matter how soothing or alpha-brainwave-stimulating it is.

Let them choose

This suggests that if well-meaning parents try and give their teen a nice Mozart CD to do their maths to when they've not heard it before, it won't help as much as if they're listening to tracks they know well – so long as these aren't too hyped, as fast rhythms stimulate the release of adrenaline: great for fast reaction times, but it interferes with abstract thinking and creativity.

The perfect calming music has 65–80 beats per minute (heartbeat rate), so see whether they would accept, say, some Ibiza **chill-out compilations** for homework backtrack purposes if you bought them. If you want to encourage them to work to classical or chill-out (as other studies suggest this can improve creativity and concentration), ensure they *get to know the pieces or tracks subliminally first* – perhaps by playing it very quietly daily in the kitchen at breakfast- or suppertime.

If you worry about the effect loud music has on your teenager's brain – whether in clubs or via an iPod – but they are sniffing in derision, it may be worth mentioning . . . the eggs. There was once a major American teen fad for taking raw ones to rock concerts, hiding them down by the edge of the stage, then eating them halfway through the gig (as they were by now hard-boiled by the intensive sound waves). Who wants a hard-boiled brain?

339. Revision – Anti-Stress, Pro-Success

This is becoming an increasingly big issue for teenagers, if the 50 per cent rise in calls over the last decade to UK helpline Childline from teenagers trying to handle exam pressure is anything to go by.[18]

New tricks for an old challenge: teenagers' parents might remember revising for hours on end without a break, aided only by vast amounts of chocolate, Pro-Plus and coffee, but this method is fast losing favour in enlightened colleges since educational experts realised that students who cram forget what they learnt within only a few weeks

Switched-on schools now suggest students revise hard – i.e. perhaps the 'learning, covering up, remembering' technique – rather than just quietly reading through notes or text, *for only 30 minutes at a stretch*, 40 minutes *max*, then take a 20- to 30-minute break to really absorb what they just read, then have another 30- or 40-minute focus session. If your child's school hasn't suggested this, talk to their head teacher, explain why it works and ask if they'd like to give it a try.

The method sounds bitty if you've not done it before, but you do get into a good and highly productive rhythm by dividing each hour of revision into 30 or 40 minutes on/20 minutes off. Suggest your teenager sets a watch beeper *each time they stop* to remind them to begin again 20 minutes later – after taking a walk, snack or having a sit in the garden. If they don't have a watch, you can buy them a cheap but reasonable one with a beeper for as little as £10.

340. Feeling Overwhelmed

The 'anti-overwhelm' remedy for intensive training, revision and catch-up sessions is **Paw Paw**. It can help you process a lot of information at once when you are short of time. It's helpful for at-home revision sessions, catch-up skills clinics at school or college and especially training courses where you are given a lot at once and feel like you're drowning in facts.

Take seven drops straight from the bottle under the tongue before you begin. Longer term, if you are going to need it over a period of weeks, make up a dilute dropper bottle, with two-thirds spring water and one-third brandy as a preservative, and take seven drops from it twice daily.

Paw Paw can be bought direct from Australian Bush Flower Essences or via Healthlines (15 ml, £8.95). For contact details, see under 'Shopping' in the Directory.

Self-Esteem and Confidence

341. Shyness

One of the best subtle ways I know to help promote self-esteem and reduce the shyness and uncertainty that cripples many 13- to 19-

year-olds is **Confid** by Australian Bush Flower Essences, available direct, from Healthlines (30 ml, £7.95) and Neal's Yard (£8.50). This mixture of essences contains, among other things, **Dog Rose of the Wild Forces** (for 'sanity in times of turmoil' and 'emotional balance') plus **Five Corners** (for self-esteem and 'opening out a crushed-in personality').

I gave it to three boys abruptly removed from a gentle, alternative Steiner school in Brighton at the age of 13 to attend a tough local comprehensive – their parents had become edgy about the lack of traditional curriculum taught and were panicking about the boys' chances of getting any GCSEs whatsoever. The first two weeks before taking the essence mix they were very nervous, didn't say a word to anyone, got pushed around and bullied. Yet after just ten days of essence-taking, one had taken on the class thug (successfully), another had signed up as lead guitar in the best band in the school, and we had to reduce the dosage for all three of them as their teacher reported they were all 'getting a bit above themselves'.

Consider also another great one for teenagers: the **Supreme Confidence** combination, especially if they happen to like, or connect well, with animals. Developed by an American ex-wilderness guide, counsellor and spiritual therapist Daniel Mapel, it's made with the energies of different animals (but without touching a hair on their heads). Supreme Confidence is a mixture of three essences, which contain energy from the **Cheetah** (for swift, decisive action), **Mountain Lion** (for 'complete confidence and self-assurance') and, believe it or not, the **Bumblebee** ('for moving beyond one's limitations and doing things one simply did not think possible': something many teenagers may well be wanting to do). In the UK, they can be bought individually or as the Supreme Confidence combination via Healthlines (30 ml, £8.95); in the US, buy them from Wild Earth direct. For contact details, see under 'Shopping' in the Directory.

See also Shyness on page 90.

Self-Harm or Cutting

Figures and Triggers

Teenagers do this more often than most of us think. For instance, when the psychiatric unit at Warneford Hospital in Oxford looked at a sample of 14 schools and interviewed 6,020 teenagers of both sexes, researchers discovered that 7 per cent – that's one in every 15 – had deliberately harmed themselves in the previous year.[19]

Self-harm usually begins during puberty and lasts on average five to ten years, says American help organisation Self-Abuse Finally Ends (SAFE), though it can go on for much longer. It may take the form of cutting (in about two-thirds of cases) or burning, scalding, puncture-wounding, hair-pulling, scab-picking, deliberate bruising and even breaking bones. Many teenagers who repeatedly self-injure also have an eating disorder such as bulimia or anorexia (SAFE suggests up to two-thirds). Four times as many girls self-harm as boys. According to news sources like the UK's Channel 4, the practice of cutting in particular has at least doubled among Western teenagers over the last 20 years.

Causes

Causes overlap with those that trigger eating disorders and include low self-esteem, anxiety, depression, bereavement, being bullied and sexual or emotional abuse (past or current). SAFE's statistics suggest at least 50 per cent of all those who self-harm have been sexually abused.

Cutting is addictive behaviour. It may begin by chance, or as a result of copying peers in a friendship group, but however it starts, it often becomes well established unless someone can be helped to learn safer ways to deal with anger, tension, frustration and distress or express what they feel inside in healthier ways (self-harmers often say they cut or burn themselves to 'make the feelings stop'). As with any addiction, just telling someone to stop it will have no effect whatsoever. They must:

1. want to stop, and they may not want to until they feel they are being heard
2. be offered, and accept, the right sort of help.

Medical Treatments

Effective help usually includes ongoing non-judgemental family support and love, and professional backup from a *specialist therapist* who is experienced in working with teenagers who self-harm – someone who can give more time and offer much more expertise than a family doctor or general psychologist. Your GP should be able to refer you to the right person.

If they are not helpful, try contacting Self-Injury and Related Issues (SIARI) for further information on self-harm, support resources and where to find good professional help. If, as the parent of a teenager who self-harms or as a teenager struggling with this yourself, you would like to talk to a counsellor in total confidence, try the Bristol Crisis Centre. This is a national helpline for women in emotional distress, but especially for those who self-harm. Background information and advice is also available from a sensible practical site, www.palace.net. In the US, try the SAFE self-injury hotline or their website, which has a directory of experts for referral across the States. For contact details, see under 'Useful Helplines, Websites and Contacts' in the Directory.

What a therapist can do

A therapist can help someone who self-harms find safer ways to deal with tension and teach positive self-soothing behaviour, such as substituting strategies to use instead of hurting themselves – depending on why they are doing it. For instance, if a teenager self-harms when he or she is angry or frustrated, to help themselves calm down or release the tension, a therapist may recommend pillow-punching, taking up kick-boxing and practising this when the anger strikes, going out immediately for a pounding run, putting on loud music for fast, aggressive dancing in their room.

If a person feels numb inside and the self-injury is to feel something, a therapist may suggest creating a relatively non-damaging but powerful sensation instead of self-harming – e.g. holding ice cubes clenched in the hand or chewing something with a hot, fiery taste like raw ginger. If the self-harm stems from the frustration of not being able to express certain feelings they have, it may be suggested they keep a private diary, draw, paint or join a drama therapy workshop to act it out. If the trouble stems from psychological damage, such as bereavement or a history of abuse, this needs to be addressed by professional counselling and support.

Complementary Treatments

There are lots of useful, supportive things to try, but they won't be enough on their own. Use any complementary health or spiritual techniques in conjunction with professional counselling.

342. The Self-Esteem Stone

A special gift for a girl who self-harms is the beautiful yellow **citrine**, to be worn on a chain round her neck at all times, says gem therapist and senior healer trainer for the National Federation of Spiritual Healers Jacquie Wilton, as this semi-precious gem can help promote self-esteem and renewed joy in life. It is also said to encourage those who wear it respond better to constructive criticism (in which case, we could all probably do with one).

343. Aroma Rescue
For teenage girls

Try regular baths in **rose absolu** – see Fix 306: Aromatherapy for Anorexia. Or put one to two drops with water in a diffuser or burner each evening in the teenager's bedroom.

Other helpful essential oils, as suggested by Valerie Wormwood, author of the seminal bestseller on aromatherapy *The Fragrant Pharmacy*, are **jasmine**, **neroli** and **rose Maroc** (for self-esteem) or **cedarwood** (for grounding, balancing and for those who are very emotionally sensitive). You can buy all of these oils from Baldwin's: Jasmine Absolute Essential Oil (5 ml, £24.95), Neroli Oil (5 ml, £26.59), Rose Maroc Oil (5 ml, £24.95) and Cedarwood Oil (10 ml, £2.95). Also try Neal's Yard and Tisserand, or the lovely Starchild, or for the very best organic ones (also most expensive!) try Florihana of Provence – see Shopping section page 571.

Suggested reading: see also Wormwood's *The Fragrant Mind*, a real bible on the therapeutic use of aromatherapy for the emotions.

For teenage boys

Two especially good oils for men are **cypress** and **frankincense**. Cypress has the characteristic of the tree itself – 'tall, strong, upright' – and is often used to help people who worry too much about what everyone else thinks of them or have difficulty resisting dominant peers. Frankincense is fortifying and uplifting, helps with fears, worries and depressive feelings. Both help strengthen self-image. Add a little **cedarwood** to the mix for enhancing self-esteem, as it's grounding, strengthening, power-enhancing, balancing and supports those who 'feel too much'.

Again, you can purchase all of these from Baldwin's shop or mail-order service: Cypress Oil (10 ml, £3.75), Frankincense Oil (10 ml, £11.45) and Cedarwood Oil (10 ml, £2.95). You can also try Neal's Yard or Tisserand. In the US, try Nature's Gift mail order or Auroma.

As with all oils, check that the person likes the smell before using them (if they don't, forget it). If you are doing a massage mix of oils, just two to three drops of each will be enough; if it's a bath with a single oil, try eight to ten drops.

For all contact details, see under 'Shopping' in the Directory.

344. Essences

Take either orally from a dropper bottle or add drops 'neat' (i.e. directly from the bottle they arrive in) at a time to a bath each night. There are several helpful ones that can support teenagers of both sexes who self-harm to feel good about themselves. The three best ones are detailed below.

Add seven to ten drops **Angelsword** to a bath. This is a terrific remover of negative energy (i.e. anger, resentment, sadness, despair, self-doubt and self-loathing) and is immensely calming. It can also be invaluable to someone who:

- feels confused but wants to understand what is really going on in a situation. Angelsword is a great truth-seeing essence, which is why you can make 'angel's word' from its name.

- is trying to decide what really is best for *them* (and never mind what everyone else is saying).

Both of the above may be very helpful for someone who self-harms but is trying to sort themselves out.

Add **Sturt Desert Rose** for a teenager whose self-esteem is low, one whom you too often hear apologising for themselves ('Oh, sorry, I'm so *stupid*'), who is a bit easily led by their friends, feels bad or guilty about the self-harming soon afterwards and who also may be feeling a bit guilty or confused about sex. Sturt Desert Rose is also, interestingly, indicated for helping heal 'fine cuts' so may be especially relevant if that is the form the self-harm is taking.

Dagger Hakea is a good one if there is anger and rage involved, or some major resentment going back a long way against one or more family members. It can help bring an ability to express buried feelings openly – and also engenders forgiveness.

All the above are from the Australian Bush Flower range and can be bought direct worldwide or, in the UK, from Healthlines (15 ml, £8.95 each).

Also try **My Body** (from Light Heart's new Urban Angels range, developed especially for troubled teenagers, £7.50 for 30ml spritzer) or the gentle flower essence **Salvia** for positive body image. In the UK, you can buy this one from from IFER (3.8 ml, £7.50) or from the Nutri Centre; in the US, direct from Petites Fleurs Essences ($18). It was developed by master herbalist and fourth-generation essence-maker Dr Judy Griffin, who works with two major cancer units in Texas and whose Petites Fleurs essences are used by both orthodox and complementary practitioners worldwide.

For all contact details, see under 'Shopping' in the Directory.

See also Fix 307: The Forgiveness Process and Teenagers: Scars on page 368.

Sexuality

345. (Over-)Assertive Male Sexuality

Sometimes teenage boys' emerging sexuality and maleness can assert itself a bit too much for the comfort of those around them. This can be balanced out by an essence remedy called **Balga Blackboy** from the Australian outback. The aborigines see the balga tree and its flowers as a warrior standing with his spear, watching over his tribe, and it is this strong, calm, mature, male quality that the essence helps bring out.

Balga seems to subtly help young men become both assertive and caring. Often used if a boy is becoming negative, aggressively sexualised or destructive – and also if he is 'too gentle' and does not yet have the masculine strength inside that he needs. Take the remedy as drops under the tongue from a made-up dropper bottle, or perhaps for the early-evening dose, you can add 20 undiluted remedy drops straight from the bottle into a warm bath – when the bath is half full, drop them directly under the water gushing out from the tap to disperse the essence properly.

To make up a 30 ml dropper bottle, add around 50 drops of Balga Blackboy, then fill up with two-thirds spring water and one-third brandy as a preservative. The dosage is six drops in the morning and late afternoon in half a glass of water.

It is available worldwide direct from Living Essences of Australia or from IFER (15 ml, approximately £8/$14).

Sleep

346. Not Enough

During term-time, adolescents all across the country are staggering out of bed after too little sleep. But 13- to 18-year-olds are *biologically programmed to sleep later and longer than adults*. This need is compli-cated by the fact that their circadian (sleep-wake) rhythms are changing so they can't help staying up later, even without the lure of socialising and MSN, possibly because their brains are getting temporarily more sensitive to light.

According to Brown University Medical School, 20 years of research confirms teens actually need 9.2 hours of shut-eye a night (compared with the 7.5–8 adults require), but three-quarters are getting less than 8.5 hours and a quarter manage on less than 6.5.

Early bed, better grades

Not enough sleep has been shown to be linked to poor concentration, behavioural problems, depression, anxiety states, ADHD and poor grades. Luckily, the reverse is also true. In 1998 Brown University surveyed over 3,000 high-schoolers and found those scoring Cs, Ds and Fs were all, without exception, *going to bed 40 minutes later and getting 25 minutes less sleep than the A and B students.*

And when the University of Minnesota looked at how 7,000 teenagers were doing after their high schools switched from a 7.15 a.m. to an 8.40 a.m. start, students got more sleep on school nights, reported higher grades, less depression and their behaviour was better.

So, if you want your teenager to get their grades up, get them into bed just 40 minutes earlier on schooldays. And if they have a punishing 7.30 a.m. start, as many US high schools do, lobby their school hard to begin later. This is catching on: in the US, the Connecticut legislature is considering banning public schools from starting before 8.30 a.m.

Sleep Tips

To help them relax so they can get to sleep earlier:

- **Baths with extras** – run *girls* a warm one and add some gently sedating organic **lavender essential oil**, 10–12 drops, which you can buy from Neal's Yard (10 ml, £8.95) or from most health food shops and good chemists. Or *for boys* add five to seven drops of the blissful **Thini-A**. Many people feel so laid-back after soaking in this one they can barely get out of the bath. Suggest they soak for a good 15–20 minutes to give

them time to absorb enough of the essence or oil to be effective, via steam inhalation and through the pores of their skin,
before bed. You can buy Thini-A direct from Araretama Rainforest
Essences in Brazil or through Healthlines (15 ml, approximately
£8). For contact details, see under 'Shopping' in the Directory.

- **Sensible stuff** – it's standard, you've heard it before, but it
  works. Cut out TV, non-relaxing music, MSN, texting, emailing,
  Net-trawling, homework and computer games *for a full hour
  before bed*.

Try and help your teenager get a bedroom routine going and encourage
them to stick to it: perhaps a warm bath or shower, a bit of reading,
even a CD story, relaxation tape or gentle time with a pet.

Pet power

Pets' physical and psychological de-stressing, anxiety-reducing and
antidepressive effects are well researched – see www.holisticon-
line.com for a taster.

Cats and other strokable animals can be great calmers-down if
they are allowed in your teenager's bedroom. And 16-year-olds
can be just as soothed by sitting in bed with a book in their hand
and a cat across their knees as a much younger child.

See also Teenagers: Energy on page 351.
For more general advice on sleep, see General: Sleep on page 92.

Teeth

347. Whiter Teeth

The colour of someone's teeth depends on genetics, their age, their oral
hygiene, whether they've been exposed to too much fluoride, taken
tetracycline antibiotics and the amount of staining substances they
consume (e.g. colas, coffee, tea, red wine and cigarettes).

Most teens, especially girls, can be pretty keen to have white teeth, but cosmetic bleaching treatments at the dentist can be harsh, only available privately and therefore expensive (usually around £300) and will need redoing once a year or so; at-home bleaching systems like the recent Crest Whitestrips, beloved of beauty editors, do a nice job on the front but can leave the back molars their old colour. You can buy the strips direct from the manufacturer (£69.99). Ordinary tooth powder is usually aimed at the stained teeth of smokers and is pretty abrasive; budget liquid over-the-counter teeth-whiteners like Pearl Drops are very short term and chemical-based.

Scrubbing up

However, a good, quick, natural alternative is an oral hygiene treatment to use every day instead of ordinary toothpaste (especially if you prefer your children to avoid sources of fluoride) called **Dental Miracle**. It is made from powdered plant ingredients: juniper berry (disinfectant and bactericidal), peppermint (antiseptic, soothing and anti-inflammatory), acacia gum (soothing), calendula (calming, antiseptic, antibacterial and antiviral) and orris root (contains vitamin C and is a breath-freshener) but no chemicals or vicious abrasives.

One small green pot is £17.99, which sounds a lot, but it acts as a toothpaste, cleaner and de-stainer in one, has a gentle, herby taste and lasts around ten weeks if used by one person, but the whole family can brush with it if they can get their hands on it. It is made by the Genesis Group and is available in the UK from Victoria Health. In the US and Canada, contact the Genesis distributor in Canada for mail order via your nearest retailer.

Note: The effect of Dental Miracle is cumulative, and it will make the very best of the teeth you have while boosting the health of your gums and helping keep cavities at bay, rather than completely changing the colour of naturally ivory- or pale-yellow-coloured ones to a fluorescent dazzle.

Tip
For an ultra budget whitening, dip a dry toothbrush in **baking soda** and brush firmly.

Whiter, brighter

Another option is the innovative American whitening toothpaste reportedly used by Kate Moss, Johnny Depp and Linda Evangelista called **Supersmile**. In the UK, you can buy it via Dealtime (£15.25); in the US, buy it direct from Supersmile (1.75 oz tube, $11). It does not contain any bleach – as the other cosmetic whitening products do – and instead uses baking soda and a compound called Calprox, which is said to work by removing the thin protein film on teeth to which bacteria and stains cling. It's not cheap, but the results are good.

For all contact details, see under 'Shopping' in the Directory.

Travel

348. School-Trip Sickness

As they become teenagers, most children are offered the chance to travel and stay away from home with their school for the first time (skiing trips, camping, adventure holidays, language-learning centres abroad). But for some, the opportunity and fun can be spoilt by travel sickness – you can feel considerably worse on a large, swaying school coach than in a family car.

If your child suffers but is too embarrassed to take any medication prescribed by their doctor because it makes them rather dopey and may have the added stigma of needing a top-up en route from a teacher, offer them a **Sea-Band**. These are discreet little elasticated acupressure wristbands (which can sit snugly with any charity bands they wear) featuring a plastic stud that presses against the **nei kwan** anti-sickness acupressure point on the inside of the wrist.

In clinical trials, the bands do the trick for 80 per cent of pregnant women suffering from morning sickness, seasick British merchant navy sailors and chemotherapy patients. They are available in the UK from pharmacies including Boots, and mail order from the Sea-Band company itself (£7.99); in the US, you can buy them from chains like Walmart or mail order from Sea-Band ($9.99). For contact details, see under 'Shopping' in the Directory.

See also Young Children: Travel Sickness on page 306, as the **ginger powder** capsules suggested there also work well for teenagers and adults.

And since they are not classified as medicines, a teenger can keep them themselves and take more as necessary without having to hand them in to a teacher.

Pets

There is so much advice to give for pets that this chapter, like the others, can only really scratch the surface. In fact, I'm currently researching another book with a homeopathic vet who uses essences, an animal healer who uses veterinary aromatherapy, an animal behaviouralist, and a telepathic animal communicator that will hopefully do the subject of natural therapy and esoteric strategies for animals a bit more justice. But in the meantime, here are as many suggestions and tips as we could fit in, many of which I've used on our own animals – at the last count, one visiting dog, four cats, five rabbits, two guinea pigs, several abandoned baby seagulls and a tank of fish.

From putting Vicks on the tail of a bitch in heat when out for a walk (to discourage the hordes of admirers) or using a programmed rose-quartz crystal for settling a mother cat who looks like rejecting her kittens, to the essences that reassure a clingy pet going to boarding kennels or a rescue animal arriving at a new home – plus how to talk to your pet telepathically (and hear them talk back) or give your dog a bit of relaxing shiatsu – there's something in here for every much loved pet.

Animals and complementary therapies

Animals are part of the family for one in seven Britons. We've got 7.7 million cats and 6.7 million dogs, on whom we spend £3.5 billion every year, much of it on animal complementary therapies, the most popular of which are reiki and healing, homeopathy and essences.[1]

Aggressive and Mistrustful Behaviour

349. Mistrustful

Bristles easily, jumpy, quick to bare their teeth or hiss . . . the dark-green **jadeite gemstone** could help here if the animal reacts this way because they are under stress or have been mistreated in the past, say natural pet-care experts and animal gem therapists Martin Scott and Gael Mariani.

Jadeite's use for animals showing this sort of behaviour has also been researched and developed by ex-wilderness firefighter turned essence-developer and healer Steve Johnson, who makes the excellent Alaskan Essences range. Cleanse and prepare the jadeite gemstone in the usual way (see Appendix 1: Cleansing and Programming Crystals and Gems on page 536) – this only takes a few minutes – then place it by your pet's bed.

You can also use **Animal Rescue**, the essence containing jadeite, in their drinking water as an accompaniment. It can be bought via Healthlines (60 ml, £11.95); in the US and Canada, it's available direct from Alaskan Essences.

However, though it's a good calmer and soother, jadeite's not magic fairy dust and you still need to exercise common sense: while it will help heal aggression that comes from stress, it won't take away, say, a mother's urge to protect her young or an animal's natural instinct for self-defence, and it works gently and cumulatively rather than instantly as a tranquillising drug would. So if you are caring for a suspicious or mistrustful animal, be cautious and use it as part of a programme, not as the only thing you do.

To find a piece of jadeite, try any New Age or gem shop. In the UK, one of the most remarkable ones I have ever come across is the Litlington Crystal Store in East Sussex (run by two sympathetic experts who are also healers and gem-therapy teachers) – call and ask to speak to Morgarian or Ru'an. In the US, try Pretty Rock (run by husband and wife gem-enthusiast team).

For all contact details, see under 'Shopping' in the Directory.

350. Territorial and Aggressive With It (Dogs Only)

Dogs may be aggressive for many reasons, but the most common reasons are because of a history of ill treatment or abandonment, or because they are in pain (with arthritis, for example). They may also have behavioural problems – a classic is showing aggression every time a visitor or postman arrives at the door – which means that they have learnt to respond to a certain situation in a certain way. It is behavioural problems that can be the hardest to treat; many animal therapists make good money helping owners encourage pets to change their negative responses to more positive ones. If you would like to contact one, try the Association of Pet Behaviour Counsellors. For contact details, see under 'Therapies and Therapists' in the Directory.

Treats

Naturally territorial, your dog may see 'strangers', such as the postman, as invaders on their patch. A simple approach to helping your dog feel differently about visitors is to encourage them to associate a visitor with a treat (offered by the person themselves) so the dog learns to welcome them, rather than go for them.

If it's the postman your dog objects to, Canine Behavioral Services of Philadelphia suggests taping a small dog-treat to the outside of the door every night before you go to bed, so the postman can put an offering through the letterbox along with the post.

If it's *any* visitor that upsets them, try keeping a box of their favourite dog-treats near the door out of their reach and ask everyone who calls to offer one as they arrive. Ensure those particular treats are not given at other times, only by visitors. As Steve Aitken, owner of Animal Behavioral Consultants, Kansas, says, it's difficult for a dog to see someone as a threat when that person's offering them something nice to eat.

See also Pets: Anxiety and Neediness on page 390.

Anti-Aging

351. Anti-Aging Treatment

Most dogs live around 14–16 years; some breeds like Labradors live nearer 10–12; and cats live an average of 16, though there are many

PETS

18-year-old felines who, with a combination of luck, love, good genes, enough exercise and a decent diet are still going stately and strong.

ACE vitamins for pets
Antioxidant **vitamins A, C** and **E** help protect humans against cancer, arthritis and heart disease and can do the same for your pet. Deva Khalsa, a Pennsylvanian vet who is also a qualified animal acupuncturist, suggests giving medium-sized older dogs:

- around 400 mg vitamin C daily (larger dogs can take nearer 600 mg), divided into two doses mixed in with morning and evening meals
- 100–400 IU vitamin E, also in two doses with meals.

Older cats can be given:

- 50 IU vitamin E, again in two doses with meals.

They may not appreciate taking the vitamins in pill or capsule form, so try the powdered vitamin C or open up the capsules, then mix in well with their food. For vitamin E, use ordinary capsules of vitamin-E oil from the health shop, pierce and squeeze into their food. Wheatgerm oil, also available in capsule form from any health food shop, is another excellent source of vitamin E.

Raw food: the gradual approach
If you don't like the idea of supplements in capsules, another great way to keep your pet healthy and help slow aging is to give them all-natural **raw food** – see 'The BARF programme' on page 408. Having said that, it is, until you get used to it, a bit of an undertaking for some.

If this is so for you, try a partway approach first: mix a small amount of lightly steamed green or orange vitamin-rich vegetables (say, a palmful for a medium-sized dog like a spaniel and half a dessertspoonful for the average cat) into their food.

A little finely diced steamed sweet pepper, one of the richest sources of vitamin C there is, is acceptable to many dogs. Cats – traditionally fussier – are often receptive to a little mashed carrot mixed well into food, which is a decent source of vitamin A. Or, if you like carrot juice yourself, give them a teaspoonful of yours mixed into each meal, as it's a tasty and concentrated source.

Sprouts for Cats

Is your cat being sniffy about taking extra vitamins in pill form? Do they eat *around* even the most imaginatively-hidden ones you've concealed in their catfood, leaving it reproachfully in the middle of their empty dish when they have finished? Many fastidious felines will in fact go for a bit of mashed lightly cooked Brussels sprout (a good source of vitamin A, C and fibre) mixed in with their usual food instead, says Dr Khalsa, and eat the lot with every evidence of enjoyment.

Anxiety and Neediness

352. Clingy Pets

Few animals are natural loners: most are paired species or pack animals. And if they do live solo without a member of their own species for company, you will be their only source of love and company, so when you go out, they may become very unhappy and uneasy, even developing a clinging, needy or downright destructive behavioural pattern that is not good for either them or you.

Friends united

The most helpful, kind and effective thing you can possibly do for a loner pet is to get them a friend of their own kind – perhaps even a rescue animal in need of a loving home – see Rescue Animals on page 425.

Remedy

If that is totally out of the question, holistic vets also recommend **Chicory** from Bach Flower Essences, which encourages feelings of being loved and of inner security. It's also used, very successfully, for clingy or possessive small children who are especially demanding.

Add a couple of drops to your pet's water bowl every day for two to three weeks and see how you go. Or, if the 'needy' state seems very acute, massage a drop into the bare skin of their ears (through which this gentle remedy is readily and rapidly absorbed). Do this three to four times a day.

Chicory can be bought from Healing Herbs (10 ml, £3.20). For contact details, see under 'Shopping' in the Directory.

353. Home Alone

Few dogs like being left behind on their own even for a few hours, and often find it particularly difficult to settle in an empty house when their humans go off to work as this is usually for a long time, anything up to ten hours plus. Unless they have a companion animal, preferably of their own kind, and/or someone who will come visit during the day to pet them and take them out for a walk, this is not a kind way to keep a dog, and the tip below is not meant to facilitate that, though veterinary research has found that it helped even with this.

What it can be really useful for, however, is when you want to go out for a shorter but still, from the dog's point of view, appreciable length of time, perhaps for an evening party. If you suspect they will pine and fret when you've gone – or worse, howl or bark continuously (your neighbours will probably have been quick to let you know about that one) try a small plug-in device called a **Dog-Appeasing Pheromone (DAP).** It releases a form of dog-soothing airborne hormones similar to those given off by a female when she is feeding milk to her puppies. These 'canine-appeasing' hormones are produced by a mother dog from the sebaceous glands round her milk teats three to five days after her puppies' birth. Their job is to deepen the loving attachment between mother and pup, and ever afterwards the scent of those hormones (undetectable by the human nose) triggers memories of reassurance, safety and comfort.

The DAP has been used successfully to help comfort dogs when they are left alone for several hours at a time. Clinical trials also suggest that the device 'improves' destructive behaviour and vocalisation' (read: ripping up the carpet and howling or whining) by 72 and 85 per cent respectively.

The device can often be bought via your local vet. CEVA Animal Health can tell you the nearest one in your area who will have it. If not, Vet UK sells it via their website (diffuser with DAP, £15.99; 48 ml refills, £10.99). For contact details, see under 'Shopping' in the Directory.

Note: the DAP is also useful for calming dogs on Fireworks Night – see also pp 404 – on long car trips if they happen to be nervous of the car rather than just carsick, for spraying comfort around their accommodation cubicle during an overnight visit to the vet (see also Vet Visit page 429) and for making a new corner of the house feel more like home to them, e.g. when you have just moved and have placed their sleep basket somewhere cosy but unfamiliar: see also Fix 435: Moving House

354. Music for Edgy Cats

Cats can be calmed by music so long as it's not too loud (their hearing's far sharper than yours), but they have their favourites. Fifty-six per cent prefer gentle classical music – e.g. Mozart, Brahms and Einaudi – to thundering Wagnerian opera or doom-laden requiems. But they also seem to be quite a cultured species: only 14 per cent like easy listening best. And one in 25 leans towards the artier and more experimental by preferring jazz of all types.[2]

Arthritis

355. Magnet Therapy

Magnet therapy has been shown by clinical trials to help with human arthritis pain, inflammation (see Fix 15: Anti-Arthritis Jewellery) and to speed human bone repair and wound healing. However, I can't yet find any similar trials with animals: just several companies who make magnetic products for pets looking for vets to participate in controlled clinical studies with them – and if there's anyone interested out there, Magna are especially enthusiastic.

What I did find, though, was a plethora of anecdotal reports suggesting magnetic therapy can help animals in the same way as it helps humans.

I also saw the apparent difference it made to a poor old arthritic Labrador (aged 11) who had been in constant pain from a degenerative hip joint for over a year despite anti-inflammatories and painkillers from his vet (so much so that they had been considering, albeit most reluctantly, putting the dog to sleep). The dog was walking more easily after four weeks of wearing the magnetic collar. I had tentatively suggested to his owner – and that wasn't a placebo effect because you don't find that in animals.

How you use it

Magnetic at-home therapy for animals is usually offered in the form of a magnetic collar for dogs or cats and as a tendon wrap or tie-on rug to promote healing for horses. If you are interested, since it certainly can't do any harm, why not try it out for a few weeks and if it's not helping, send it back – reputable companies always offer a money-back guarantee. Try **Magna Therapy**'s pet collars (£17.99), which carry a 60-day money-back scheme, or **Bioflow**'s cat collars with bell (around £27) and collars for small- to medium-sized dogs (around £30), all with a 90-day money-back-if-not-happy guarantee. For contact details, see under 'Shopping' in the Directory.

Magnetic therapy is usually at its most effective if the magnets are worn (all the time) *near to the site of the injury or pain*. So a magnetic collar worn round the neck is likely to benefit, say, arthritis in the front legs more than in the back legs, and arthritis or upper-back pain more than pain around the pelvic area or tail base.

In the case of the latter, it might be helpful to try a magnetic mat for the dog's basket, which your pet could lie on all night. It can be covered with their usual smelling-of-them blanket. These mats are slim, flexible and waterproof, have small magnets placed inside them at regular intervals and cost approximately £60. Again, choose a supplier offering a money-back guarantee.

Note: the nutritional route can help prevent arthritis from developing and may help alleviate it to some degree if it's already biting. Talk to a holistically minded vet about using fish oils and also more natural foods – see Pets: Anti-Aging on page 388 and Pets: Food on page 407.

Birthing

356. Aromatherapy

Rose essential oil is wonderful for anything 'female' (for humans as well as animals – see Fix 167: How to Stay Calm – The Fast Natural Fix.

'After birthing, most mothers and their newborns are keen to take in the aroma of rose. For the mother, it helps balance and regulate her body; for the babies, it can help clear any birth-trauma memories,' says international animal aromatherapy pioneer Caroline Ingraham. She suggests that one drop in a drinking bowl or in a full drinking bottle (for rabbits and guinea pigs) is enough.

> Always offer another plain source of drinking water by the side of the one containing even a drop of aromatherapy oil, so the animal can choose how much they take.

Use *only* organic oils for animals. For supplies, try Star Child's Organic Rose Absolute (trial bottle, 1 ml, £7.95) or Florihana in Provence. For contact details, see under 'Shopping' in the Directory.

> **Cat caution**
>
> For cats, never, ever put essential oils in their water, food or in a diffuser or burner, as their systems cannot metabolise the oils and this would be toxic to them. Instead, offer the open essential-oil bottle from about a metre away for them to come forward and sniff if they wish. See also Fix 382: Cat Aromatherapy and 'Is it the right one?' on page 414.

Problems?

For an animal who is upset after her birth, or is showing signs of neglecting her young, give her a comfortable, secluded environment, lots of privacy (prevent the rest of your family from 'having a look' to see how she is or peeking at the babies) and place a small **rose-quartz crystal** (see Appendix 1: Cleansing and Programming Crystals and Gems on page 536) near her bed. This one is the 'love stone', and it has a gentle, reassuring, softening, loving influence on all living creatures. Females of all species like it especially.

Chewing and Scratching

357. Chewing
Animals can be forgiven totally for not immediately understanding why it's all right to go for a chew-toy but not your best stilettos, so explain it to them, behavioural-style. Every time you catch them gnawing something they shouldn't, say, 'No,' firmly and immediately replace the object with something appropriate. When they start to worry that instead, praise and pet them.

Hot stuff
If that doesn't work, or it's an object you can't really remove (like a large piece of furniture), Bob Gutierrez, the animal-behaviour coordinator of the San Francisco Society for Prevention of Cruelty to Animals, recommends putting a splash of **Tabasco** sauce on the forbidden object — those handmade brogue shoes, the leg of a designer coffee table, the corner of your best black leather briefcase . . . but always do a small spot-test first. Though Tabasco usually wipes off as easily as it goes on, it may leave an orangey stain on more porous, lighter-coloured items like pale leather.

358. Scratching the Furniture
Cat scratching your sofa base to shreds? Buy some double-sided industrial tape from a DIY or professional decorating shop. Stick the tape on the area they usually go for at the height where the claw-marks begin, in two bands separated by about 5 cm of clear space, one above the other. It is important that it is set at this distance because your cat will be unable to scratch either above or below.

Wait quietly until your cat approaches the sofa, chair or table again and tries to lock on as usual. Allow them to discover the surface has changed, then take them gently to something they *are* allowed to tear at (such as a doormat or a scratching-post), encourage them to put their paws on it and have a rip.

Do this every time you notice them get their claws out near your furniture. If you find your cat is managing to scratch above the taped area and spot a few claw-marks, place another band of tape over the new marks. They'll soon stop as it will be uncomfortable to stretch higher.

After a couple of weeks (the time period varies somewhat, depending on how used your cat is to sharpening their nails there) you will usually be able to remove the double-sided tape because they're choosing the permitted scratch area instead.

For a more subtle, but equally – if not more – successful approach, see also Animal Whispering, below.

Communication

359. Animal Whispering

Telepathic (or psychic) animal communication is an amazing, loving and respectful way to bond even more closely with an animal you care for. It also has many immediate practical applications based on crossing the human-animal language barrier, so you can, when necessary:

- explain things clearly to your pet, so as to encourage their more willing cooperation – 'Why does the damn vet have to poke about in my sore mouth like that?'
- find out why a happy, confident pet has suddenly become defensive or timid – 'It's that new cat over the road: he's going for me every time I step out of the cat-flap.'
- know exactly how and where they have hurt themselves. For instance, if your dog is limping but the vet can't tell quite where the trouble is coming from, your dog can 'show' you by perhaps allowing you to scan mentally along his spine until you come to the very vertebrae that's been misaligned by a recent tumble you never realised he'd had.

- 'send' your pet daily messages of love and reassurance, when you leave to go on holiday, telling them exactly when you'll be back. Pets can count days and have a good internal clock – if you have a dog or cat who's at home when you're out at work, how often have you found them waiting for you on the windowsill or by the front door when you arrive home? Sending love home helps them feel more secure, so they are less likely to pine or be worried you'll never return. This a very common fear for animals as they are not told any different.

- find out why they have gone off the food they've always wolfed down before and what they fancy having instead to start them eating again. Again, you can do this by sending visual images of suggested foods plus the taste (if it's something you don't mind eating too, such as tuna) and smell – e.g. you could offer a cat who's gone off Whiskas a mental picture of a bowl of those glistening salmon chunks in oil, plus an impression of its smell or taste and see if you get a 'Yeah, not half!' or a 'No' coming back. Your pet will usually respond immediately in matters of food preference.

- explain why certain sorts of behaviour are not allowed in such a way as to help ensure they willingly act differently for you in the future. The conventional 'No' each time and removing them from the scene usually works eventually, but it's quicker, more polite and gentler to show an animal what you'd like them to do via a mental picture, followed up with a sensation of love, praise and thanks coming from you as a reinforcement of good behaviour.

Anyone can do it

You don't have to be 'special' to do this. You don't need to see yourself as psychic either. So far as communication goes – especially with someone you like or love, like a pet – *everyone is psychic*.

Have you ever had the experience of, say, the phone ringing and you know exactly who it is even before you pick up? Or you take your child to the doctor, who says there's nothing wrong but you just *know* there is and are later proved right? There you go. You're picking up on things on a telepathic level and probably do it all the time without realising.

Telepathy as film

According to top US animal psychic and communicator Amelia Kinkade, who teaches pet owners and animal carers from refuge staff to vets worldwide, when you are in contact with an animal or person you establish a line of unspoken two-way communication with them. They hear your words, see the gestures you make and the expressions on your face – and they also pick up on the silent visual images you are sending them while you talk with their mind's eye (third eye, if you like).

Perhaps you are telling a friend about your holiday. You describe the blue of the sea, the soft, sugary feel of the powdery sand, the heat of the sun, the taste of the tomato salads you ate, the smell of the sea, the crying of the gulls – and all the while you are also automatically sending them a mental film of it, the better to help them understand. That's why we use phases like 'I can see what you mean', 'Yes, I can picture that' and 'I get it.'

Telepathic communication between people and animals is essentially based on sending them these messages and seeing in your own mind's eye the messages they send back. The messages aren't restricted to the visual, however – they can be physical sensations like touch (tickly, rough, pressure or even pain), smells (fish, raw red meat or the scent of grass) and emotions (fear, anger, puzzlement, joy and contentment).

Talk to the animals

But it's not possible to just go up to an animal and start bombarding them with images. That's like walking into someone's house without knocking: it would be intrusive, even intimidating: most animals would at the very least blank you right away, others might even become distressed or aggressive. So Amelia Kinkade always teaches a gentler, step-by-step method:

1. First, you need to ground, calm and relax *yourself*. Many people prepare themselves in the same way as they would for a simple healing or session of therapeutic touch. For a quick and easy method, see page 290.
2. Next, you need to rid yourself of any negativity (e.g. cross thoughts, impatience and sadness) so you are in a positive, clear and receptive state to both hear your animal and be heard by them. They won't

want to listen if what you send them is tainted with your own irritation, fear or distress.

3. Finally, send them waves of love and affection, wrapping them gently in it as if it's a soft, golden light, so they know you mean them well. Essentially, simply look at them and send them love from your eyes – and also, if you can, your heart.

4. When you have established this calm, loving contact, 'ask' if you may talk to them. Wait to see if they say, 'OK.' They may not, though – well, sometimes we don't feel like talking either. If that's the case, accept gracefully; gently stop sending your love and just try again another time. However, if you get a 'yes' feeling, proceed to Step 5.

5. Send your pet a visual image from your own mind of what you'd like to ask them. Make this image as simple and clear as you can. For instance, if your dog's gone off their usual food and you want to know what they *would* like to eat that evening, first send a sense of evening (the world getting darker, cooler). Next, send a picture of their bowl in their usual eating place filled with something different. Perhaps a juicy bone? No? OK, some chopped raw meat? No? How about some lamb chunks, half raw, with a few pieces of chopped-up veg? Or a bowl of crisp Winalot biscuits? Try and imagine the scent and, if you can, possible taste or texture of each one and 'send' that too. You will probably get a 'yes' for one of the options you suggest; sometimes you might get a 'yes' for two options, but one is likely to be more enthusiastic – e.g. for the Winalot.

6. Now you have your answer, withdraw, thanking them for their help. Gently 'detach' your thoughts from the animal. Breathe deeply, rub your hands together, stretch – that's it. And make sure you come up with those biscuits for supper.

Checking for hurt

You can also check your pet for illness and harm by asking them, firstly, if you may mentally inhabit their body for a few moments and, secondly, if they will allow you to see into their body like an X-ray, working your way along bit by bit to see if all's well. **Animal medical gestalt** works in this way, and it's the technique that forms the basis of animal communicators' work with vets, zoos and animal refuges. It enables you to find, say, if an animal has toothache, which tooth is the problem and even which bit of it. Or if they have a digestive problem, whether there is an area of blockage or inflammation and, if so, where. This skill can be invaluable when it's used in a veterinary context.

It can be a bit of a surprise when it first happens, however, because you will be seeing through the animal's eyes, feeling what they feel. The first time I tried this (with a rabbit of ours who was unwell), I suddenly, without warning, found I was looking at the world through the chicken-wire mesh of their run, the long grass they were peering at me through tickled my own nose, and I got an instant perspective of the world looking huge as it was being seen from about 25 cm off the ground.

Remote viewing – Lassie, come home

Another important facet of animal telepathy is controlled **remote viewing**, which is used to find missing or lost pets (and has also been used to track down missing persons). It involves taking a fix on the animal concerned by thinking about them and picturing them in your head (if you know them) or linking into them via a photo (if you don't), then sending your senses ranging out there to see where they are. This often enables the animal communicator (AC) to find them and tell their owner. Usually the information requires some interpretation of local geographical landmarks. For instance, it may be along the lines of:

> **AC:** They seem to be behind a bus shelter – looks like clear plastic with a red trim – next to some sort of thick hedge. There's a big brown building with a red sign nearby. It's got a hammer on it – maybe it's a DIY-store logo.
> **Pet owner:** Yes! I know it, that's the Drayton Road one, at the other end of town.
> **AC:** Excellent. Get down there in the car, quick.

The animal communicator could also relay a message to the animal to ask them to wait – perhaps by offering a picture of them lying down calmly where they are – and indicating that help is on its way by sending them a 'film' of being picked up and cuddled by their owner in the place where they are at present. Every single instance is different, but you get the idea.

Proof

Remote viewing does work. The US government takes it so seriously that it was used and taught by the CIA as a counter-espionage technique for many years. The project, initially called Stargate, had $20 million spent on it. Its practitioners got results that were 65 per cent accurate on average, but often far higher, sometimes nearing 80 per cent.

Telepathic animal communication may sound like a subject for several years' study. In fact, the rudiments (ready to use right away, at home) can be taught in a day's professional workshop with anything from a dozen to 200 participants, though like any skill the more you do it, the better you get.

Finding out more

In the UK, the organisation **Animal Communication Training (ACT)**, which teaches both animal reiki and telepathic animal communication, offers one-day introductory workshops and longer courses leading to professional certification. In both the UK and the US, the excellent **Amelia Kinkade** does regular workshops – I have done some with her – (from around £50 a day). In the US, see also animal psychic Carol Gurney's ($150–$200 a day). For contact details, see under 'Training Courses' in the Directory.

Recommended reading: try *Straight From the Horse's Mouth* by Amelia Kinkade for a step-by-step how-to approach to communicating with animals, plus illustrative anecdotes and some background explanation. This is also available on CD from Amelia Kinkade's website ($15.99). Her book *The Language of Miracles* is also recommended, as is Carol Gurney's *The Language of Animals. Heart Talk*, an animal-communication teaching programme, is available from her website. She also offers a CD-Rom, *Beginner's Guide to Animal Communication*.

Constipation

First, take your pet for a check-up with the vet, as constipation may sometimes be a symptom of a more serious underlying condition. Next, have a look at how you are feeding them. Packaged pet food can be a common culprit, and a natural raw-food diet – or at least an improved diet (see Pets: Food on page 407) – can often banish constipation for good.

The Top Three Anti-constipation Tips:
1. Always have fresh water down for your pet.
2. Add a little mashed vegetable, organic if possible, or plain fibre to their food at every meal.
3. Ensure they get plenty of exercise (see below).

Useful things to try
Bulk it up
Add half to two teaspoons, depending on their size, of **psyllium husks** to their food as this absorbs water and helps bulk out stools, making them softer, bigger and easier to pass. Or add the same, depending on their size, of **linseed** to each pet meal, which act like ball-bearings on the stool, easing their passage out of the body.

For psyllium husks, try Solgar (200 capsules, £11.96); in the US, call Solgar toll free. For linseed, try Linusit Gold from any local health shop – e.g. Holland & Barrett (250 g, £3.95). For contact details, see under 'Shopping' in the Directory.

Exercise
Play with your cat, trailing laces and tinkling balls all over the home twice a day for at least ten minutes at a time, and walk or run with your dog. Walking, running, tumbling and jumping movements cause the gut muscles to contract, which helps move food waste along and out.

Homeopathy
Nux vomica can often help. If the problem is a 'shy' stool (i.e. one that comes a little way out only to disappear back in again), try **Thuja**; but if it is big, passing seems painful and the anus looks red, try **Sulphur**, suggests the veterinary dean of the London Faculty of Homeopathy, Christopher Day. Give the remedy at potency 6c two to three times a day. If the situation is *really* acute (i.e. your pet is straining fruitlessly to empty their bowels or becoming distressed), it is best to give the remedy you have chosen up to every ten minutes until you notice a change.

360. Suitcase Panic

Does your dog or cat get upset at the mere sight of you bringing out a suitcase? Try bringing one out more often, put toys or treats in there, let them sleep or play in them for half a day now and then. It helps break the exclusive association between luggage and what they see as abandonment while you go away, and can reduce their anxiety when it really is time for you to take a trip, suggests Karen Overall, specialist in behavioural medicine at the University of Pennsylvania School of Veterinary Medicine.

361. Farting

This may often be the subject of daft jokes and much amusement, but a pet passing wind regularly is no laughing matter – some can clear a room in seconds. There are some fairly extreme flatulence-deodorising appliances on the market that help, but look pretty silly on. (Seen the Dogone Gas Neutralising Dog Thong, 'a snip at $19.99', which the pet has to wear over their rear end at all times? If you want to, it's on www.flat-d.com/thong.) However, naturally-minded pet owners might prefer trying **yoghurt** and **charcoal**.

Yoghurt

Natural live yoghurt contains 'friendly' bacteria (probiotics) that help balance the workings of the gut and can cut down smelly flatulence a treat for both animals and humans. You can also get these bacteria in freeze-dried powder form, which may be best for dogs as they are not too good at digesting dairy products and it might merely contribute to farting problems in their own right. BioCare has been supplying this for years in powdered form. For contact details, see under 'Shopping' in the Directory.

If you'd like to give yoghurt a try, the suggested dosage is a quarter of a teaspoon of plain live yoghurt for cats or small dogs, one teaspoon for dogs weighing 7–9 kg and one tablespoon for big dogs once a day mixed in with their food. If using the powder, the bacteria are very concentrated so just an eighth of a teaspoon for small dogs and cats, a quarter for medium-sized dogs and half a teaspoon for big dogs, mixed in with their food once a day.

Charcoal

If your pet's gas problem is pretty dire, also add a little activated charcoal to the food – in the same amounts as above. The substance is available over the counter in most pharmacies. However, because it can absorb certain vital nutrients as well as gas from the digestive tract, it ought not to be used for more than five days at a time.

Fireworks

362 Making Bonfire Night Bearable for Dogs

Holistic vets recommend the following:

• Feed your dog a really good meal rich in carbohydrate, which is calming, with added vitamin B6, which supports the nervous system. Give this mid- to late afternoon so your dog has a full belly. Don't do this, however, if they tend to experience diarrhoea when they are nervous or at other times. To ensure they eat really well, perhaps give only a small snack in the morning.

• Try the **Dog-Appeasing Pheromone (DAP)** device. When used to comfort dogs during Bonfire Night, owners reported an 80 per cent reduction in the dogs' displays of fear (panting, trembling and hiding). For more information about the DAP, see Fix 353: Home Alone. They are available on request from the vet. Contact CEVA Animal Health for the nearest one in your area who will have it.

- Take your dog to a blacked-out room (to screen out flashes, which they can find alarming) at sundown with their favourite blanket, the DAP device plugged in, some toys and some things for you to do. Stay and keep them company for as long as you can.
- Put some music on – either gentle classical or something with a regular, constant drumbeat to distract from the bangs.
- Ignore the noises yourself and try to engage your dog in a game or tummy-tickling marathon. However, try not to fuss over or pet your dog each time they jump – just keep up regular friendly attention and company.
- Offer **Animal Care** essence in their water (two to three drops for a small dog, five to six for a medium-sized one and seven or more for a large one), plus a plain bowl of water, so they can choose whether to take it or not, and regulate how much they have. You can buy Animal Care in the UK via Healthlines (7.5 ml, £8.95); in the US and Canada, buy it direct from Alaskan Essences.

For all contact details, see under 'Shopping' in the Directory.

Fleas

363. General Flea-Busters

Chemical flea control is the last resort for a pet owner who prefers to look after their animal naturally, as those products contain some very powerful substances, like organo-phosophorous compounds, which have been linked with a variety of health problems for animals and humans alike.

But you don't want an infested house – and this can happen quickly in the heat of summer or in a cosy centrally heated winter home – so if you gotta do it, you gotta do it. However, here are some sensible, and often highly effective, DIY and natural measures to try first.

Your home

1. Every two to three days hoover all carpets and rugs in rooms where the pet goes. This gets any flea eggs that will otherwise hatch out

within a matter of days and start the whole thing off again. Wash rugs on the hottest cycle on your machine.

2. If your pet sleeps on your bed, or another, hoover mattresses; then wash all the bed linen, blankets, duvets if they contain cotton or man-made fibre and underblankets on as hot a cycle as they can stand. Spray with an anti-flea product then send pillows off for dry-cleaning. Ditto for feather/down duvets. When they return, peg them out on the washing line in the garden or out of a window for the day (weather permiting) to help get rid of the chemicals.

3. Hoover all sofas and soft upholstered chairs for the same reason, using a nozzle attachment.

Your pet

For a cat or small dog, add one small capsule of **garlic oil** to their food each mealtime (pierce and squeeze over), plus half a tablet of **brewer's yeast** from the chemist. For a medium-sized dog, make it one and a half capsules plus a whole tablet of brewer's yeast. For a large dog, give two or two and a half capsules of the oil, plus one and a half tablets of brewer's.

This 'may create a hostile environment for fleas', according to Christopher Day, veterinary dean for the London Faculty of Homeopathy in the UK, since both substances can alter the scent coming from the animal and also change the taste of their blood, neither of which fleas like. (Humans can use a similar tactic with garlic to help repel mosquitoes.)

Garlic essence (a homeopathically dilute remedy) can have the same effect. You can add a few drops to a bowl of your pet's drinking water, or sprinkle them over their food. Originally designed as a general protective essence, it can apparently also help repel fleas but doesn't smell or taste of garlic – or upset their stomachs, which, occasionally, garlic oil may. Try the one from American company Flower Essence Services (¼ fl oz, $6.60), which can be bought in the UK via IFER (approximately £6). For contact details, see under 'Shopping' in the Directory.

364. Natural Flea Collars for Dogs

There are literally scores of different ones available, most impregnated with insecticide and containing organo-phosphates, a group of chemicals linked with a wide variety of health problems for both humans and animals. However, the Pesticide Action Network has come up with a good alternative: a natural flea-collar mix you make up yourself using organic essential oils.

1 drop lavender
1 drop cedarwood
1 drop citronella
1 drop thyme
4 crushed garlic cloves or garlic oil squeezed from 4 capsules

Mix together the above essential oils and garlic. Then just soak a soft, padded dog collar in it, let it dry naturally and put it on the animal. The effects last about a month.

You can buy organic essential oils from Star Child. For contact details, see under 'Shopping' in the Directory.

Cats and collars: warning

Because the above collar mix contains essential oils, *do not use it for cats* (see Fix 382: Cat Aromatherapy), only dogs. And watch the dog carefully for the first few days to ensure they are comfortable, as not all are happy with essential oils vaporising under their nose 24 hours a day.

Food

365. Raw Food for Cats and Dogs

Many of today's 'modern' pet diseases, especially allergies, eczema, arthritis, weight problems and general lack of vitality are thought to be exacerbated, or even caused, by the convenient but low-quality tinned and packaged pet foods we feed them. Numerous studies support this, such as one carried out over several years by the Karolinska Institute in Stockholm, which compared the health of animals fed on packaged and processed (i.e. ordinary) pet food with that of those who were fed on **raw food** all their lives. The former developed heart disease, arthritis and other degenerative diseases now common in Western-owned pets; the latter were mostly free of these degenerative illnesses well into old age.

Another piece of research published in the *British Journal of Small Animal Practice* in 1995 found that packaged pet foods suppressed the animal's immune system and also led to liver, kidney and heart damage – this research was later repeated and confirmed by the Australian Veterinary Association.

Unfortunately, this does rather mean that concerned pet owners have just three choices if they really care about the health of the animals they love:

- Start improving what your pet eats by small additions and simple strategies
- Go all out by feeding them a good-quality, natural, raw wholefood diet.
- Pay extra for a better quality pre-packaged pet food (see page 410), which will probably need to be delivered by mail order.

If you want to go all out, the raw wholefood diet is based on meat, bones, vegetables and organ meats like heart that mimic the natural evolutionary diet of a feral animal. Most ingredients you'll find at your local supermarket, the rest at the butcher's. You can further enhance that diet with:

- **essential fatty acids** like evening primrose oil from the pharmacy or supermarket, especially if the animal has a skin problem like eczema or a coat in poor condition
- **probiotics** to help keep their balance of healthy digestive bacteria (e.g. from BioCare)
- **alfalfa-sprout powder** from the health food shop
- **vitamins and herbs.**

The BARF programme

One such eating programme for animals is called the **BARF (bones and raw food) diet.** Launched in Australia in the early 1990s, it swept through America and Europe. It is accredited with not only producing healthy, energetic, happy animals in excellent condition, but also improving the health of those with:

- diabetes
- early-onset arthritis
- orthopaedic disorders – e.g. hip dysplasia, appearing in young animals
- continence problems
- behavioural problems (there is a major link between food and behaviour in humans for similar reasons – see Fix 297: Nutritional Approach).

Natural feeding the easy way

If you want to try your pet on the BARF programme, but cannot face regular trips to the butchers, how about buying the raw food food pre-packed? If you have internet acess, search for **Nature's Menu online** for the nearest stockist that offers vacuum-packed sachets that are 60 per cent oils, rice and seaweed. Nature's Menu also offers frozen BARF meals consisting of pellet-sized chunks of meat and vegetables meant to be defrosted and eaten raw. For contact details, see under 'Shopping' in the Directory.

If you'd like to go for a simpler, more straightforward approach, see Pets: Anti-Aging on page 388, which includes an easy way to give your pet raw food.

Further information

Recommended reading: see *The Barf Diet for Cats and Dogs* by Australian vet Ian Billinghurst and *Give Your Dog a Bone* by the same author. In the US, look out for *Raw Dog Food: Making It Work for You and Your Dog* by Carina Beth MacDonald.

Note: this method of feeding has tens, maybe even hundreds of thousands of fans worldwide, but it also has its critics, who have concerns both about splintering bones and any parasites or bacteria that may be lurking in untreated (uncooked) meat intended for pet consumption. Bones can be ground, however, and Billinghurst suggests that occasional bone-splinter problems and the possibility of food-borne infection are far less of an evil than the damage that commercial, additive-packed pet food made from rendered-down, low-grade animal carcasses causes. Guess this one's a decision for pet owners and their animals themselves.

366. Positive Packaged Pet Foods
Ordinary pet foods

Packaged pet foods are not generally very nice. Even if you see the words 'real meat' (what other sort is there, then?) on the label, by law manufacturers can get away with putting in as little as 4 per cent. The major ingredient is water (90 per cent) and what's known in the trade as 'animal derivatives', which covers everything from nutritious bits like kidneys, liver and brain to udders, windpipes, hair, ground-up beaks and claws, even, in some documented cases, diseased carcasses and animal excrement.

These are turned into pet food by rendering (high-temperature boiling), resulting in a sludge that can be fashioned into small squares as 'meat chunks' covered in gravy or into dried food.

The final product also tends to contain preservatives like butylated hydroxyanisole (BHA) that have been shown to affect the nervous system and an antioxidant called ethoxyquin – used in pet foods in the US but banned in Europe – which can cause liver problems and cancer. In fact, one survey of American pet foods found that most of them contained cancer-causing chemicals.[3] Manufacturers also add vitamins and minerals, but this doesn't make up for the more negative ingredients – and a medium-sized dog fed exclusively on ordinary commercial pet food is thought to get up to 4.5 kg of additives with their meals every year.

Positive pet food

Food-aware pet owners can try one of the below packaged pet foods, all of which got top five-star rating from *Proof* magazine's panel of pet-testers and their owners. (*Proof* is an alternative *Which?*-style publication offering excellent consumer information.)

For cats

Try Eagle Pack Adult Cat Formula, available from Postal Pet Products (3 kg, approximately £12), and James Wellbeloved Turkey and Rice Cat Food from Crown Pet Foods (2 kg, approximately £10).

For dogs
Try Eagle Pack Holistic Select Lamb Meal and Rice (1.8 kg, approximately £7) and Fromm Family Adult Gold Dog Food (3 kg, approximately £10), both from Postal Pet Products.

For all contact details, see under 'Shopping' in the Directory

Fur and Hair

367. Condition
When an animal has been malnourished or its immune system has been under attack and it has become rundown, its coat may become dull, lose condition and not lie well. There is an essential oil called **wild carrot seed** that restores lost condition beautifully. For animals, only ever use the organic variety. In the UK, you can buy it from Star Child (5 ml, £6.75); in the US, try the Simplers Botanical Company (5 ml, $18.85). For contact details, see under 'Shopping' in the Directory.

Horses adore this oil (possibly because of their innate fondness for carrots) and it can do a great job on their coat and hooves. Dogs are less keen but will take it when they need it. For horses, international animal aromatherapy pioneer Caroline Ingraham suggests five to ten drops, depending on the severity of the condition, in 5 ml base oil or water daily taken by mouth, or 10–20 drops in base oil for applying to the hooves daily. For dogs, give one drop in their water bowl daily for small ones, two for medium to large ones.

368. Hairballs
Hairballs can be more than a nuisance that means cat sick on the carpet – they can cause potentially life-threatening blockages of the intestinal tract. There are several commercial remedies that can help ease fur through the gut, such as J's Hairball Remedy, available from Pet Planet (50 g, £2.99), Katalax or Malt Bit Treats by Beaphor, which is available in many pet shops (35g, 99p). For contact details, see under 'Shopping' in the Directory.

If your cat is prone to hairballs, these remedies need to be used for three days at a time at regular intervals.

But what if your cat's already starting to hack fruitlessly and you don't have any special hairball treats available?

Petroleum jelly (Vaseline)

Put a quarter of a teaspoon of **Vaseline** either on your cat's front paw or just under their nose. Being fastidious, they'll lick it off. Follow up by doing this once a day for three to four days.

Butter

Most cats actually like the taste of **butter** (an advantage over Vaseline), so if they are beginning to cough, dab some under their nose and they'll usually lick it off right away in between the coughing and spluttering. Even better, according to James Dalley of the Michigan State University College of Veterinary Medicine, as well as being a natural lubricant to help ease up a hairball, butter also makes the gallbladder contract and empty out bile (which is a powerful digestif and mild laxative), which will help with any fur on its way down the gut tubing.

Hens

369. The Eco-Pet

If you thought chickens were messy and required a farmyard, think again: they are apparently, in the UK at least, the rising urban eco-pet. Easy-clean, brightly coloured plastic **Eglus** (sort of Habitat meets hencoop, or iMac for chickens) plus two hens are available for city and small-garden fresh-egg fanciers. Contact Omlet for a starter package of one Eglu, two hens and delivery in the South and Midlands (approximately £400). Farm-bought chicks and a home-built hencoop are far cheaper, but don't look so cool. For contact details, see under 'Shopping' in the Directory.

> **Energy levels**
>
> **Marmite on toast** is an excellent way to boost a chicken's energy levels if they are feeling a bit low – it's the B-group vitamins – according to the organisers of National Chicken and Egg Day, which is on 2 February every year and earmarked for those who have chickens as garden animals or pets to spend extra quality time with their feathered companions.

Extra advantage

If you keep hens, you'll not only get about six eggs (organic if you feed them organic, free-range providing you let them run about plenty) a week per bird, but they're also great garden-pest foragers (see also Fix 415: Pest Patrol) and produce good-quality organic-waste fertiliser.

Holidays

370. Catteries and Kennels

If your pet has to spend time boarding out (perhaps the house is being renovated or you are off on a few weeks' holiday and cannot take them with you), as well as installing them with their favourite blanket and toys, try taking along an **amethyst crystal** as well.

It can be a small one, as little as 8 cm across; this would cost around £5–£6 in a gem or New Age shop. First cleanse and programme it (see Appendix 1: Cleansing and Programming Crystals and Gems on page 536), which only takes a few minutes, then place it near where your pet sleeps.

'The amethyst is the key crystal for treating separation anxiety,' explain Martin Scott and Gael Mariani, who are pioneer therapists in natural animal care. 'A classic example is when a pet is spending time in a kennel, cattery or quarantine pining for its owners.' Besides being natural therapists who work exclusively with animals, Scott and Mariani are also fellows and tutors at the Institute of Homeopathy in London, tutors at the UK's Animal Care College, have a regular holistic column in *Dogs Monthly* and are co-founders of the Society for Animal Flower Essence Research, which also investigates using crystals for animal well-being.

Recommended reading: *Crystal Healing for Animals* by Scott and Mariani.

371. Going Away

If you are going away for a while and leaving your pet with a different carer in your own home (instead of at boarding kennels or a cattery) who may perhaps only be coming in once or twice a day for brief periods, and you know that your animal is shy or very strongly bonded with you, there are three things you can do to help reassure and settle them when you're not there:

1. **Check in with them** at the same time once or twice a day (early morning and bedtime are good times), 'sending' love and reassurance to them with an 'I'll be back in X days' message – see Pets: Communication on page 396.
2. **Ask the temporary carer to give them Separation essence** in their bowl of water or on their food daily. It contains the energies of plants such as white bleeding heart, morning glory, St John's wort and goldenrod, and has a calming and reassuring effect. It is made by Green Hope Farm Essences and can be bought from Jembush (15 ml, £8.45). For contact details, see under 'Shopping' in the Directory.
3. **Place a rough amethyst crystal near their sleeping place** – see Fix 370: Catteries and Kennels.

See also Fix 360: Suitcase Panic.

Infections

372. Silver for Infections (and grunge)

As the incidence of antibiotic-resistant bacteria rises, and some owners prefer not to give their animals antibiotics anyway unless absolutely necessary, next time your pet has a minor to moderate infection, consider a good old-fashioned mineral remedy called **colloidal silver** – a liquid holding fine particles of silver in suspension.

What silver can do

Silver can kill bacteria most effectively. In fact, up until the 1940s, when antibiotics were mass-introduced, colloidal silver was used for humans for the same purposes – in throat-gargle form for sore throats, as a douche, applied directly on the skin as a topical remedy and also taken by mouth. To this day, it is still applied to the eyes of newborn babies to prevent infections developing, and its popularity for animal use is on the increase. Pet owners are using it to:

- Clean grungy aquarium tanks.
- Treat minor infections and ailments. Pigeon-fanciers, for example, are finding that if they add some to the water for the first round of

chicks, those baby birds are no longer prey to many of the common ailments usually seen in nestlings.

• Clear up ear infections, laminitis, sweet itch, mange; improve chronic kidney and liver problems and even clear up some digestive disorders altogether in dogs and horses in the US.[4]

Colloidal silver is not an instant get-better-immediately remedy, more of a slow but steady measure.

You can buy it from Higher Nature, who offer a pump spray (100 ml, £14.90). Spray it directly on to the area of infection externally, or unscrew the cap and measure out a teaspoon per saucer of water. Higher Nature also stocks *The Colloidal Silver Report* (£2.50).

For cats and dogs, keep the saucer of water down at all times and change the water each day. Use for two to three weeks for stubborn infections, allowing the animal to drink their usual amount of water in this way. For rabbits, give half a teaspoon in a clean water bottle or dish, changed daily, for a couple of weeks. For other animals, see *The Colloidal Silver Report* or contact Higher Nature and ask to speak to one of their advisory team, who if they are not sure of exact amounts for a specific animal, should be able to put you in touch with a vet who knows about colloidal silver and can help you by phone or email. For contact details, see under 'Shopping' in the Directory.

In Heat

373. In-Heat Cats

Play some soothing music, as pets in heat will often settle down when you switch on something classical – especially Mozart, says Nashville-based animal behaviouralist Pam Johnson (who wrote the splendid *Twisted Whiskers: Solving Your Cat's Behaviour Problems*).

But lay off the sexy, funky James Brown soul and energising rock – in fact, anything with a driving beat that could evoke thoughts of 'mating rhythms', advises Michael W. Fox, who's vice-president of the Humane Society of the US, as apparently these evoke sexual arousal. Just like in humans, in fact.

Oh, and keep your windows closed. Male cats can sniff those 'Hello, boys . . .' messages in the air from up to a mile away.

374. In-Heat Dog-Walking

Taking a female dog in heat to the park for a pee? Good luck. A dog's romance range is nearly three miles

However, you can help mask the 'come and get me' pheromones your pet's exuding with a little **Vicks VapoRub** dabbed on the fur just above her tail, where it meets the start of her upper back: those menthol and eucalyptus fumes are pretty camouflaging. But wipe it off when you get home: if she tries to lick it, it'll make her tongue burn.

Itching

375. Oatmeal Baths for Itching Skin

The fastest way to soothe a pet with itching skin is to give them an ordinary cool bath or, better still, for animals who will stay in there for a bit, even reluctantly, add **colloidal oatmeal lotion** from the chemist's – e.g. Aveeno, which is widely available in the UK and highly recommended. 'Oatmeal baths can be just as helpful to animals as they are to people,' says Tam Garland of the Texas A&M University College of Veterinary Medicine in College Station.

Try the Soothing Bath Treatment, made by Aveeno and available in Boots, which comes in individual one-bath packets (8 sachets, approximately £5). This is a viable option for dogs, hamsters, guinea pigs and rabbits, but when it comes to cats, most would sooner fight than bathe. For helpful advice, see Pets: Washing on page 430.

376. The Scratch-Soother Drink

If your pet suffers from itchy skin, try a single drop of **yarrow essential oil** in their drinking water for a few weeks, suggests animal aromatherapist, kinesiologist, ex-show-jumper and specialist animal healer Liz Whiter.

To check if an essential oil is right for your animal and how to give it to them if it is, see international animal aromatherapy pioneer Caroline Ingraham's advice in 'How to offer oils safely' on page 424 and 'Is it the right one?' on page 419. Recommended reading: also look out for her excellent book *Aromatherapy for Animals*, which is the acknowledged bible on the subject for practitioners and public alike.

As to where to get the very best and purest organic essential oils – which they need to be if they are going to be used for animals, since their sense of smell is so very acute – in the UK, try Materia Aromatica's Yarrow Oil (1 ml, £5.15); all their oils are certified organic by the Soil Association. In the US, see the Essential Oil Company (5 ml, $26.05). Star Child also do good-quality organic oils, but they don't have any yarrow. For contact details, see under 'Shopping' in the Directory.

> **Cat caution**
>
> If it's a cat who has the itchy skin, you cannot give them yarrow essential oil in water or food as they can't metabolise it and it could poison them; however, they're safe to take it by sniffing it at a distance instead. See Fix 382: Cat Aromatherapy for how to give oils to them safely.

377. Itchy Paws (Dogs Only)

Dog with allergies also tend to get itchy paws, but soaking the area in a gentle infusion of **Epsom salts** can bring good, if temporary, relief.

Jim McDonald, associate professor of dermatology at Auburn University College of Veterinary Medicine in Alabama, suggests you fill a plastic washing-up bowl (or a bath) with just enough cool water to cover your dog's paws if they stand in it, dissolve several cups of Epsom crystals in there (enough to taste appreciably), then encourage your dog to stay in this for five to ten minutes. Keep your dog calm and still by stroking and talking to them.

Note: make sure they don't drink any. The salts can have a laxative effect.

Mourning and Bereavement

The death of a mate or companion hits animals very hard indeed, since their emotional responses are the same as those of humans.

378. Essence Comfort

Besides giving extra love, keeping your pet near to you (if they will allow this) and trying to find another companion for them after a decent interval (absolutely essential), offer them some **Red Suva Frangipani** essence, perhaps one or two drops for small animals in their drinking water. Or put drop five drops into a bowl of water, dip your hands in it and run them gently over your pet in loving, stroking motions twice daily.

Red Suva is an Australian Bush Flower essence that's used for the first phase of deep grief and sadness that comes at the death of a loved one. It is available direct or via Healthlines (15 ml, £8.95).

You could also try Bailey Flower Essence's gentle combination **Grief** (10 ml, £5.15), made from the plants of Yorkshire's Ilkley Moor and gathered by their maker in the early-morning mists when there is plenty of dew still on the plants.

I gave Red Suva to our beautiful black Rex rabbit, Lavender, after her mate was beheaded by a fox. For three days she had simply sat, hunched in the corner of her cage, staring at nothing, eating little. Within 24 hours of having the essence in her drinking water and being stroked with it, she started to look around and eat a little more. Within ten days she was almost back to normal, and after a month was able to welcome another (exceedingly cocky and handsome) young mate.

For all contact details, see under 'Shopping' in the Directory.

379. Life-Force Stone

If the loss of a mate seems to have taken away the remaining partner's will to live, it helps to place a cleansed and programmed **carnelian** (see Appendix 1: Cleansing and Programming Crystals and Gems on page 536) in or very near their sleeping quarters.

This stone boosts energy, vital force, stimulates their mental and physical faculties and boosts the will to survive, say animal-healing pioneers and homeopaths Martin Scott and Gael Mariani, who also treat animals with crystals and research the effects upon them.

New Home

380. Essential Oils for Moving Home

An essential oil made from the **leaves of violets** is a lovely one for animals who feel shy, out of place, not at home, anxious and cannot seem to fit in. 'This is good to use when you are introducing a new animal to others who live in that house and for the rehoming phase in general,' says animal aromatherapist, kinesiologist and healer Liz Whiter, who works extensively with animal refuges and small zoos as well as individual domestic animals and horses from her practice in Streat, Sussex. 'It gives inner strength – the very opposite of a shrinking violet.'

Essential oils are given very differently from the much subtler and homeopathically dilute essences, as essential oils are the plant in its most concentrated form. 'Hold the bottle of the essential oil you feel may help the animal near to them, without putting it right under their nose, as their sense of smell is so very, very much more sensitive than ours,' advises Liz.

> People have 10 million sensory nerve endings in their nose; animals have an average of 200 million.

Is it the right one?

'Watch for their reaction. If they want that oil and know it's right for them, the signs can be subtle – a twitch of a whisker, a slightly flared nostril, cocking their heads slightly, a narrowing or widening of the eyes or pupils, but in some cases they may actually move nearer and stay there, sniff closer or even try to lick the bottle, so you'll know it's for them. If they back off, turn away, show other signs of dislike or just act disinterested, forget it. And please' warns Liz, 'ensure you don't follow them around asking them to give a second try to a bottle of essential oil they've already rejected! That is a *really* offensive thing to do to an animal.'

Using it

Put just a single drop of the violet-leaf oil in their drinking water and always offer another drinking source right next to it that contains no oil so they have a choice as to whether they take it or not and how much they use, says Liz. 'Make sure you don't push essential oils given in their drinking water on animals. Never force it. They're very smart and will know how much they need instinctively.'

For animals, as with small children and babies, always use organic oils. The one place I can find a good organic violet-leaf oil (which is not very common) is from an excellent French company called Florihana, Provence. They speak good English too if your French is a bit wobbly.

Note: this oil is semi-solid at room temperature, so when you use it, heat up the bottle a little very gently beforehand. You can do this on an extremely low temperature in the microwave for 20 seconds or even by placing it on top of a radiator.

Cat care

Cats cannot take essential oils in drinking water, food or via an air diffuser or burner. See Fix 382: Cat Aromatherapy for how to give them safely.

If they don't like it

If your pet does not like the smell of any of the 'new home' oils you offer, go for a tried and tested Bach Flower essence for moving and change of all types – **Walnut**, which you can buy from Healing Herbs (10 ml, £3.20).

Last time we moved we gave it to everyone – adults, children, cats, rabbits, guinea pigs, even watered the house plants with it and put it in the water of the tropical fish tank – and we've never settled in so fast. Within 48 hours it was as if we'd always been here, animals included. And this family's had a few moves: one year (best forgotten) we had five homes in 12 months. Wish we'd known about Walnut back then.

For all contact details, see under 'Shopping' in the Directory.

See also Houses and Gardens: New Home on page 470.

Overweight

What helps? After you've taken your pet for a check-up to ensure there is no underlying health problem that explains why they are putting on weight (such as diabetes), it's back to looking at the food they eat (what and how much of it) and exercise.

There are a lot of overweight animals about. According to a recent RSPCA survey in the UK, one in three people think their pet's too heavy, a quarter of these have not yet done anything about it, and three-quarters of all veterinary surgeries are running 'fat clinics'.

> **Taking the rib test**
>
> If you want to confirm whether your pet is overweight, a bit stocky or just nicely covered, then for dogs, stroke your hand along their side. If you can't feel their ribs, it's the former. For cats, see if their tummy protrudes below their ribcage or their face seems overly plump.

Easy Holistic Weight Loss Tips for Pets
If your cat or dog is too heavy, try the following:

- **Go for garlic.** According to Ann-si Lee, a practitioner of Chinese veterinary medicine from Oakland, California, raw garlic helps regulate the liver and gallbladder, thus encouraging the digestive system back into line. For small pets, crush a quarter to half a clove and mix into their food; bigger animals can have one or two crushed cloves daily.
- **Feed them little and often.** If they're on a diet, to stave off hunger, feed your pet four to six very small servings a day, say at two-hourly intervals. It keeps their stomach busy, provides a food comfort hit, and they may not be so conscious that they are actually eating much less than usual.
- **Hide and Divide**. If you can only feed them twice a day – perhaps you are out at work the rest of the time – divide each meal into 3

or 4 separate bowls, then place those all around the kitchen plus one other adjacent room (on a big piece of newspaper to prevent spattering if it's on a carpet).

This means it takes your pet longer to eat as they have to *find* it all first, which in turn encourages gaps between helpings. That helps them feel rather fuller than if they had bolted all their grub down in one go, and also promotes natural foraging behaviour, i.e. searching for their feed and being rewarded by another helping of it, which is both fun, and satisfying for an animal in a way that 'having it all on a plate' isn't.

- **Cut out snacks and treats.** Give extra love instead.
- **Exercise** (see page 402)

Relaxation

381. Animal Shiatsu

Animals like **shiatsu (acupressure) treatment** as much as people do, and again, as with humans, shiatsu can be purely relaxing or problem-targeted. It is also, like any form of touch therapy for animals, a wonderful way to bond with your pet. A 'full-body once-over' treatment takes around 30 minutes, but may require as much as an hour; specific issues can sometimes be addressed with sessions as short as five minutes.

> **Tip**
> Use shiatsu only when your pet is calm, not to quieten an angry or irritable animal, or you may get snapped at.

Quick sample routine

One gentle way to help introduce your pet to the idea of shiatsu and see if they like it is a brief ear routine, which many find relaxing and pleasurable.

Animal-shiatsu expert Pamela Hannay, who is a senior instructor at the Ohashi Institute in New York City and co-author of *Touching Horses: Communication, Health and Healing Through Shiatsu*, suggests the following routine on a dog's floppy ears, which I've adapted for this book (for the full-body routine, see her lovely, clear book *Shiatsu for Dogs*):

1. Sit down comfortably next to your dog and take three deep, easy breaths.
2. Warm your hands and imagine them filling with a beautiful golden light.
3. Gently slide your hand round their ear so your index finger's at the front of it, the other three fingers behind it and your palm against their head. Use your free hand to support the other side of their head.
4. Rotate that ear carefully to the left two or three times, then carefully to the right two or three times. Feel the skin moving slightly as you do so.
5. Hold the ear in both hands and press from its base to its tip with your fingers, gradually pulling the ear outwards – but not so hard you move their head.
6. Repeat, only this time pulling the ear slightly forwards instead.
7. And again, but this time drawing that ear backwards.
8. To finish, stroke both ears at once with your hands firmly but lightly a slow three times.
9. Let your hands hold their ears gently for a count of a few seconds, then release.

Further information
There are few professionals who specialise in animal shiatsu as yet, but one or two good-quality courses for both the therapist and the pet owner are now available in the UK and US. In the UK, try the Institute of Complementary Animal Therapies, which offers courses and diplomas in canine massage and equine shiatsu, and has a list of their qualified practitioners around the UK. Or contact animal-shiatsu pioneer Jacqueline Cook at the Roseheart Kingdom Therapy Centre for Animals in Shropshire. In the US, try the Northwest School of Animal Massage at Fall City, Washington, or the Bancroft School of Massage, Massachusetts, and ask about their animal-massage and shiatsu programmes. For contact details, see under 'Training Courses' in the Directory.

382. Cat Aromatherapy

Cats like **lavender essential oil** and find it very soothing. However, *felines cannot metabolise essential oils* so it would be *toxic* to them if these were put in a burner to diffuse near them, dabbed on their body or added to their water or food. The same goes for the more dilute, steam-distilled variant of essential oils called hydrosols, which are often promoted as being fine for cats. It also needs to be *organic essential oil you use for them*, not the standard variety.

Try Neal's Yard Organic Lavender Oil (10 ml, £8.95) Star Child's (10 ml, £5.95) or even better if you can afford it, the Lavender from Florihana of Provence, whose oils are of an especially high standard and purity. For contact details, see under 'Shopping' in the Directory.

How to offer oils safely

The truth is that essential oils can be incredibly healing for cats, but those oils need to be very pure and offered at arm's length. 'Merely sit about a metre away, take the top off the oil bottle and offer it,' says international animal aromatherapy pioneer Caroline Ingraham, who goes all over the world teaching vets, animal breeders, trainers and therapists how to use essential oils safely for animals.

'Give them time, be patient. If they want it, they'll sniff some and absorb what they need. They may move closer to do so, or they may be getting enough for their needs from where they are, so don't take the bottle nearer, just stay still. If it's not right for them, they'll know and will simply turn away.'

She adds, 'If the cat makes a sort of gurning face, this doesn't mean they don't like it, but that they are expanding their breathing passages to take it in.'

See also 'Is it the right one?' on page 419.

383. Thirsty Pets

If your dog or cat doesn't seem to be drinking enough, check what their water bowl's made of and where it is. If it's shiny metal, some animals are put off or downright alarmed by their reflection suddenly appearing in the bottom as they drink. And if it's by a radiator (again, many drinking bowls are, as it's often the one place in the

kitchen that affords a slight alcove without fitted cupboard units
and thus protects against humans treading in it), they may be
getting hot, dry air in their eyes or face as they try to drink.

Rescue Animals

Caring for a rescue animal, or one who has been abandoned? As well
as love, care, warm and comfortable living quarters, the right food, medication or clinical treatment if necessary, and patience, the special holistic
measures below can greatly enhance what you are already doing.

Crystal Care

384. Smoky quartz
This one is grounding, calming and soothing – often used to help both
animals and people adjust to life-changes or new surroundings and for
'Help needed now!' relief from shock and trauma. It is suggested by
animal homeopathy, crystal-healing and natural-therapy pioneers Martin
Scott and Gael Mariani.

Place a piece of newly cleansed and programmed **smoky quartz** very
near where the animal sleeps. For how to cleanse and programme, see
Appendix 1: Cleansing and Programming Crystals and Gems on page
536. This one is very inexpensive, and you'll only need a piece around
5–10 cm across (which is likely to cost £2–£3). You can buy it from
New Age or gem shops.

385. Helping Heal a Damaged Spirit
A great all-rounder essence combination for helping animals who have
had a troubled or abused history is **Animal Care** (originally named Animal
Rescue). Part of the excellent Alaskan Essences range, this one is used
by several animal refuges and charities in Canada, and both North and
South America to very good effect as it helps the animals to settle, then
to process and eventually begin to let go of some (or often, the whole)
of the trauma they have been exposed to and remember their former
natural positive behaviour. Made from the plants and minerals of that

vast area's lake and mountain country by Andrea Freixeda, a biologist and flower essence therapist who works with animal refuges, shelters and ecological parks in the greater Sao Paulo area of Brazil, the mix was developed for any animal who has:

- been abandoned
- been abused
- lived in petshops or other unsuitable conditions for too long and so lost natural behaviour patterns and either developed dysfunctional coping strategies (rocking, gnawing, self-biting, obsessive grooming, head-shaking) or become very withdrawn or aggressive
- due to injury or disability, need to be kept either temporarily or permanently in a zoo, animal shelter or refuge (including wild animals in temporary captivity for medical treatment)
- been exposed to man-made toxicity e.g. seabirds caught in an oil slick, river animals such as otters or water rats suffering from the effects of industrial pollution. Animal Care is usually used much diluted in water and either given in drinking water, dripped into their mouth or, if they will let you, rubbed in (in acute circumstances, in neat form) onto the hairless insides of their ears. In the UK it's available via Healthlines (60 ml, £11.95); in the US ($12.45 for 1oz bottle) and in Canada, direct from Alaskan Essences.

Longer term, when they seem far more settled, try spraying **Pet Calm** around their sleeping quarters. You can buy this direct from Living Essences of Australia worldwide (125 ml, £8.95/$15). Alternatively, in the UK, you can buy it from Healthlines (£10.95). For more information about Pet Calm, see Fix 389: Vet Visit.

For all contact details, see under 'Shopping' in the Directory.

Timidity and nervousness

386. Tellington touch
This technique is often called the 'teaching touch for animals'. Derived from the Feldenkrais method of massage for humans (which shows how

certain patterns of movement can become restrictive and habitual, thereby causing chronic pain, irritability or tension), it was originally used on animals by San Francisco Feldenkrais practitioner Linda Tellington for her horses.

The Tellington method isn't animal massage in the usual sense at all, as it uses only the very lightest of pressures and softest of touches; practitioners say this is all that is needed to help realign the nervous system (which for years may have experienced brisk pats and back rubs, poking, pulling, etc., and won't respond in the same way to firmer corrective touch any more).

It has been successfully used to combat stress-related behavioural problems in all sorts of animals from iguanas and parrots to sheep and cats. The **Confidence Course** based on the Tellington system and run by practitioner Mark Simmons helps dogs focus and overcome both aggression and timidity, while concentrating on an activity they are constantly praised for. There are also workshops to teach simple techniques from this gentle but effective animal therapy to pet owners and animal trainers (a day's introductory course for one person with one dog, from £49). For contact details, see under 'Training Courses' in the Directory.

387. Confidence – in a bottle

There are two gentle but really helpful essence combinations in the Bioforce range for underconfident or timid animals – and another one in the same range for those who are a bit pushy and over the top. Called '**Timid**' and '**Over-Dominant**' (30 ml, £4), they were developed by top naturopath Jan de Vries and can be used either on their own as a good first step approach, or as as an adjunct to Tellington Touch. Give three times daily, either directly into their mouth from the dropper bottle, put into food, or rubbed gently into the hairless insides of their ears. For very small animals (such as hamsters), give four drops each time in food or water; for medium-sized animals (such as cats, dogs and rabbits), give seven drops in food or water; for large animals (such as horses), give 12 drops in food or water. For contact details, see under 'Shopping' in the Directory.

See also Pets: Aggressive and Mistrustful Behaviour on page 387.

Travelling With Pets

388. Car Sickness

Just as miserable – if not more – for pets as for people. With animals, travel sickness might be accompanied by actual vomiting, but is usually expressed by drooling lots, a miserable or anxious expression and a desire to remain very still.

The gentle homeopathic remedy **Petroleum 6c** can be very effective here, especially if travelling by car, and your pet doesn't like the smell of the vehicle either. Give this to them every ten minutes or so until symptoms begin to subside. You can buy it by mail order from Ainsworths (£5.55). If you know your pet gets carsick, give them their remedy for the first time an hour before your journey begins, then another dose 30 minutes before you leave, then the next just before you put them in the vehicle. Continue every 10-15 minutes for the next half hour, after which, stop for a bit and watch them to see how they are doing. If they show no motion sickness symptoms, fine, just continue topping up with another pillule each hour (unless they are peacefully asleep, in which case leave them be).

Animal Anti Travel-Sickness Do's
Always
- keep the window nearest your pet open
- ensure no one smokes in the car
- have your pet travel at least on the back seat instead of in the luggage area right at the back of the car (very queasiness-inducing).

Calm-promoting tip
Use **PetCalm** spray around the area where your pet is sitting, to encourage a bit of tranquillity; see Fix 389 below.

Vets

389. Vet Visit

Before a visit to the vet's, it helps – apart from giving love and reassurance – to spray **Pet Calm** in your pet's travel carrier or just in the car if they're travelling without one. Pet Calm is a combination of several essences made from the wild plants of Australia and is designed by Living Essences. Vets working on the 'pinkie programme', a major wild-animal rescue programme in New South Wales, picked up on the usefulness of Pet Calm for distressed animals and began using it as part of their initiative.

What are pinkies?

Pinkies are baby kangaroos (joeys). Kangaroo young are born tiny and barely formed, so small they have not even grown hair – they're effectively very premature babies. Once born, they crawl up into their mother's pouch and remain there, suckling at need, warm and protected until they are strong enough to face the world. If their mother has been killed, however, either in the wild or on the roads, pinkies are so immature that they cannot leave the pouch, and need to be removed and raised by hand, or they will perish with their mother

Before and After

Before using Pet Calm, the project staffers found 80 per cent of these tiny pinkies died despite everyone's best efforts, yet after using Living Essence of Australia's formula, 90 per cent survived and most could be released back into the bush. Those early deaths were caused not by having insufficient food or care, but by the sheer trauma of being removed from what is in effect an external womb and having to survive outside it long before they were ready.

For your pet

In the same way, the essence combination is able to help animals of all types and in all stressful or worrying situations where they feel vulnerable, exposed or insecure, whether it's a vet visit, a long car trip or trauma recovery after an accident or fight.

> **Tip**
> You can also rub Pet Calm on to your pet's paws or the hairless flaps of the inside of their ears as it will be well absorbed via these routes too.

Pet Calm's available direct from Living Essences of Australia worldwide (125 ml, £8.95/$15). In the UK, you can also buy it from The Essence Shop, or via Healthlines (£10.95). For contact details, see under 'Shopping' in the Directory.

390. Unnecessary and Unsafe Treatments

What Vets Don't Tell You, a book produced by the apparently fearless *What Doctors Don't Tell You* magazine, is a mine of useful background and 'Why didn't anyone tell us that?' information, invaluable for any holistically minded pet owner.

This book looks at pet vaccines and how to avoid unnecessary ones, commonly used veterinary drugs and their safer alternatives, the issues around tinned pet foods and what options there are to use instead, plus a listing of many of the holistic and homeopathic vets in the UK. You can buy it direct from *What Doctors Don't Tell You* (£12.95 including postage and packaging). For contact details, see under 'Shopping' in the Directory.

Washing Cats

391. Bathing one

Not easy, with most. The following can help:

1. Put on gardening gloves and enlist a helper. Wear a sleeveless old top: you're going to get a bit wet.
2. Wrap, or swaddle, your cat gently but firmly in a thin towel or a bit of cotton sheeting to stop them flailing and scratching. Leave their head free and stroke and talk to them lovingly and reassuringly.
3. Still holding them, lean over and place them in the bath.

4. Carry on holding the cat and ask the other person to spray warm (*not* cold – it's too much of a shock) water from a showerhead on *low power*, soaking first the towel, then the cat's fur and finally their skin.

5. When you've finished washing your cat, dry their fur lightly, leaving it and their skin damp. Then, since they'll probably be deeply offended by now, if it's not cold outside let them go into the garden, if you have one, to dry off slowly.

You could also try some animal whispering first to explain why you are subjecting them to this indignity (see Pets: Communication on page 396) and that it may help them feel more comfortable.

It can help reduce your chances of being lacerated by putting a non-slip rubber bathmat in the bath for your cat to hang on to: some owners also attach their cat to a lead and fasten one end round a bath tap or handrail.

> If you are washing a cat – or, indeed, any animal – ensure that their face stays dry. Cats especially will usually lose it completely if it gets wet.

392. Smelly Cats: the no-bath wash technique

Has your cat rolled in something disgusting (or possibly been liberally sprayed by some un-neutered tom) and smells – *really* bad ? If they detest being bathed, an effective but non-confrontational option is to put something they love in a bowl for them (e.g. tuna, cat-treats or rice pudding – whatever it takes to keep them still for a moment), drip a little natural non-scented shampoo on to a warm, damp flannel and stroke them gently clean in the direction their fur grows. 'Rinse' well with another warm, damp cloth, then gently blot their fur dryish with a towel. This one works on all furry animals

Houses and
Gardens

Houses and gardens can benefit greatly from complementary therapies and esoteric strategies, just like their owners.

Try aromatherapy in the hall to calm you down the second you step inside from a hard day's work, feng-shui the bedroom for better sex and deeper sleep, discover which wall colours enhance mood and appetite; discourage slugs with natural copper wire and Vaseline, rather than death-dealing insecticides, or try a basic spiritual healing technique to supercharge your seedlings (proven results) instead of the usual artificial fertiliser.

We've also included many go-green and eco tips, since a holistic house is a happier and healthier house – and looked at some major geomancy issues, such as what to do if there's a big power line or pylon belting out electromagnetic emissions just across the road from your home.

Aromatherapy for your Home

393. Scents and Scentsibility

After a long, hard day, airborne aromatherapy can start the emotional rescue process the second you walk back in your own front door. The scent that greets you in the hall, or which subtly pervades the sitting room as you flop down on the sofa, can start gently working right away on any negative experiences or problems you have had during the day.

If you've been out for hours, first open the windows, then place a few drops of essential oil in a water vaporiser and light the candle beneath it (dedicating the flame to the Angels of Peace if you feel so inclined). Ceramic burners are best and can be bought in health and New Age shops (from £4). As to the little tea-light candles to put underneath, buy in bulk from supermarkets – e.g. Asda (100 lights, £2.50) – otherwise these tend to be sold individually at 10–20p each, which is a bit of a rip-off. What to put in it? UK aromatherapy queen Maggie Tisserand suggests the following:

Hallway
Melissa is just the thing to greet you if you've had a tiring day, especially if it's left you feeling emotionally hypersensitive, as it is both calming and uplifting. It is expensive but lovely and is available from several sources. Try Neal's Yard (2.5 ml, £35.75).

Orange is good if you find you've been coming home feeling a touch glum as it spreads a bit of sunshine, like the small sun its source resembles. Try Neal's Yard Orange Essential Oil (10 ml, £5) or Tisserand's, which is a little cheaper (9 ml, £3.99/$7.85).

Sitting room
If this is where you head to relax as soon as you get home, try the sweet, slightly musky, herbaceous scent of **angelica**, available from Baldwin's (5 ml, £18.19). Angelica acts, among other things, as a fillip to the nervous system, says Tisserand, so can help relieve exhaustion and stress (helpful for post-commuting syndrome). Or use **geranium**, which helps lift the spirits and bring the mind back into balance. It can be bought from all aromatherapy oils suppliers, including Neal's Yard (10 ml, £8.55).

For travel rage
Just experienced road rage (yours or someone else's) or general 'Three bl***y trains were cancelled on me' travel rage while battling home after work? Try the woody, clear, refreshing **cypress**. Tisserand says it's useful for calming 'talkative, irritable people' in general and can help soothe rage of all types. Cypress is available from many different essential-oil companies, including Tisserand (9 ml, £5.99/$12.25).

Kitchen

Try aromatherapy (broadly defined as affecting the emotional or physical well-being through the power of natural scents) of a different kind for this room. Pop one of those part-baked baguettes from the supermarket into the oven, bake, then leave the oven door (and kitchen door) partially open. The quick-bake takes five to six minutes, smells heavenly, lingers for an hour or two and is one of the most welcoming, homely scents on the planet. Hot fresh bread's pretty good to eat, too.

For all contact details, see under 'Shopping' in the Directory.

Ambience

394. Peace

There is a wonderful way of spreading pure, lasting peace throughout your home. Like most good ideas it is simplicity itself. It was suggested by Diana Cooper, the UK's most prolific and respected author and teacher on the subject of angels, spiritual enlightenment and Atlantis.

It takes just a few moments a day, or even every few days, if this is the only time you have, so is available to even the busiest person. You don't need flowers, you don't need candles, you don't need any other esoteric bits, pieces or ceremonies – just a peaceful thought or two every day.

Creating your home's Peace Place

1. Choose a quiet corner of your home to be your special Peace Place. It can be a chair on your upstairs landing, a big cushion in a corner of the sitting room, a nook in the bedroom – one person I know chose the far end of her kitchen table, as she liked to perch on it and look out at the view over the valley.
2. As you approach it, get your mind into a calm, peaceful state *before* you sit down there. Put aside all worries and hurried thoughts – just for a little while. You can always go back and sort them later. *Note:* only do this if your thoughts are peaceful. If you are feeling fed up one day and cannot shake it off, leave it for the time being and try again later.

3. Now, sit down in your Peace Place and get comfortable. Start thinking your favourite peaceful thoughts. One person I know imagines a big circle of adults and children of all races, ages and colours with flowers in their hair, sitting on a lawn holding hands with their eyes closed. Another sees herself on a beautiful deserted beach she once found in western Australia. Another holds a mental image of herself, her partner and her young children asleep together in a big, feathery bed with white covers. Yet another sees herself sitting in her grandfather's big armchair by a top-floor bedroom window looking out on to a park: she used to curl up there when she was small. It can be whatever you want.

4. Sit here on your own for a little while every day if possible (from a minute or so to many minutes if you have them).

5. When you've finished, take a deep breath, bless the place or send it love in whatever way you are comfortable. And that's all there is to it.

Your peace thoughts will begin to build up: first in that special area (you'll start noticing it feels good as soon as you sit there), but then the tranquil atmosphere will begin to spread outwards from your Peace Place, like the warmth from a small log fire that's just getting going – first throughout the room and eventually throughout the whole house, filling it with loving calm.

Note: only let other people sit in your Peace Place if they are prepared to think calm thoughts too.

395. Atmosphere – Not Great

If the atmosphere in your home – or even in a particular room – remains uneasy, no matter what you try, but you still want or need to stay in this particular place, it may be time to think about a different approach.

In some homes, many of us who are faced with a 'difficult' nest have tried the lot (me included) – extra radiators to warm an inexplicable chill in the room, redecoration with brighter or lighter colours to cheer up a heavy atmosphere, changing the lighting because a room feels less than relaxing to be in, feng shui, smudging, essences; geomancy and electromagnetic-pollution checks because we always felt inexplicably tired after a night sleeping in our bedroom – without lasting results. Yet often a simple spiritual approach can succeed – and *last* – where other strategies have failed.

Another indication for spiritual action is if there's nothing specific but your life simply hasn't gone well since you moved in, or there's been one life problem (whether health, work, love or with children) after another ever since you arrived.

If this sounds familiar, one direction to try is to check whether there is a spiritual problem either in the whole house or just in this particular part of it. Perhaps something unfortunate happened here once (possibly a long time ago), or maybe someone lived here who was unhappy, lonely or ill – and the distress energy still remains. Possibly there is even an earthbound spirit around who's become stuck there and wishes to leave but cannot find their way.

If you are now wondering whether this might possibly be the case – and it is, in fact, reasonably common – there is a good, down-to-earth and very practical organisation called the Spirit Release Foundation that is well worth contacting for advice. If after talking to them you both reckon it's advisable, they could either come and have a look at your place for themselves and see what they can do or work on it at a distance (which can be just as effective).

The Spirit Release Foundation was founded in 1999 by a medical doctor called Dr Alan Sanderson. Its worldwide membership includes other orthodox clinicians, such as medical doctors, complementary therapists and healers. It runs sensible training courses for those working professionally in this area and can also put you in touch with your nearest qualified practitioner. For contact details, see under 'Therapies and Therapists' in the Directory.

Note: if the cause of the odd atmosphere *is* a spiritual one, don't worry, as this is very fixable – and often quickly so – providing you get someone who knows what they are doing to deal with it. However, if a person is not properly trained or sufficiently experienced they're likely to make matters worse – in the same way as if you had, say, a burst boiler, you'd be in far safer hands with an experienced plumber rather than his junior apprentice, no matter how keen to help the latter was.

396. Making Your House Sing

There's feng shui, and there's Karen Kingston feng shui. She uses the beautiful traditional Balinese techniques of space-clearing and environment enhancement to remarkable effect and has trained practitioners all over the world.

Kingston creates a warmer, more loving and somehow friendlier energy than the rather more mathematical, traditional Chinese style of feng shui (which also works very well). If you can afford a once-over for your home with one of her people, this seems to lift the atmosphere like nothing else. It costs approximately £350–£450 for an average-sized, three bedroomed house (standard for an ordinary Feng Shui person, too, see page 459) You can find practitioners who have trained with Karen in countries all over the world via her website, www.spaceclearing.com.

Recommended reading: see her book *Creating Sacred Space With Feng Shui* for general principles and some make-a-difference tips you can use immediately.

397. A Little of Everything That Helps

One of the best, most practical and widest-ranging books on homes and improving atmospheres I have ever come across is Denise Linn's *Sacred Space.* Though its title sounds a bit rarefied, its upbeat, broad and imaginative approach treats cleaning up the vibes of a home as a perfectly logical extension of spring-cleaning with housework and elbow grease (which indeed it is).

Linn, who gives home-enhancement seminars worldwide, uses several different approaches – some drawn from her Native American heritage, others from Chinese, Balinese and traditional Celtic cultures. It's all in here, something for everyone: smudging with sage sticks, invocation, crystals, feng shui, sound and spirituality . . . a smorgasbord of techniques that invites you to go for the ones that attract you most and make a start. Thoroughly recommended for anyone with esoteric home improvements in mind. Another good book to check out: *Clearing* by Jim Pathfinder Ewing (2006, £6.35, via Cygnus Books, see Shopping: or £7.99 on order via any local bookshop).

See also Fix 439: Clear a Room.

398. Muck and Magic Hands

Serious gardeners or allotment enthusiasts can often be spotted a mile off by the ingrained dirt in their hands. The usual way to remove it is by using harsh, if businesslike, bloke-soap – which can lead to dryness, soreness and cracked skin, especially in winter.

If this is so for you, try a gentle but effective dirt-remover that's possibly the best-kept secret in the South: **Gardener's Hand Soap**. Hand-made in small batches, and gentle without being effeminate or ineffective, its cleaning power is enhanced by the pumice-stone grains it contains. The shea butter and olive oil are great moisturisers; it contains lavender essential oil and chamomile-flower extract to soothe sore skin; and, reassuringly, its makers say it's 'tested on husbands, not animals'.

Note: For a healthy treat for non-gardeners with sensitive, rash-prone skins try **Heaven Scent**: generously high in essential oils and respectful of an easily-irritated epidermis, (several friends, both male and female, with mild to more moderate recurrent eczema report being able to use both these with no problem). It's also good value (both are £2.95 per bar, by New Forest Soaps). For contact details, see under Shopping in the Directory.

Bedrooms

Top Ten Tips for Great Sex and Sleep Feng Shui-Style

Different feng shui (FS) practitioners, depending on their training and personal inclinations, will often tell you different things: 'Always do your bedroom all in cream – very sensual', 'No, no, sexy, warm, earthy colours are best.' But there are three principles that they all agree on:

- The master bedroom occupied by the owner of the house *has* to be right or the entire home suffers.
- A bedroom should be an oasis of calm and comfort meant for

sleeping and sex only. So get the computer, TV, desk, multiple shelves of books and knick-knacks, work files and sports equipment out of there.

- De-clutter before you do anything else.

Some of the following were shown to me by Arto, a down-to-earth ex-Black Hat Tibetan Buddhist monk who for many years was one of the leading FS practitioners in the UK; some come from international space-clearing expert Karen Kingston, who uses the Balinese FS methods (see also Fix 396: Making Your House Sing) and others are based on very traditional Chinese FS principles as explained by international FS master Lillian Too.

399. De-Clutter (No. 1)

- Throw out anything you don't much like, seldom wear, hope to get back into one day or think could come back into fashion. If you can't bear to give it to the charity shop or a friend, bag it up in bin liners and put it in the loft (or garage, or someone else's box room) for further consideration in six months' time. After which, you'll probably find your attachments to the garments have weakened or dissolved altogether, so it's far easier to give them away. To help you get started, see Fix 411: The Mr Motivator of Spring-Cleaning.
- Remove all knick-knacks and ornaments that aren't beautiful, beloved or useful.
- How little furniture can you get away with? Take out anything remotely extra – e.g. that chair by the window as you've already got one for clothes in the corner, the padded, rather scrotty blanket box at the end of your bed: perhaps you could relocate the blankets it held in the linen cupboard, and put the blanket box out for recycling?

Less is definitely more.
See also Fix 420: Have a Major Clear-Out (No. 1).

400. Out of Sight (No. 2)
Tidy all clothes away so you can't see them.

If you don't have cupboards or built-in wardrobes, a quick and inexpensive option is to get a cheap clothes rail (approximately £40) and hang a plain, ironed cotton sheet over it that tones with the rest of the room, or get an inexpensive canvas cupboard (wooden frame, thick calico stretched over the sides, plain hanging curtain in front) – Next and Ikea do some decent ones.

Strict FS fans also leave their dirty clothes in the bathroom laundry basket at night and put shoes outside the bedroom door. *Really* strict ones won't have clothes cupboards in there at all and instead use an external closet (e.g. built into the upstairs hall), which is fine if you've got the space.

401. Relocate Photos (No. 3)

. . . any, that is, which don't show either you and your partner together – or you, or your partner, on your own.

These include photos of your partner's mum, your brothers and sisters, even your children and certainly, advises Graham Gunn, former chairman of the UK's Feng Shui Society, hearty single-sex 'group-event' pictures like the First Eleven cricket-team line-up. Put these, with respect and kindness, downstairs in the 'family corner' or 'helpful friends corner' of the house – for how to find this, see Fix 423: Bagua Your Space (No. 4) – with a small flower in a vase or glass jar beside them to enhance and energise them.

This is because the bedroom is *your* space, so it should be protected from other people's energy imprints. To put it another way, do you really want to have sex under the photographic gaze of his mother or the local rugby-club First Fifteen? One woman I know hung a large portrait of her (dead) sister, of whom she had been very fond, right opposite the end of the marital bed and found her sex life with her husband plummeted. It took her three years to make the connection, by which time their marriage was really floundering.

402. Your Bed (No. 4)

If you're starting a new sexual relationship, your bed or mattress should be new as well, advises international space-clearing expert Karen Kingston. This is also a good idea if you've had a series of one-nighters or short, multiple relationships but have now met someone really special. Under FS lore, it's not auspicious (the rather circumspect Chinese expression for 'lucky') to sleep with a new partner in the bed you shared with someone from a former failed relationship, or a relationship in which you were not valued, as you may attract more of the same. If a new bed is a bit of a tall order (they're expensive), get a new mattress.

If that's out of the question too, perform the powerful spiritual **Silver-Violet Flame** three times over the bed and mattress to help transmute all former negative energy. For how to do this, see Fix 310: Their Room – a Fetid Teenage Pit? It can also help greatly to get new bedding – say a duvet set and sheets – in honour of the new person in your life.

Bed Tips

Choose, or make with love, a wooden base around 45 cm off the ground, which gives plenty of room for circulating air and energy.

Ensure underneath the bed is kept clear – i.e. no under-bed drawers or boxes full of stuff.

Mattresses matter

Never, ever buy a second-hand mattress if it's one you'll be sleeping on all the time. It will be steeped in the energies of its previous owner(s) as they'll probably have spent eight to ten hours a night, every night, on it. You'll be spending too long in physical contact with it if their vibes aren't good (e.g. if their relationships were troubled, if they had poor health or financial troubles). However, second-hand *barely used* ones are a possible option for spare rooms where people will only sleep on them for a short while.

403. Bedroom Furniture (No. 5)

Bedroom furniture should ideally be new (i.e. you're the first owner) or have come from a source you know to be positive and happy. Second-hand or even antique furniture will have some of the energies of its previous owners and you don't know their 'luck', as the Chinese say – i.e. were the previous owners happy, did they struggle with relationship problems, or ricochet from one financial crisis to another? If you take on someone else's belongings, you are bringing their energy, and the atmosphere they created in their own home, into yours.

404. Decorate to Sexualise (No. 6)

If you want to encourage a quiet, unbothered, asexual existence, go for chintzy prints and Impressionist pictures or a very plain, neutral effect. If you want to enhance your relationships and sexual energy, however, specific FS tips from international expert Arto include the following:

- Have at least one positive, erotic (or loving without being either cutesy or painfully pornographic) picture you both like on the bedroom wall.
- Place soft lighting at floor level (no overhead lights) and draped muslin or mosquito netting around the bed. Bulbs (40 watt) with a hint of pink are terrific, inexpensive enhancers of women's looks, also putting one in mind of soft, rosy flesh and . . . sex. Take care not to have them *too* pink: you'll look like you are setting up a suburban brothel. Remove any big light fittings or lampshades hanging down over the bed: these create potentially harmful 'cutting' energy. See also Fix 405: Ban Those Beams (No. 7).
- Get rid of any photographs or pictures that aren't either erotic or of the pair of you. See also Fix 401: Relocate Photos (No. 3).

405. Ban Those Beams (No. 7)

If you've got an old house with attractive wooden beams on the ceiling in your bedroom, FS practitioners believe this is a problem (which is a pity if you're living in a dream 17th-century country cottage). They strongly suggest either covering those beams with a false plasterboard layer or at the very least painting them the same colour as the ceiling so they stand out far less. This is because long, straight beams, which look so cosy and atmospheric, are said to create what the Chinese call 'poison arrows', which send cutting energy at you and are thought to adversely affect both relationships and health.

Dividing line

Beware especially of having an exposed beam running along the centre of your bed from top to bottom. It symbolically divides you and your partner, and 'can wreck a good marriage', says Karen Kingston, adding that one running *across* you where you sleep 'can result in medical problems' in whatever part of the body it traverses. For the same reason, avoid those beds made with two adjacent single mattresses and a narrow wooden strip down the centre where they join. Again, this represents division between you and your partner.

406. Mirror, Mirror . . . (No. 8)

A mirror can be fantastic for erotic games or to watch your lovemaking, but make sure that it's not positioned so it reflects you sleeping in bed, or directly facing you as you get up. If it does, drape a cover (e.g. a soft, sensual voile curtain) over it when not in use.

According to Lillian Too, the reflection of someone in a wrongly placed bedroom mirror can represent infidelity, 'a third person coming between you and your lover'. Mirrored tiles are not thought to be good either – they fragment your image, representing harm being done to you.

407. Books – the Write Stuff (No. 9)

If you like to read in bed, build bookshelves elsewhere nearby (in the hall or stairwell) and just bring a couple in at a time. If you have bookshelves in your bedroom already, FS consultants usually advise people to take them down, as shelves tend to be angular and so give out cutting energy. See also Fix 405: Ban Those Beams (No. 7).

From an FS point of view, a master bedroom's magic works best when it's used exclusively for lovemaking and sleep: reading takes you away from both these activities. Also, books, because they contain so much of the energy of both their writer and the story or material itself, may send out vibrations that disrupt the calm, sensual feel of a 'good' (from an FS point of view) adult bedroom. Instead, keep some erotic or love-orientated picture books to both your own and your partner's taste, sexy literature or love poems around.

408. Love-Power Details (No. 10)

According to Lillian Too (one of the pioneers in bringing FS to the West), a picture of a lush red or purple peony 'is a wonderful symbol of fidelity between lovers', as is a pair of little Mandarin ducks (carved wooden, jade or pottery) placed in your home's 'marriage corner', but 'stick to one pair of ducks unless you want multiple marriages. You could also set up a group of the following:

- a picture of you both looking happy together
- a small vase of two one for each of you beautiful red or purple flowers. Red and purple are the colours of love and passion. The flowers can be good-quality artificial if you don't want to keep replacing fresh ones.
- a piece of rose quartz. *Note*: it only takes a few minutes but this must first be cleansed in salt water, then programmed with loving thoughts to be effective. For how to do this, see Appendix 1: Cleansing and Programming Crystals and Gems on page 536.

These things need to be placed in the 'marriage corner' of your bedroom. This is easy to find: just put the bagua grid over a diagram of your room, marking major areas like the bed, window, door, etc., and it will show you the position of the marriage corner. For more information, see Fix 423: Bagua Your Space (No. 4).

However, it's important to make sure that the arrangement is to scale – i.e. don't put a whopping pair of foot-long Indonesian wooden ducks or a big vase of tall silk peonies in a small alcove in the hope that bigger will bring better luck. It won't. In fact, the overwhelm factor can cause the reverse effect, as it creates disharmony.

Cleaning and Housework

409. Keeping It Green

Keeping the cleaning green is an excellent way of cutting down the level of chemicals in our own environment and our children's (and being eco-sorted into the bargain). There are lots of effective holistic cleaning methods, but the truth is that not everyone has the inclination – or the time – to mix cream of tartar with essence of this and that, then scrub like a fiend. Because, as it says in Allison Pearson's *I Don't Know How She Does It*, for most women: 'Busy has got busy since my mother's day. Busy has gone global.'

So why not buy an eco-friendly pre-packaged product? You may have tried them in the past and been put off because many aren't that effective. However, two that do work properly are:

- **Orange Cleaning Concentrate**, given five-star rating by *Proof*. It is distributed by Earth Friendly (650 ml, £3.50).
- **Multi-Purpose Organic Citrus and Geranium Cleaner** from Green People (200 ml, £6.99).

Note: both the above have been tried and tested by a panel at the excellent *Proof* magazine, which is similar to *Which?* and is produced by the publisher of *What Doctors Don't Tell You*. A year's subscription to their Web magazine costs £12 in the UK and $21 in the US.

For all contact details, see under 'Shopping' in the Directory.

If you do need to use chemicals . . .

For especially mucky jobs you may reckon that a high-powered, pre-packaged chemical SWAT product is called for, so here are some tips from *Proof*'s report on the subject (June 2005) to help reduce the harmful effects:

- Wear rubber gloves.
- Use less product than it says on the packet: manufacturers tend to overstate.
- Do not mix cleaners if they both contain bleach.
- Go for liquids over sprays: a fine mist of chemicals is easier to inhale.
- Ventilate the area you're working in well.
- You won't need cleaning agents every time you wipe down a surface: often just a clean cloth and hot water do the trick.

410. Polished Tricks – Budget Beeswax

Beeswax is great for maintaining and improving the condition of all types of wood, especially antique furniture, and smells wonderful; but it's not cheap.

If you are feeling budget-conscious or have run out of wax, mix together half a cup of **lemon juice** and a teaspoon of **olive oil**, and apply to the wood with a soft cloth, being careful not to put too much on at once so the wood gets soaked. Rub with strong movements, preferably in the direction of the wood grain. This gives a lovely soft sheen – much nicer than the aerosol coat 'em and cover 'em spray 'polishes'.

411. The Mr Motivator of Spring-Cleaning

Anyone who likes a tidy house and becomes despondent when they open cupboards and things cascade down on their heads but who finds it hard to summon up the necessary impetus for a really good under-the-beds, drawer-emptying classic spring-clean might be interested in the remarkable essence **Red Henbit**.

Red Henbit gives any desire to tidy up and reorganise serious impetus. Before you know it, you are zooming about purposefully with bin liners and damp cloths, thoroughly *enjoying* the process of putting your environment in order and really getting into it, whether it's a reorganisation of a workspace or tool shed, or a total top-to-bottom clean of your entire house.

Red Henbit is available from Healthlines (10 ml, approximately £7) and direct from its makers, Bloesem Remedies, in the Netherlands; in the US, you can buy it from the United Field (10 ml, $8). For contact details, see under 'Shopping' in the Directory.

Note: it seems to be best not to take this for more than about three to four days in a row, as it's a true focus remedy. Some people I have given it to achieved such excellent results within just a couple of days that they wanted to keep using it, but taking it for too long made them feel restless and driven (like one art therapist and potter who reorganised her entire studio, which had been stuffed to the gunnels for years and then found she couldn't stop decluttering).

412. Loo Rings

One of my gran's: if you don't want to resort to aggressive chemical cleaners every time, try dropping three or four big **fizzy vitamin-C tablets** into the toilet bowl, let them dissolve, then bog-brush the rings away with ease.

Garden Pests

413. Ants Out
A favourite place for an ants' nest in the garden or conservatory seems to be in the rich earth around big plants housed in attractive earthenware pots. Unfortunately, ants get very comfortable here and can be quite hard to get rid of. If you'd rather not flood the pot in question with boiling water (the usual advice, which will kill them and won't do the plant roots much good either), use persuasion – ant-style.

1. Get another big pot or bucket and fill it loosely with a mixture of soil and compost.
2. Place it next to the infested one.
3. Balance a stick across the rims of both, to create a bridge from one to the other.
4. Slowly flood the affected pot – repeatedly if necessary – with cool water. You will shortly see the ants belting to the surface carrying their pupae to get away from the deluge.
5. It won't take a few of them long to find the bridge and start crossing it; the others will follow. This should clear the entire pot. However, if some have taken refuge in the leaves, remove the stick (so the first lot of ants don't return), wait an hour for the ants that are hiding in the leaves to come back down again and repeat the process.
6. Take the newly colonised pot out into a corner of the garden where you would be happy for the ants to live and tip it out gently.

414. Greenfly – Get 'Em Off
Greenfly are possibly one of the least favourite creatures for any gardener as they multiply like wildfire, coating roses and other precious plants in what looks like a heaving green carpet of tiny, ravenous bodies. But instead of spraying them with toxic death, why not deal with it naturally and instigate a fun family project that younger children (and maybe older ones too) would enjoy?

Make a **ladybird farm**, watch them grow and develop, then release your holistic red-and-black protection squad on to the roses, stand back and watch them go to work.

The Organic Gardening Catalogue has ladybird breeding kits with which you nurture them from egg to insect, checking their progress with a special wall chart for 30 days until they're all ready to go (50 eggs and kit, £19.50). Or, more simply, the Organic Gardening Catalogue also do a pack of 30 eggs (available from April to August) that can be sent by post and, when sprinkled on to infested areas, will start a colony in 30 days. The breeding kit may be a better bet as 80 per cent of the eggs will be eaten by pupae stage. For contact details, see under 'Shopping' in the Directory.

415. Pest Patrol

Hens and ducks are delightful to watch, companionable to have around and are multi-purpose gardeners' friends, even in quite small urban backyards.

Fowl play

As a method of holistic garden-pest control, they come highly recommended by the internationally acclaimed Centre for Alternative Technology (CAT) in Wales. Ducks and hens nibble up invasive grasses and weeds, eat snails, bugs and slugs, reducing the population so far that it can be kept down well with natural sprays and you'll never need chemical killers again. They supply good-quality manure too (if you don't mind shovelling a little avian excrement: ducks produce 150 g daily) and also provide delicious eggs.

> Hens adapt easily to towns. But think twice about getting a rooster if you want to stay on speaking terms with your neighbours.

The duck must-have

Ducks are usually easy-going and undemanding, but they need a pond – even a small paddling pool a metre wide filled and emptied each day will do at a pinch – because if deprived of water they find it much harder to keep clean and groom themselves in the usual way, may become depressed, develop behavioural problems like head-shaking or aggression and are far more prone to eye problems.

Getting started

Ask your local council if it's OK to keep ducks or hens (some ban them in gardens). Kahaki Campbells and Indian Runners are the breeds best suited to domestic life; however, experts warn that the former can be a bit territorial and scare neighbours' children. Barred Rock hens are especially recommended as garden-dwellers, as they are attractive, sturdy, quiet, non-aggressive and good layers.

For health and bird-keeping advice, fox-proof coops (adaptable foxes are now found in many urban areas as well as in the country), duck and hen feed, and the hens themselves, try the Surrey-based enthusiasts and breeders Perfect Poultry, plus Regency Poultry, Omlet (manufacturers of the Eglu) or your local farmer, provided his birds are healthy free-rangers. For contact details, see under 'Shopping' in the Directory.

For advice about ducks, try the Indian Runner Duck Association for specialist information, or the British Waterfowl Association. For contact details, see under 'Useful Helplines, Websites and Contacts' in the Directory.

Recommended reading: in the UK, try *Small-Scale Poultry-Keeping* by Ray Feltwell. Or, for accurate information and inspirational colour pictures, see *The Domestic Duck* by Chris and Mike Ashton (available via the British Waterfowl Association); in the US, a really practical and comprehensive one on hens is *Chickens in Your Backyard* by Rick and Gail Luttmann.

See also Pets: Hens on page 412.

416. Rats in the Rubbish

Spotted a scaly tail whisking round your rubbish bins or compost area? Here's how to get rid of rats without harming them or resorting to poisons – get yourself a **wormery**.

The worms (usually tiger worms) eat any kitchen scraps going except citrus skins; the unit seals tight shut, so whiffs can't get out and rats can't get in. All you get out of it is an excellent organic liquid plant feed that, diluted with water, flowers and vegetables thrive on. And if you're mildly squeamish about wriggly things, don't worry – you tend to never even see the worms.

Try the wormery from Original Organics, which can handle all the scraps left over by a family of four (£49.95). For contact details, see under 'Shopping' in the Directory.

417. Slug Off

No one wants slugs waxing fat on their lettuces, but every time you mention natural slug-off methods people urge you to create a 'slug pub' (essentially a beer-filled saucer that they crawl into and drown in: messy, very messy). Or a slug 'milk bar', which is the same principle but the milk-bloated little things are then, following sustainable horticultural principles, fed to the birds, which you can't do if they've been at the beer.

However, the following **copper** trick works a treat and simply sends them off elsewhere: no mess, no fuss. It is based on the fact that slugs will not cross copper tape or wire. This is because the water content in their slime reacts with the metal, producing a small electrical charge that they find uncomfortable.

There is no need for the wire to be connected to batteries of any kind. Simply lay it around the area you wish to protect – builders' yards and electrical suppliers will be able to sell you some. Or, more cheaply, do the same with copper-backed tape, which also looks pretty and is effective when placed round potted plants, garden furniture and pet-food dishes (slugs adore a bit of cat food) that are placed outside. You can buy copper-backed tape from the Organic Gardening Catalogue (4 m x 3 cm, £6.95). For contact details, see under 'Shopping' in the Directory.

418. SnailStopper

Stop them crawling up to feast on your lovingly nurtured potted plants by wiping **Tiger Balm** around the pots' rims in a one-inch slick. This:

- stings a bit, because of the camphor, peppermint and cloves it contains
- is slippery, so they can't get a grip.

Tiger Balm's stocked by most health shops and many independent chemists. You can also buy it from Express Chemist (19 g, £4.39). For contact details, see under 'Shopping' in the Directory. If you can't get any Tiger Balm, however, use a thick coat of Vaseline instead, smeared in a 5 cm band. *Note*: this tip also works for slugs.

Heating

419. Cutting fuel bills

Want to see your energy bills slashed by 50 per cent, and your CO_2 emissions down by three-quarters, straight away?

If you have high fuel bills but are worried about potential toxic leakage from foam-injected insulation there's a solution that's both ecologically sound, and money-saving. There are at least two types of natural materials that are not only effective at preventing heat loss, but will also save most efficiently on winter heating costs – and won't leach dodgy chemicals into your home. One's made from sheep's wool (Thermafleece), the other from cellulose (Warmcel). Both have very low heat conductivity and are fire- and insect-resistant.

The terrific Centre for Alternative Technology (CAT) in Wales can tell you about them, as it runs eco building courses that include their use: some are weekend tasters and week-long comprehensive introductions; others will take you to professional standard (e.g. CAT's tuition is part of the University of East London's MSc in architecture: the advanced environmental and energy studies module). For contact details, see under 'Training Courses' in the Directory.

CAT also offers a very good range of books on the subjects of energy conservation and innovative, sustainable building and design, and has leaflets on Thermafleece and Warmcel. Recommended reading: for more detailed, wider-ranging information, take a look at *The Energy-Saving House* by Thierry Salomon and Stephane Bedel, and *Eco Renovation* by Edward Harland, both of which can be purchased direct from CAT. For contact details, see under 'Shopping' in the Directory.

CAT can even find you an eco-energy consultant who can advise you and, if you want to go ahead, will install the stuff as well. Call CAT's consultancy services for advice on everything from solar power and sustainable construction methods to low-energy design and alternative materials. For contact details, see under 'Useful Helplines, Websites and Contacts' in the Directory.

Home Improvement

The Top Ten Feng Shui Tips

> Every single thing in your home has a particular energy of its own. Therefore every single thing can, and does, affect you. FS can help ensure it does so in the right way.

You don't need an all-out redecoration or a load of expensive new furniture to make your house feel fantastic: try a spot of home improvement, feng shui style, instead. The following suggestions on pages 454 to 466 are quick, simple and can make a world of difference, creating a friendlier, happier atmosphere, an impression of more space, and improving inhabitants' sleep, mood, relationships and even their health.

You probably know already that feng shui is the traditional Oriental system of designing an area, whether it be a house, skyscraper garden, park or single room, so that it utilises the universal energy (chi) available. You may well also already know that this involves:

- using the positive, helpful chi that flows into your living space in such a way as to make the very most of it. The Chinese believe this is the main thing that nourishes and energises your home.
- protecting your place from any negative external chi that would otherwise enter it
- getting rid of, or neutralising, any negative chi that is already in the house to create a harmonious, happy, protected and balanced space that's a pleasure to be in.

However, since the proper study of FS can take several years, the many different ways of working with it can seem so complex – often unneccessarily so – and different practitioners and teachers may tell you different things, it can be difficult to know where to start if you are interested in, say, just making one or two positive changes to enhance your home, then seeing how you go from there. So coming up are the **Top 10 FS Tips** suggested because they are some of the easiest to do, and the most effective.

The suggestions come from a variety of sources. Some were shown to me by Arto, formerly one of the leading FS workers in the UK; others are used by Karen Kingston, who is an expert in Balinese FS; and several come from world-famous practitioner and author Lillian Too, who teaches the traditional Chinese system.

Note: these measures can work very well indeed, but homes are complex and multidimensional, even when they're just a single multi-functional room, so these are tips and guidelines only. If you have on-going problems or something that is not responding to straightforward first-base measures, consider a proper professional on-site consultation: see 'Calling in the professionals' on page 459.

See also Atmosphere: Not Great on page 435, Electromagnetic Fields on page 480, Bedrooms on page 453 and see Fix 396: Making Your House Sing.

Does it work?

It's believed that feng-shuied workspaces are happier and more profitable, feng-shuied houses are more agreeable and healthier to live in, feng-shuied gardens grow better and enhance the luck of the house they are attached to . . . and so on.

Think that sounds like a load of Oriental designer bunk? Could be. But just from a (very small) personal perspective, having used it to great effect for the first time ten years ago, our family now have an FS consultation (and follow most of the suggestions made) for every new home we buy. Far more impressively, major businesses and multi-million-pound corporations (see below) including Western ones – none of them known for wasting their hard-earned cash – spend millions on this ancient system of spatial energy manipualtion, insisting that it improves and energises both profit and workforce and is well worth the money.

FS and big business

Many huge corporations have had their reception areas, board-rooms, entrances and even entire buildings designed along FS principles. This includes the $1 billion HSBC headquarters, the offices of the *Wall Street Journal*, Harvey Nichols, Virgin Airways, Microsoft and the Morgan Bank.

420. Have a Major Clear-Out (No. 1)
What?

Drawers, kitchen cupboards, clothes cupboards, sideboards, the glory hole below the stairs, even (if you have a loft with storage space and can face it) the eaves.

See also Fix 411: The Mr Motivator of Spring-Cleaning.

Why?

Rubbish holds stale energy like a soggy old flannel holds stagnant water. If you make any FS changes to re-energise the house without first clearing rubbish, all you will be doing is energising what is already in there – i.e. the space itself *plus* all the mess in it. On an esoteric level, accumulated junk like this may make one feel more muddled, and it can become harder to get things done outside the home as well as inside it. If there's anything negative there, it needs to be cleared or any FS measures may also turbocharge that, which can create further problems – i.e. encourage anything that's not going right to get worse.

421. Mend and Repair (No. 2)
What?

Mend anything that is broken, complete everything that's unfinished (e.g. that half-painted wall over there).

Why?

This sends out the message that *you are effective*, and everything you do is going to work properly and be taken to completion.

Any FS realignment you then undertake will amplify this. Unfortunately, if you leave the broken and unfinished stuff around, the reverse is also true.

First clear up – then move on up

Interestingly, both No. 1 (de-cluttering) and No. 2 (repairing), the rocks on which FS is built, echo universal spiritual lore: which is that if people want to develop themselves spiritually (perhaps through healing or reiki training, learning about on basic shamanism, doing an introductory essences or meditation course) and want to raise their consciousness (i.e. become more intuitive, sensitive, practise communicating with beings on other levels, such as angels or animals), they first need to purify *themselves*.

This sounds a bit saintly, but it's just practical and sensible since purification in this sense just means sorting out your own mental or emotional dross and negativity – which we all have by the bucket-load – so your way is clear for moving forwards and raising your awareness by meditation or other esoteric practices.

If someone tries to practise self-development without first doing the above, they are likely to get into difficulties. So a bit of extra time spent on clearing out will pay dividends.

422. Don't Love It, Don't Use It? Pass It On (No. 3)
What?
Throw out or give away undistinguished knick-knacks or second hand things, unless they mean something special to you or you like using them. And think about whether you really do want to keep any antiques which are in your home, unless they used to belong to someone positive whom you loved or liked, or they have a good feel about them. This includes that large china dog from Auntie Gladys (whom you've always loathed), the spare, rather temperamental lawnmower that has yet to come in useful, books you half read and weren't impressed with, furniture that's just 'there', kitchen appliances you've never worked out how to use . . . In short, give away anything that isn't:

- loved
- useful
- good to look at.

Why?
Antiques because you don't know 'the luck', as the Chinese say, of those who had them before you, and the unique energy of previous owners will be soaked into them. We instinctively know this anyway. It's partly why someone may be delighted to have, say, the rocking chair that used to belong to their much-loved grandmother and will find it comforting to sit in, but a sideboard inherited from a bullying uncle they disliked

may make them feel a bit uncomfortable and they wouldn't want it in their bedroom.

Once you've done this, you will be left only with those things that send out positive signals to you. And a house full of positive signals is a very good place to live in.

423. Bagua Your Space (No. 4)

What?

The bagua is a simple diagrammatical grid derived from *The I Ching* (the Chinese *Book of Changes*) that can be placed over a plan of your home or office to show which areas of it relate to various aspects of your life – love, health, wealth, etc.

Why?

The grid is central to the science of Chinese feng shui. Once you see it, everything in your house takes on rather more significance – 'There's mould on the wall in my "wealth corner". Wonder how that relates to that overdraft I can't seem to shift?'

So where's my 'love corner', then?

One very attractive, divorced friend of mine in her mid-forties whose romantic life had been bumping along on rock bottom for a long time found that in the 'relationships corner' (the part responsible for your love life) of her West London mews house there was a dying fern she kept forgetting to water and a badly cracked windowpane hidden by a scruffy, rather grubby roman blind that blocked out most of the sunlight. She replaced the desiccated fern with a splendid fluffy plant, repaired the windowpane, junked the blind and hung a beautiful crystal there to create rainbows from the sun when it came in – and, possibly quite coincidentally – the next time I met her, she had not one but two men on the go.

Not everything's that cut and dried. For one thing, you usually need to tackle the entire home. Some results are instant – e.g. the area feels clearer, brighter or somehow 'bigger' – but positive life-changes usually take longer to kick in. So if an FS practitioner is promising you instant, fabulous results, don't use them. Good practitioners don't need to exaggerate.

How?

1. Draw a sketch of your house on a large piece of paper, roughly to scale. Include all the different rooms and mark doorways and windows. If you have more than one storey, draw each floor on a separate piece of paper.
2. Copy the bagua grid (see illustration) on to a piece of tracing paper. If your house is square or rectangular, draw two diagonal lines from the corners, quartering it. If there are areas 'missing', square them off with dotted lines.
3. Put the centre of the bagua grid exactly over where the two diagonal lines cross. Just by taking the lines out further, you can make the grid shrink or grow to the size to fit your home.

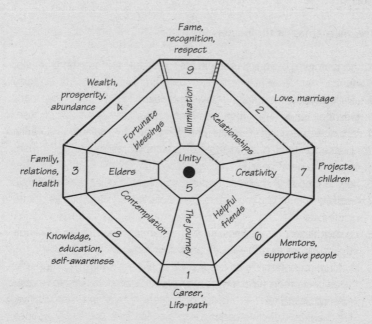

4. Turn the bagua so its lower edge is flush with the entrance that most people use, as this is where energy that flows into your home from the outside world will also enter. Usually this is the front door, but for some it could be the side or back one. If you live in a bed-sit, a studio flat or have a room in a shared house, the 'front door' is the one leading into your bit of personal living space. If your home is on two or more floors, on each successive floor above ground level, align the edge of the bagua grid with the direction you face as your staircase brings you up to that floor.

5. Check each portion of the bagua, described below, against the diagram of your home, and see what is in each area. Decide whether they need clearing, energy enhancement or the contents repositioning for better effect.

Note: the numbered sections don't follow each other clockwise around the grid starting at the 'one o'clock' position as one might expect, but tend to jump about. This isn't an error: it's just how the system works.

The nine areas of the bagua

1. **the journey** (i.e. your journey in life) – career and personal development
2. **relationships** or **marriage** – love and sex
3. **elders** or **family** – parents, relations and ancestors
4. **fortunate blessings** – wealth, prosperity, money matters, and general abundance (which is not just to do with money)
5. **unity** – general health
6. **helpful friends** – mentors, backers and 'useful' people who help you
7. **creativity** – anything you make, create or give birth to, such as children or projects
8. **contemplation** (inner knowledge) – learning new things, self-knowledge, wisdom and the development of intuition
9. **illumination** or **fame** – covers a wide brief from charisma , reputation, the respect others have for you, and personal achievement to whatever lights up your life

Mistakes?

If things take a turn for the worse soon after you have made an FS adjustment or change, chances are you have the grid placement or its interpretation a little wrong (though the grid looks simple, this isn't uncommon). Check it again and talk to a professional *if more than two* even moderately unfortunate things occur in the two to three weeks after you have done so: things may just need a professional tweak.

Calling in the professionals

A consultation from a good professional is a very worthwhile investment, but it will cost from around £400 for an ordinary three-bedroom house – and if the practitioner isn't very good, they may get things wrong, which could well make matters worse. If you are looking for a qualified FS worker, word of mouth is usually best. If no one you know has got any good contacts, then try the Feng Shui Society as a starting point; in the US, try the American Feng Shui Institute. For contact details, see under 'Therapies and Therapists' in the Directory.

Practitioner check

- Always check their professional qualifications.
- Ask to see their certificates. If they can't show you, ask the name of the organisation they trained with and where it is, find the telephone number via the Net or directory enquiries and contact the place to check whether this person did indeed qualify there (and when).
- Ask to see written references or testimonials from other clients. These should be relatively recent and written by people you may contact yourself, if required, rather than Xeroxed letters from people whose phone number the practitioner does not appear to have a record of, which could have been written by anyone.
- Get a written costing or ballpark quote accurate to within £50 *before* work starts.

Professionals should be willing to provide all of the above. If you are not happy with the information they give you, are simply not quite comfortable with the person, or if they promise you overly shiny results, get someone else.

Further information
There are literally hundreds of books on feng shui. Two of my favourites are *The Complete Illustrated Guide to Feng Shui* by Lillian Too, which is straightforward, practical and beautiful to look at, and *The Feng Shui Handbook: a Practical Guide to Chinese Geomancy and Environmental Harmony* by Derek Walters. Both are oldies but goodies.

424. Where's Your Loo? (No. 5)
What?
The discreet and controlled Chinese won't call something 'bad' or 'unlucky'; the furthest they will go is 'inauspicious'. But over many hundreds of years it has been seen by generations of FS practitioners that where the toilet goes matters.

Why?
If it's in the 'fortunate blessings corner' of the house, this is considered particularly inauspicious as it's thought to affect your prosperity and wealth – you are symbolically 'dumping' on your money-making potential, then flushing wealth down the toilet every time you use it. People with their WC here often feel they 'should have' plenty of money coming in but that somehow it all seems to go straight back out again.

How?
Apart from moving the loo to a less problematic siting (which is expensive, and, let's face it, there is probably no aspect of your life that you would want compromised by the esoteric influence of sewage plumbing) or not using it if you have another less sensitively sited one elsewhere in the house, there are several suggested FS solutions to this one. It seems to work best if you do them all simultaneously.

1. Always keep the loo seat down when not in use.
2. Always keep the door to the toilet shut.
3. Put a mirror on the outside of the door to deflect energy away. This can be any shape or size you feel comfortable with.

4. If there is a window, hang a rainbow crystal in front of it.

5. If there is room, put a healthy, round-leaved, upwards-growing plant in there to introduce some positive energy into the space. If the space is too tiny, hang up a picture or poster of healthy-looking trees or some flowers in bloom.

Worst places for your WC

According to Lillian Too, these are:

- by or near to the front door (as it affects the energy coming into the house)
- in the 'fortunate blessings corner' or 'journey (career) corner' of the home, closely followed by the 'marriage corner'.

425. Mind the Gap (No. 6)

What?

How to fill in the missing areas of your living space.

Why?

If you look at a plan of your home against the bagua grid – see Fix 423: Bagua Your Space (No. 4) – and can see your house has a missing area (i.e. it's square or rectangular but has a chunk taken out of one corner), it's important under FS lore to square this off representationally, as otherwise you may lack the luck symbolised by this part.

According to space-clearing and Balinese FS expert Karen Kingston, many people find that their lives take a downturn after they've built an extension or conservatory on to part of the back of their house, especially if the house was a square or rectangular shape and the add-on square or rectangular conservatory has left an area at the back with nothing in it.

How?

It is easy enough to energise or square off (i.e. put something there to fill the area) a missing chunk of space using mirrors (see diagram), a hanging crystal, a splendid, healthy outdoor potted plant or shrub and also by lighting the area from outside at night, say, with an angled garden light or a flat-fronted one set into the ground.

426. Front Entrance (No. 7)

What?

Keep the front entrance to your house and the entrance hall as clear, bright and clutter-free as possible.

Why?

If the first thing you see as you open your door is a load of stuff, your energy level will sag before you even come in, warns Karen Kingston. Also, keeping the house entrance and hallway clear represents your approach to life (a clear entry equates to clear purpose and personal effectiveness). It also affects how much uninterrupted energy can flow into your home from the outside world to nourish it.

How?

Don't:

- Stack up stuff to recycle at the front door, hallway or porch, as this represents constant recycling of the past, says Karen Kingston – e.g. past problems, past relationships (ever wondered why you keep getting the same sort of partner?) and past ill health – which makes it harder for your life to move forwards. Recycling is excellent and necessary, but keep it at the back or side.
- Cram all coats, shoes, etc., into a tiny cupboard right by the front door. Only keep a few in there that are in constant use. Better still, keep nothing there and dismantle the cupboard.
- Pile things to 'remember to take out' around the front door that then hang about there for ages.
- Place a mirror so that it faces you as soon as you open the front door. It deflects the incoming energy straight back out again.

Do:

- Keep your hallway light, bright and welcoming.
- Keep it clutter-free.

427. Front and Back Doors (No. 8)
What?
Ensure front and back doors are not in direct line with each other.

Why?
According to FS rules, the energy that would usually be flowing in to nourish your house comes in the front, then swiftly disappears straight out the back. A bit like eating a nutritious meal but not being able to digest it properly so you receive no goodness from it.

How?
It can be expensive to reposition a door, but is there another side entrance you can use to get into, say, the garden?

428. Ceilings – Hint of a Tint (No. 9)
What?
This fix can change the feel of your house fast. According to top FS practitioner Arto, white ceilings are the scourge of Western decoration.

Why?
'They seem to suck up all the energy in a room,' he complains. 'I am always telling clients to paint their ceilings a light but warm, or pale, colour. Again and again I do it. The energy in the room changes immediately.'

It does too. After I'd had Arto round for a consultation ten years ago, being unable to face painting every ceiling in the house I cheated and resorted to fast colour-washing.

A decorater friend told me that the quickest way to do this is to heavily dilute some water-based paint, dip a rag in it, then squeeze out almost every last drop ('it's what you take out, not what you put on that does it'), and give the ceiling a rough once-over that tones in with whatever colour the walls are. To my amazement, this worked beautifully and didn't take long (two hours flat for an area 14 ft x 12 ft: way quicker than giving it the standard couple of coats of a single new colour which would have taken nearer 6 hours). And afterwards? The house glowed, its energy levels shot up, and the entire atmosphere seemed to smile.

This was probably partly a reaction by the human brain to the different light frequencies and wavelengths sent out by the new colours, yet it didn't seem to account for the whole of such a major change. So it's likely that colour also works on a spiritual and esoteric level (the chakras are, after all, associated with specific vibrational frequencies expressed as different colours – red for the base, orange for the sacral, yellow for the solar plexus, and so on) especially if there is such a large uninterrupted area of it (in this case a ceiling). I now do this in every new home we have.

Fuss-Free Tips for Fast Work

- Tie a damp cloth on to a broom and clean the ceiling you're going to paint first. The colour goes on better and faster, and you are not sealing in old dirt, which would be unhelpful from an FS point of view.
- One ceiling measuring 12 ft by 16 ft takes approximately three hours, depending on how fussy you are. You only need one application, unless you are going for a very subtle, more artistic two-toned look.
- If you want a bolder look, do it to rock music. If you want something subtler, pick gentler music – ambient country, mellow jazz, chillout, a Mozart violin concerto . . . It makes a major, automatic difference to the way you work.
- You don't need special colour-wash paints: they cost more and the colour ranges are limited. Merely dilute – and dilute again – in a big container, in which you have put a little ordinary emulsion of the shade you like, plus water.
- It's a good idea to make that a really big container (e.g. a cheap bucket). Don't try and do it with a little paint you have left over from earlier decoration days. If you need to make more to finish one ceiling, it is almost impossible to get the concentration, and hence the colour, the same twice.
- Keep a clean, damp J-cloth tucked into your belt to wipe off any smears on dado rails or other walls the instant they are made. This saves a lot of time later.

Note: it's impossible to colour-wash with gloss and not easy with vinyl silk. Emulsion paints work best.

Soft ceiling colours

Keep ceiling colours pale as a rule, so they continue to reflect as much light as possible and do not bring the ceilings lower down, unless that's what you want. A room needs lots of light for a stronger ceiling colour, though some (e.g. orangey-yellow) can do a great job of warming up a chilly north-facing room as long as it's not too low. Quick rub-on ceiling shades that work best include:

- washed-out orange (warm)
- palest yellow (sunny)
- palest blue (a blue-sky infinity feel)
- palest green – only use to 'cool' or 'freshen' if the walls are in very warm or dense shades (e.g. terracotta) or it can be a depressant
- soft pink
- washed-out orangey-pink
- hint of lilac.

429. If It Ain't Broke, Don't Fix It (No. 10)
What?

Oscar Wilde said that too much of a good thing can be wonderful, but this does not apply to FS.

Why?

Twenty FS adjustments are not necessarily more effective than two, and it is possible to overdo it. Making changes to things that were OK before in the hope of enhancing certain areas of your life still further may result in a backlash if you've disrupted existing harmony or are perhaps being a tad greedy.

Many years ago I had the bright idea of putting a Pa Kua mirror (Chinese FS mirror) on my front door to 'defend' the house better. But the Pa Kua is a very powerful symbol indeed and should be used with care. And since the front-door area was actually fine already, after a few weeks the place started feeling a bit flat, my freelance work was inexplicably dropping off, friends were calling detectably less often, and I realised I was deflecting *away* the nourishing outside chi that should have been coming into the home. It took months to recover.

So go easy on the wind chimes, rocks, round-leaved plants, crystals, Pa Kua mirrors and furniture replacement. Have a good think about how your life really is at present and what you truly need – you may only require a couple of subtle FS adjustments here and there. If in doubt, talk to an expert – see 'Calling in the professionals' on page 459.

Furniture

430. New-Sofa Tip

Buying a new sofa or easy-chairs? If you can, let them 'out-gas' outside your home, freed of any plastic covering, for three days – maybe in the garage, shed or back garden if the weather's fine, covered in a light cotton sheet overnight to help absorb dew.

> Ever sniffed the distinctive aroma of a brand-new sofa? Then you'll know what out-gassing smells like.

According to six years' research (1979–85) by the US Environmental Protection Agency, air chemicals are five to ten times higher inside a house than out. And we're not talking about the odd leaking gas pilot light here, but emissions of the myriad of new chemical substances used in paints, building materials, floor coverings and soft furnishings.

The biggest group of out-gas baddies are volatile organic compounds (VOCs), which are made from petrochemicals, known to cause cancer in humans, and have also been linked to impaired fertility, constant headaches, fatigue, joint pains and asthma. So if you've got a posh new three-seater, why not let it breathe before you make it part of the family?

Household Pests

431. Fly Away, Flies

When summer is a-coming, so are flies seeking a bit of cool and shade. If you don't want to spray insecticides at them (especially not in a kitchen, where food's prepared) and remember old-fashioned sticky fly-paper with disgust, grow **window boxes of lavender** (or fast-track cheat by buying the plants ready fluffed up and putting them straight in). Alternatively, if you can get them, cut some bunches of **elder twigs** with the leaves on and place those on the windowsills. Flies dislike both and tend not to cross these botanical barriers.

432. Moths Out

Camphor balls tend to keep them away but they don't smell great, and once you've got a moth infestation they can be very hard to get rid of even if you don't resort to Rambo-style chemical methods (or sometimes even if you do). And moths aren't just a bit annoying – their ravenous larvae can leave carpets, curtains and wardrobe contents in tatters. But according to the expert moth-sorters at Pest Control Direct, you can deal with larvae and eggs by putting clothes affected in a plastic bag, squeezing out the air and freezing the lot for 72 hours. For contact details, see under 'Useful Helplines, Websites and Contacts' in the Directory.

Traditional housewife lore also states that you can deal with infested areas by ironing them (put a light cotton cloth over the top if the fabric is delicate or liable to melt).

Mouse Traps

You can avoid needing them by religiously wiping all surfaces free of food fragments at night, making sure bin lids fit well, blocking up suspected mouseholes and putting all scraps of food away in the evenings. But if you do all this and they are still treating your house like their own, and you want to catch them without hurting them (i.e. no poisons or traditional traps), what can you do? Consider the humane mouse-house approach.

Basically, these are plastic tubes with a trapdoor at one end that you bait with a mouse-enticing scrap. Once you have your mouse, just take it to a patch of open ground (e.g. a park, local recreation ground or the far end of your garden) and gently let it go. You can buy the Live Catch Mouse Trap from the Organic Gardening Catalogue (£7.10). For contact details, see under 'Shopping' in the Directory.

However, there is a far cheaper but very similar device from Rentokil that is sold in hardware outlets (approximately £1.35) – and you can also ring Rentokil for sound advice about humane rodent discouragement for free. For contact details, see under 'Useful Helplines, Websites and Contacts' in the Directory.

> Bait traps with *really* smelly food like tuna: it works way better than the traditional lump of Cheddar.

433. Rout those Roaches

Cockroaches sure are hard to get rid of. Tread on one – and it merely shakes itself irritably and strolls off. They're said to be so tough and adaptable that they're the one life form predicted to survive a nuclear disaster. However, you don't need to resort to strong pesticides to get rid of them if they've moved in, and an increasing number of householders are preferring not to, since these chemicals can find their way into the food chain and are dangerous to have around pets and children. Instead try the **Natural Roach Motel**.

The Natural Roach Motel
'They check in, but they don't check out.'

1. Take a piece of white sandwich-style bread.
2. Place it at the bottom of a high-sided bowl.
3. Sprinkle over a little sugar.
4. Coat the inner rim, and 5 cm below the rim on the inside of the bowl, in Vaseline.
5. Place it on the floor of the kitchen near where you've seen the roaches sauntering.
6. Leave overnight.

Next morning there should be several roaches in there, unable to escape because of the Vaseline. You can dispose of them either by pouring boiling water over them or, less drastically, putting them in a sealed plastic bag and placing this in the freezer. Remove 24 hours later and bury it in the garden or place in the rubbish bin. Do not release live roaches somewhere in the interests of being kind. They breed like mad and you will just be responsible for a new infestation.

434. Woodworming

This may need to be done if you don't want your house to be eaten away. There is, however, something well worth knowing that the DIY manuals and woodworming companies don't tell you but which is very relevant if you want to have children at some time in the future or are trying to get pregnant: anti-woodworm treatments often contain the known reproductive-hazard chemicals permethrin and lindane.

> Homeowners whose places have had woodworm treatment are invariably told that the chemicals used drop down to safe levels after just eight hours. They don't.

These chemicals can also cause eye and breathing-passage irritation, and even seizures after short-term exposure; longer term (e.g. substantial traces of it lingering in your home) can affect the immune system, liver and increase your likelihood of developing cancer.

Research by the Fraunhofer Institute of Toxicology and Aerosol Research in Germany suggests one way that permethrin and lindane can find their way into your body is via ordinary house dust – the particles pick up these chemicals, then deposit them on food and kitchen surfaces, so you may end up both breathing and eating it.

Wise woodworming

The Institute's advice is not only to move out while the job's being done, and then ventilate ferociously before you move back in, but also:

1. **Move** all foodstuffs not in unopened tins or sealed packets out of the house as well. You could store them in boxes in the car boot, a friend's place or the shed.
2. **Hire** protective masks and gloves from the local DIY shop and damp-dust or wash down *all* surfaces in the house, including walls and wooden floor afterwards. If that sounds just too much, take a chance on the walls but do the rest, especially in the kitchen and bedroom.
3. **Vacuum** all carpets while still wearing a mask. Ensure you have or can borrow a sealed-unit model that doesn't blow dust back out.
4. **Dispose** of the used cloths and carpet debris in a sealed bin liner in the dustbin.

New Home

435. Moving House

This can unsettle everyone from the potted plants to the guinea pig (not to mention adults and children) for many weeks; but certain essences are terrific at helping you bed in and feel as if you really do live there, fast.

Feeling safe

If you are feeling a bit uneasy and uprooted – often presenting itself as not feeling as 'safe' as you did in your old neighbourhood (children especially) – try **Guardian** combination, which is a grounding mixture of mineral and plant essences from the Alaskan wilderness, particularly if you tend to be very sensitive to your environment anyway.

It's good to use as either drops in water or, for children especially, in a warm, soothing bath for the first few nights or in spray format to spritz around rooms. For animals, add a couple of drops to their water bowls or on their food; for people, take three or four times daily in a small glass of water; for plants, especially if you've had to dig them up and replant them, put four to eight drops in the average-sized watering can and use that to moisten them. You can also sprinkle or spray it on their leaves for a week.

Guardian is made by Alaskan Essences and available in the UK from Healthlines (spray, 60 ml, £11.95; stock bottle, 7.5 ml, £7.95) or, in the

US and Canada, direct from Alaskan Essences (spray, 2 fl oz, $11; stock bottle, ¼ fl oz, $7.45).

Another good one is **Walnut**, available from Healing Herbs (10 ml, £3.20). Use as above, or, if taking orally, take four drops in water three times daily.

For all contact details, see under 'Shopping' in the Directory.

For pets, see also Pets: New Home on page 419.

---

436. Tile-Shine

When you want a natural, chemical-free way to stop bathroom or kitchen tiles fogging up, cut a medium to large potato in half and rub it on in circular motions, removing any watery, starchy residue with a soft cloth.

Painting and Decorating

437. Clever Colours

You'll probably already be well aware that colour – which is essentially light of different vibrational rates and wavelengths – can influence your mood, health, behavioural habits and energy levels. But in case you are thinking of redecorating, the following 'what does which, where' tips from Alexander Schauss, a clinical psychologist and director of the American Institute for Biosocial Research in Tacoma, Washington, might come in useful:

- For a sense of well-being, paint some (not all) of the walls a **warm pale pink**. This is good for bedrooms and classrooms or school corridors if the children are disruptive – see Fix 241: Colour and Décor. I've also seen this shade used in the waiting rooms of Marie Stopes Well Woman clinics (often inhabited by unwell patients or unhappy and anxious women waiting for pregnancy-test results or terminations) as it both calms and lifts the mood.
- Relaxation spaces: **light blue** is one of the best. Use it on a couple of walls but not all.

- Children's bedrooms? Schauss reckons it ought to be their own choice – however unappealing adults think it looks – as the shades they like will help them feel more content.
- Studies and office spaces: use some **yellow** – how much is up to you. This colour increases heart rate, respiration and stimulates the left hemisphere of the brain, the side that controls judgement, writing skills, reasoning, logic and right-hand movements like hand-writing.
- Eating areas (e.g. dining rooms and kitchens): use **orange**, as it stimulates the appetite and enjoyment of food. Something that's not lost on fast-food chains, who use it extensively in their interiors.

Eau de nihilism

Green is the *worst* colour to live with, says Schauss, especially for someone who has any type of mental disorder, as it tends to have a depressant effect. Ever seen those old-fashioned pale-green walls of the sort beloved by the traditional and slightly shabby British upper classes – a shade known in the decorating trade, because of its gloom-inducing effect, as 'eau de nihilism' (as opposed to 'eau de Nil')?

However, green can work well as an accent colour or for a section of wall, or even a feature wall, especially if you are creating a natural effect with wood, plants and stone in a very urban environment.

Prison pink

There is a very specific shade that has been likened to bubblegum or Pepto Bismol called Miller Baker Pink, which is also a temporary appetite-suppressant. Dieters have been known to look at big squares painted this colour when trying to squelch chocolate cravings.

Miller Baker pink also has a temporary calming effect. This was first noticed when two naval officers, Miller and Baker, painted the walls of their detention cells this colour on the advice of a local psychologist, then observed that it calmed down aggressive and often drunken men at the US Naval Correction Center in Seattle. Its effects ('sort of tranquillising – it saps your energy,' said one prisoner) wear off after a while, though, and people exposed to it for too long become even more aggressive than they were in the first place – so think twice about painting a bedroom this colour.

438. Eco-friendly Paints

Cheap or even 'ordinary' petrochemical-based decorating paints have been linked with a wide range of potential health issues, including allergy, breathing problems, skin and eye reactions, headaches and general fatigue. But eco-pure paints that are both petrochemical-free *and* have a decent range of colours that actually look nice on the walls (ideologically sound paints often come out a bit dull) are not easy to come by.

However, the Auro range appears to be both. Voted 'Best Buy' by *Ethical Consumer* magazine, their undercoats, emulsions, silk finishes and glosses are all water-based, and the colours are made from natural plant and mineral pigments. Auro's wood products are good too (as the coating for their varnishes is porous so they don't blister or flake). They have stockists countrywide and will export to Europe and the US (tester pots, 30 ml, £2; emulsion to cover 19 m², approximately £20).

Try also Ecos Organic Paints. They have a range of 108 colours and were voted 'Best Buy' by *Which?*.

For all contact details, see under 'Shopping' in the Directory.

See also Houses and Gardens: Bedrooms page 438 and Houses and Gardens: Home Improvement on page 452.

439. Clear a Room

To keep the atmosphere of a room clear and light, place an **amethyst crystal** or a **clear quartz crystal** (it doesn't have to be big) in it to soak up any negative atmosphere (e.g. after a row or an illness) and next to it place a fresh flower in a vase.

Plants

440. Repotting Trauma Tip

This can shock and upset plants and it may take the more delicate ones a while to recover. Minimise repotting trauma by adding some drops of **Walnut** essence to their water for the first few days (around four to five to an ordinary domestic watering can, seven to eight to a big 'garden' can). They perk up far faster and more often than not adapt right away without any sign of distress or droop.

You can buy **Walnut** from Healing Herbs (10 ml, £3.20). Also, homeopathic products company Nelsons' version of Bach's Walnut is sold by most big chemist branches, such as Boots, and the majority of health stores. For contact details, see under 'Shopping' in the Directory.

441. Super-Size Your Seedlings

Healing energy can be used most effectively to enhance seedling growth and ensure the resulting plants have additional protection against pests and fungi. There is a good deal of research to show this 'hands-on, chemicals-off' approach to gardening and farming works.[1] With a bit of practice and preparation, you could supercharge your seedlings with a little universal energy too, and this practice is growing among biodynamic farmers and esoterically aware gardeners.

Lettuce pray

For the last three years the Psi Research Centre in Glastonbury and the Center for Indic Studies at the University of Massachusetts have been carrying out field trials on lettuce crops on organic farms in the UK and have found that after the first generation of healer-treated seedlings, the plants were more resistant to fungi, then after the second, they generated faster and grew stronger and healthier.'

How to do a little healing on your seeds

1. Sit down quietly where you won't be disturbed for a while, with the packet of seeds on your lap.
2. Breathe easily and deeply with your eyes closed – in for six, hold

for six, out for six. Imagine you are sending strong roots down from your feet into the ground.

3. Now imagine a gentle golden light growing around you in a big ball, getting stronger with each out-breath you take. Breathe in golden light, breathe out golden light. Feel it becoming denser and brighter.

4. Ask whatever spiritual source you feel comfortable with – God, the Universal Source of Love and Light, Mother Nature or perhaps the devas and angels of all plants (who help all kindly intentioned holistic gardeners) – to remove all and every bit of negativity from you, otherwise this can *contaminate the healing energy you pass to the plants.*

5. Feel that negativity – whether it's a bit of bad temper, an old feeling of resentment, worry, physical aches or pains – dissolving and lifting.

6. Next, ask that healing energy for the seeds to be sent *now* through you to them. Place your hands roughly 5–15 cm from the packet. Feel warmth building in your palms and allow this to flow to them. Another technique is to try and send them 'love and kindness' with your eyes (as with the Therapeutic Touch technique used by nurses for patients and sometimes taught to parents of sick children – see Fix 274: The Touch That Soothes).

7. Allow this to happen for perhaps three to four minutes, asking that the seeds be made strong and healthy.

8. Now ask for the energy to stop coming through you, and let it fade gently. Take your hands away and say thank you.

9. Ask that you be de-attuned (disconnected once more) from the energy source and closed down safely, so you are no longer 'open' to allow the energy to come through you. *This last point is very important or you may feel spacey and wobbly afterwards.*

10. Take a deep breath, stretch, rub your hands together, rub your feet on the floor to ground yourself, perhaps have a drink of water or a snack if you are feeling a bit dreamy and un-together – and go plant those seeds.

Healing training

This is only a very brief description of how to pass healing energy to plants. If you would like to find out more, or develop your healing skills safely and professionally not only for plants but animals and people too, contact the National Federation of Spiritual Healers, which runs good training courses and support groups countrywide.

Reiki healing is another method: the courses are far shorter – often a day can teach you the basics and a weekend can bring you an initial basic certificate – but these short courses will be much less detailed and are not usually supported by ongoing supervised practice sessions or support groups, as the NFSH's are. For reiki teaching, try the Reiki Association and, in the UK and US, try the International Association of Reiki Professionals.

For all contact details, see under 'Training Courses' in the Directory.

461. Bigger, Better Fruit and Vegetables ('*My Radishes Are in Virgo*')

What's one better than organic gardening? Going biodynamic. Produce grown by this method is larger, more colourful, nutritious and flavoursome than even equivalent organic foodstuffs: if you were ever considering entering a biggest or best marrow competition or flower show, this is the holistic secret weapon you could use to win.

Biodynamic gardening and agriculture involves organic growing methods *plus* additional measures including herbal- and quartz-based plant feeds, special wonder-manure methods and planting, pruning and picking schedules based on the phases of the moon (the sophisticated ancient Greeks and the Romans both used lunar planting to excellent effect).

Pedigree and research

Biodynamics has been around in its modern form for about 75 years. It is based on a holistic, spiritual approach to agriculture, plus the philosophy of Rudolf Steiner, the man who started the worldwide Steiner school movement. There are only a very few studies to show biodynamic food is better for you, but one that did make a media splash in 2004 was undertaken by a group of nuns in a German convent at Heiligenbrunn in the Black Forest, who found that after just four weeks of eating only biodynamic ingredients headaches disappeared, their ability to work on challenging logic-based problems improved and their energy and well-being increased.

Results

If you want to check out what biodynamic methods can do and have a branch of **Fresh & Wild** near you (there are several in the UK, including Edinburgh, Bristol and all over London), pop in and look at the biodynamic goods lined up next to the organic produce. The latter is up to a third larger than organic stuff, glowing with health and practically jumping off the shelves. It is also more expensive, but the good news is you can produce some for yourself in the smallest of urban backyards. Unfortunately, the odd how-to hint isn't much help here because this is a total system, and instigating a couple of one-off biodynamic wheezes will make little difference. However, doing even a brief weekend course *does* enable you to make the cornerstone changes to your growing methods, which will.

As well as at Fresh & Wild, ready-grown biodynamic food to try and enjoy can be bought from health shops and farmers' markets countrywide. Look for the worldwide **Demeter** label, which certifies that the product has been produced biodynamically.

Finding out more

In the UK, the Biodynamic Agricultural Association offers information and training courses: everything from a weekend for interested gardeners ('Biodynamics for the Backyard', £75 for the weekend, plus £15 B&B per night) to a three-year certification, taught at Emerson College in East Sussex. In the US, see the Biodynamic Farming and Gardening Association. There are also courses for beginners to serious biodynamicists all over the US, such as those at the Pfeiffer Center in New York. For contact details, see under 'Training Courses' in the Directory.

Recommended reading: for what to do when, see *Gardening and Planting by the Moon* by Nick Kollerstrom. *Note:* you need to get the edition for the *current* year, or the year before which also has the following year marked up in it.

443. Fertiliser-Free Growth-Enhancer

There is something that has been shown in rigorous scientific trials to double plants' growth rate, but it's neither natural manure nor chemical fertiliser. It's sound.

If you want your plants to be healthy, strong and grow twice as quickly as everyone else's, play them classical music quietly *all day*, especially if it majors in violins. Bach's Brandenburg Concertos also work really well.[2]

Plants don't respond well to just any type of music, however – rock for instance, stunts them. In fact, it usually kills them off altogether if it's left on long and loud enough. And if they do survive, they're spindlier and have grown at an awkward angle, leaning away from the source of the sound as far as they can.

Research by the head of the Botany Department at Annamalia University in India, Dr T. C. Singh, has confirmed the doubling effect of classical music on plant growth and he has also discovered why. Apparently, the sound waves generated by harmonious classical music increase motion in the plant's cells' protoplasm. What's more, the seeds taken from the musically enhanced plants produced healthier ones in the next generation too, which were larger, grew faster and had more leaves: it appeared that sound had improved their very DNA.

Some commercial greenhouses use the music effect, though not necessarily all day, to excellent effect (the famous garden centre in Lillington, Sussex, for instance). And there is no reason why this can't be done in a greenhouse – or wherever your seedlings are propagating – at home too, using a CD or tape player.

See also Houses and Gardens: Garden Pests on page 447 and Houses and Gardens: Weeds on page 486.

Ponds

444. Proactive Ponds

A healthy pond in the right place is said to bring great good luck and wealth to a home, according to feng shui principles. And seeing as you can feng-shui parks and gardens as well as indoor spaces, if you'd like to try this, why not use the bagua grid to, say, work out where the 'fortunate blessings (wealth) corner' of your garden is and enhance it with a fishpond? – see Fix 423: Bagua Your Space (No. 4).

Big isn't necessarily better here; in fact, it is important that it's in keeping, size-wise, with the scale of your garden. For lining it up with the front door (as you'd do if you were using the grid on an interior space), the garden's 'doorway', where you place the bottom of the Bagua, is usually the area where you go into it from your house.

Positive pond pointers

- Circular is good (auspicious). Pa Kua-shaped – octagonal – is *very* good.
- Keep the pond clean, tidy and clear of mud and clogging weeds. If it goes stagnant or gets bunged up, that is said to do the reverse of bringing you good fortune.
- Some of the luckiest, or most auspicious, fish are Koi carp. These can be a bit expensive though, so healthy goldfish will do fine instead.
- How many? Ensure you have nine fish in all: eight golden or orange and a black one. The latter is said to absorb any bad luck coming to you.
- If one dies, remove and replace it right away.
- Never have a fishpond on the right-hand side of your main front door (right as you look out of your doorway towards the street, that is). It may bring success or wealth, but traditional FS practitioners warn that 'The man of the house may develop a tendency to stray.'

Power Lines and Pylons

The question of whether power lines and the strong electromagnetic fields (EMFs) around them are a health hazard, and if so, how much of one, has come in for a lot of British media attention in the past decade, and some of the studies carried out on the subject are contradictory.

But although this area remains controversial in the UK and in many other countries, in the US the situation is rather different. At least ten states have limits on the levels of EMFs emitted by power lines that are permitted in people's houses – and there is plenty of litigation in progress relating to both homes and workplaces.

How much is too much?
A **tesla** is the measurement of the strength of a magnetic field. The average household has around 70 nT (nanoteslas). The level around power lines is 1,000 nT. Of those studies that found a link between health issues and raised EMFs, it seems anything over 200–300 nT presents a potential problem.

EMF-related health problems

Perhaps the most high-profile potential health risk from the strong EMFs generated by the presence of power lines and pylons too close to homes is childhood leukaemia. The studies have not all been consistent, but according to Dr Leonard Sagan of the Electric Power Research Institute in Pao Alto, California, this may be because some researchers were looking for an association between the power load from the lines and how far away these were from the children's homes, while others were checking measurements *inside* the homes.[3] However, pooled results from three strict Scandinavian pieces of research showed a doubling of this form of paediatric cancer.[4]

Other studies have suggested links with depression, ME, heart attack, cot death and suicide, as well as insomnia, recurrent miscarriage, low energy, irritability and sleeplessness. Often one or more of these may occur at once, and in health-savvy Sweden, electromagnetic sensitivity (EMS), the most common symptoms of which are mood disturbance and sleep disorders, is now an officially recognised health problem estimated to affect around 250,000 of the country's 9 million inhabitants.

What to do

If you've got a pylon or a power line near your house, the following suggestions come from Dr Roger Coghill, a UK research scientist who has spent 20 years tirelessly investigating – and agitating about – the potential health problems EMFs may cause. He is a member of the Department of Health's Mobile Telecommunications and Health Research Programme and is director of Coghill Laboratories in Wales.

1. If you've got a pylon near your home and are suffering from irritability, headaches, low energy, insomnia or if you have babies or young children living there, the best-case scenario advice is to move. People do so an average of seven times in their lives as it is. If you really need to stay there, sleep in bedrooms on the far side of the house from the pylon or power line. The field is not at its strongest right underneath the power source but spreads outwards like the ripples in a pond that's had a stone dropped in it and can be at its most troublesome some distance away from its original source (how far depends on the electrical load it is carrying). As houses are generally further than 9 metres from a pylon, the strength of the EM field has already grown a fair bit by the time it reaches the house and has started to get, from an electromagnetic point of view, stronger. It is important therefore to sleep as far away from the source as possible. There will also be more solid objects (such as furniture and walls) to absorb some of the EM fields. This bedroom suggestion applies to children especially. In fact, sleeping *downstairs* and on the far side of the house is best, as the EMF fields seem to be stronger off ground level.

2. Sleep at right angles to the power line. Its magnetic field comes out perpendicular to the line itself, and in this way you can minimise your exposure to it.

3. Avoid sleeping with any metal objects near you – e.g. next to a radiator that's on the wall or on metal bedsprings. These may amplify an EMF field.

4. Plant some fast-growing trees or shrubs like leylandiis between your house and the power line or pylon, as these can help screen out the worst of the EMF.

5. Get any suspect areas properly checked. You can get a portable device called a Gauss meter that measures the strength of magnetic fields. It is more accurate to take measurements over several days and at different times. Prices range from £70 to around £500. However, it is also possible to hire one particular type called the Enfield Pro Meter for £35 a week via Powerwatch. Powerwatch is a respected independent organisation that has been researching the role of electromagnetic fields in health and advising consumers on safety and protection strategies for the last 17 years.

6. Read and research. For information about power lines, electricity substations, mobile phones and their masts, there are many different publications available, but a sensible starter book on the subject is *EMF and Microwave Protection for You and Your Family* by Alasdair and Jean Philips of Powerwatch. You can buy it direct from Powerwatch.

For contact details, see under 'Shopping' in the Directory.

415. Crystal Protection

A good-sized chunk of **amethyst** – big enough to cover the palm of your hand – can help with EMFs too. Cleanse it first, and to empower its effect, you could also programme it to transmute all negative energy that passes through it using the powerful **Silver-Violet Flame** technique. (For how to cleanse and programme, see Appendix 1: Cleansing and Programming Crystals and Gems on page 536, and for how to do the Silver-Violet Flame, see Fix 310: Their Room – a Fetid Teenage Pit?) Then put the amethyst on the windowsill so it is between you and the pylon or power line. Cleanse and re-energise the crystal weekly for maximum effect.

If your bed is in the pathway of any EM emissions from that power line/pylon (e.g. next to the window, and you can see it from your bed when you lie down, first turn it crossways to the field (imagine this field as spreading out with the pylon or power line's base in its centre, like the ripples in a pool after something's been dropped in it). Then either move your bed as far away as possible and place the crystal next to the bedhead on the pylon's 'side' – or better still, if you possibly can, move bedrooms, preferably to the other side of the house or better still, the other side *and* downstairs (see page 481). If your sleep quality, health or general energy levels have not been good since you started to use that bedroom, it should improve considerably right away.

Ski story

A bit of crystal stopping something as powerful as a strong EMF may sound pretty unlikely. But this year our family stayed in an Austrian ski apartment in Söll right on the slopes which looked out over beautiful snowy vistas – and also, as we discovered when we arrived, something else not featured in the brochure – a great fat pylon, not 20 m away. My son's sleeping area was on a sofa-bed right by that wall, and the EM energy coming in through there was a tangible force if you held your palm up to feel it.

The first night, despite being exhausted from a much-delayed journey, he couldn't sleep properly and was haggard the following morning. Fortunately, the village had a tourist shop that sold, alongside the party-sized Suchard bars and postcards showing the resort's annual Naked Skiing Day, crystal chunks.

By turning our son's sofa-bed crosswise to the EMF field, then cleansing and programming the amethyst and putting it on the windowsill next to him, he was able to sleep more or less OK there for the week. Obviously, this is by no means conclusive, but it was certainly interesting, and a solution we'd use again in similar circumstances.

Further information

Recommended reading: *Electro-Pollution*, a very useful specialist report from *What Doctors Don't Tell You* magazine (£12.95/$15). It looks at EMFs at home and at work, power lines, mobile phones and mobile masts, VDUs, geomagnetic stress from the earth. Subscription to the magazine itself costs around £52 per year. The magazine is also available electronically. For more information, also see any of Powerwatch's excellent books, which can be bought via their website. For contact details, see under 'Shopping' in the Directory.

Stain removers

General

For holistic housework, the Low-Impact Living Initiative's downloadable fact sheets (www.lowimpact.org) offer the best free collection of *effective* natural cleaning tips that are both less likely to upset sensitive skins and noses in the family and won't wage war on the ecosystem as soon as they swirl away down the plughole.

Low-Impact Living make creative use of substances such as **white-**

wine vinegar, baking soda, essential oils, potato (a good gentle stain-remover), lemon juice and borax (which is good for carpet stains) – if you can't find any borax around, see traditional laundry suppliers Dri-Pak's website or the Green Shop.

Recommended reading: for the many housekeeping uses of good old-fashioned bicarb of soda, see Vicki Lansky's *Baking Soda: Over 500 Fabulous, Fun and Frugal Uses You Probably Never Thought Of*, if you can get your tongue round the title. It can be bought from the Growing Lifestyle website.

For all contact details, see under 'Shopping' in the Directory.

446. Red-Wine Stains

The following is an old trick from your grandmother's (or great-gran's) household in the 1930s – when they didn't have products like Vanish and biological washing powders, which our generation are now trying to avoid for a more holistic household approach. To banish red-wine stains:

1. Make up a solution of a quarter milk and three-quarters water in a saucepan.
2. Add the stained fabric.
3. Bring to the boil.
4. Simmer for three to four minutes, after which time the stain should have gone.

Note: if it's a fabric that cannot take this level of temperature, this tip's not suitable.

Televisions

Electromagnetic fields (EMFs: see page 479) are not only generated by power lines and pylons; they are also produced by electrical appliances. These may disrupt health – the extent to which they may do so depends on how strong they are, how much time you spend close to them, your age and sensitivity – women and young children can be especially reactive to them.

Research (see page 480) suggests that potential EMF-related health problems may vary from low energy levels and headaches to, at the very worst, brain tumours.

So if you like to enjoy all Sky and cable have to offer but also have an eye on your health, it's sensible to:

- sit at least 2–2.5 m from a large or widescreen TV, 1.5 m from a little one
- switch your TV off – *at the wall socket, not just using the remote handset* – when not in use. This applies especially to big plasma TVs, which use as much power as the average refrigerator.
- avoid having a TV in the bedroom – or even next door to the bedroom
- put your TV on two or three of those cheap cork flooring tiles, rough side upwards. Cork has been found to help suppress EM fields for both TVs and computers.

447. Green screening
According to the Dulwich Health Society in London, who have researched this area quite extensively, put lots of evergreen plants, like ferns or cacti, round the TV. They look good and are also thought to reduce the de-ionising effect of strong magnetic fields. The **torch cactus** (*Trichocerus spachianus*), which can grow up to 1.8 m tall and has lovely white flowers that open at night, is especially useful for this.

448. Teen TVs
Banning TVs in bedrooms may not please teenagers – over 90 per cent of British teens have sets in their bedrooms – but perhaps try and instigate a teen den to have their TV in, such as a converted garage, cellar or part of a big downstairs laundry or rumpus room.

Shed chic
Or how about a fully insulated garden shed 'office' or small summer-house for a teenager to watch television in? There is room for one of these small sheds even in the standard 9 m inner-urban backyard. You can get 2.5 m² ones with full insulation, carpeting and electricity from

around £2,700. The teen-shed option may sound expensive, but parents say it is well worth the investment as its benefits are many and long-term.

It not only means your child is not sleeping in the same room as a television, it also gives the growing-up children their own much-needed territory and allows you to reclaim some of *your* living space. As a result, the home is likelier to be harmonious than if it's permanently a-simmer with teenage hormones crashing into (menopausal) parental boundaries.

Washing

449. Give Laundry a Lift
Instead of using environment-bashing, skin-irritation-causing, chlorine-based bleaches in a whites wash, lift whites the DIY eco-friendly way: just put half a cup of **washing soda** in the first wash cycle, then tip in half a cup of pure **lemon juice** during the rinse cycle – this has a gentle bleaching effect, as any blonde will tell you. Then, if you can, hang the washing outside in sunlight – it dries to an improved shade of white and smells lovely.

You can usually buy washing soda in the laundry-products aisle of your local supermarket, but if you can't find it, try Dri-Pak (3.5 kg, £12). For contact details, see under 'Shopping' in the Directory. Peroxide is also available in bottles in any supermarket.

See also Fix 412: Loo Rings and Fix 436: Tile-Shine.

Weeds

450. Death to Dandelions
Catch them young and deal with them the pesticide-free way with the **vampire method** – i.e. run a knitting needle into their centre, then shake salt into the hole you just made. If you've got rabbits or guinea pigs, remove the leaves first – they regard these as a major gourmet treat.

Holistic Weed Discouragement Tricks

Natural tips on everything from dealing with whitefly using homemade eucalyptus-oil spray to deterring garden pests the pretty way (i.e. putting flowering plants they can't stand round greenery you want to protect), plus creating beautiful drought-resistant and ultimate low-maintenance urban gardens, can be found in the inspirational, full-colour *Creative Sustainable Gardening* by Diana Anthony.

Work and Office

Want to know how to calm down an angry colleague without saying a word, use laughter therapy to increase your chances of promotion, feng-shui your workspace for career success or which leafy plant to put on your desk for reducing work stress and headaches? It's all in here, as are the body-language and NLP tricks that'll turn you into a networking goddess, the best fast-forward lunch for upping creative brainpower, how to deal with clinical burnout, and the exercises that'll protect your eyes from computer damage. Who says you can't get holistic at work?

Burnout

Burnout is the millennial scourge of anyone who loves their work (or even those who don't but are trapped with no alternative – see page 53, Stuck or Stymied and New Jobs on page 524). Though it's been given many clinical definitions, in a nutshell burnout's when you've come to the end of your physical, emotional and spiritual resources and there's just no more left for the moment.

In 2006 a survey of over a thousand workers and management members for the British human-resources consultancy Hudson found over half of all employees had experienced burnout symptoms in the last six months, and six out of ten workplaces had no support system whatsoever to help deal with this. 'Burnout is almost entirely a recent, Westernised, middle-class, professional, post-industrial and post-war phenomenon,' says Stephen Wright, associate professor at the Faculty of Health and Social Care at St Martin's College and chairman of the Sacred Space Foundation.

Are You Burnt Out?

Burnout's not the same as nervous breakdown, but it can lead to it if you don't heed the warning signs. It's not quite the same as stress either, though it's caused by prolonged work (or carer) pressure. You may be burnt out if you:

- can't stop your mind racing at night and find it hard to get to sleep
- wake up tired, regardless of how long you've been in bed
- feel dissatisfied with your life, no matter how good it may look to an outsider
- are no longer satisfied by what used to be absorbing work
- want each day to be over so you can go home and get some peace
- want people to leave you alone
- feel trapped, stymied and stuck at work
- make too many stupid mistakes in usually simple tasks
- are easily irritated – and others seem to be getting cross with you more often too
- feel drained
- are not that interested in sex, or emotional closeness, any more
- have difficulty finding time for friends, loved ones and interests outside work
- can't relax and switch off like you used to
- increasingly go for, as one Michigan-based work psychologist put it, 'quick crap fixes': more junk meals, more booze, more drugs, more rubbish TV, more casual sex
- can't seem to get on top of your workload
- feel a bit disconnected from those around you.

According to a recent report in *Nursing Times*, if more than three of the above apply to you, be careful. You are in imminent danger of burning out. So:

**Stop NOW,
Rest . . .
Get help.**

Medical Treatment

Tell your GP how you feel. Ask them to sign you off work for as long as you both feel is sensible. If you should get the sack, so be it. Because if you don't do something, you risk losing rather more than your job. Tell your superior at the office, having got your GP to write to them first, and try and get a return-to-work strategy worked out with them – if, that is, you want to go back. You may not.

Complementary Treatments

What helps? *Anything* that helps you step back, relax, give yourself time and prioritise what you really want from life on all levels – financially, professionally, emotionally and esoterically (if you've got that 'Is this all there is, then?' feeling, as so many people with burnout do). The range of help available is very wide: it potentially includes everyone from a really good life coach, psychologist or skilled neuro-linguistic programming (NLP) practitioner (some therapists offer all three) to an experienced shaman or an inspirational meditation teacher.

Actual natural 'treatments'might range from laughter therapy (see Fix 480), tai chi, using nutrition/essences/herbal remedies to strengthen, de-stress and calm, to investigating esoteric philosophy, or taking a new look at western religion (as offered by the Alpha courses currently running all over the UK), going on a five-month overland trip to Kathmandu in a four-by-four, or perhaps just sitting looking at the sea every day for several weeks.

> If you've temporarily burned out, here are two factors that will underpin every recovery effort you make: **sound sleep, and good nutrition**. If you can get these sorted first, you'll have the mental energy to retreat, rethink and fix your life. If you can't – you won't.

451. Restoring Sleep and Relaxation

If you aren't sleeping properly and are constantly tired, it is very difficult to do anything other than doggedly carry on what you are already doing.

All sort of natural strategies from self-hypnosis (taught by a professional hypnotherapist) to aromatherapy, can help: it's a case of finding one that suits you.

Fast, deep, efficient relaxation

If you like the sound of a well-researched hospital-validated therapy that has a good clinical track record and gives rapid results, a course of **Auto-genic Training** might suit you really well. It's a very simple system of deep self-programmed relaxation that is much quicker to learn to do effectively – and seems to bring faster results – than ordinary meditation. It's taught in groups or on an individual basis in six to eight sessions.

Generally, the very first thing you notice, often after a single session, is that you start sleeping a bit better. After a couple more, people are usually sleeping soundly *all night* and not waking up at 4 a.m. with their brains in overdrive. To find a trained therapist who can teach you the method, try the British Autogenic Society or the British Association for Autogenic Training and Therapy. For contact details, see under 'Training Courses' in the Directory.

Medication from your doctor can help you sleep, but unfortunately it may also leave you a bit disorientated and dopey for a couple of hours after you wake and not feeling that refreshed either. Something that is natural, yet can be strong enough to work, doesn't give the hangover effect and starts working right away is **Magnolia Rhodiola Complex** by LifeTime, available via Victoria Health (60 capsules, £19.95). It also contains the excellent de-stressing herbal combination **Relora**, plus **L-theanine**, an amino acid that promotes muscular relaxation, which is very helpful if long-term stress has left you with permanently stiff muscles round the neck, shoulders, back and scalp (leading to headaches that always seem to be hanging around, even when you wake in the morning).

Take two to three capsules with food or on an empty stomach an hour before bed at night and – very important – give it a chance to get going by spending the *last half-hour before bedtime* relaxing in a warm bath, not in front of the TV or computer or being talked at by anyone.

If this doesn't work, it may be best to see your GP after all for a short course of medication – you really need that sleep.

If that doesn't help within a week or so, top UK nutritionist, osteopath and applied kinesiology practitioner John Taberman-Pichler says, 'If you can't *get* to sleep, it's often the adrenals. And someone who manages to go to sleep but wakes up a few hours later and can't get back to sleep – that's the adrenals again. The person's had a bit of a rest but because they're always stressed they release adrenaline ready for the *next* stress. And it's that adrenaline which keeps waking you up so early. Try taking vitamins B5 and timed-release C (see page 37) for adrenal support.

'I would also suggest feeding the pineal gland [which controls sleep]. The product to go for is **Pineal Support Formula** from Metabolics [250 ml, £14.50]. Take 20 drops an hour before you go to bed. You may also need another ten drops with breakfast, but see how it goes. Too little or too much of this will disrupt sleep even more, but the right amount can be just the job. Also, look to the usual culprits: i.e. don't eat late or let yourself become dehydrated, nix the caffeine or other stimulants, turn off the TV an hour before bed, have a warm bath then lie under your duvet and read or listen to a tape, or something reassuring like the BBC World Service on low so your mind is relaxed . . .'

For all contact details, see under 'Shopping' in the Directory.

See also General: Sleep on page 92 and Work and Office: Sleep on page 529.

452. Increase Energy with Nutrition

Trying to make major life-changes without energy reserves is like trying to do the Paris-Dakar run without petrol.

Better-quality sleep (see above) will help tremendously. However, you will probably need an energy boost as well. If you possibly can, making a visit to a good professional nutritionist could really pay off. Because stress depletes not only the adrenal glands – which can end up feeling like a pair of squeezed satsumas and will need support to recover in the form of the relevant good-quality supplements – but it also drains many vital nutrients from your entire body, such as vitamin C.

A good nutritionist should ideally send off a blood or sweat sample from you to a reputable biochemical assay laboratory: in the UK, Biolab in London is one of the very best. If it's not Biolab, ask your practitioner exactly where your samples will be sent for assessment, and about the firm's pedigree. Those test results can be invaluable as they will tell your practitioner precisely which nutrients you are short of and to what extent, enabling them to customise the perfect rescue programme for you. To find a professional nutritionist, try the British Dietetic Association, the Institute of Optimum Nutrition or the British Society for Ecological Medicine who can supply a list of members for the area where you live. For contact details, see under 'Nutritionists' in the 'Therapies and Therapists' section of the Directory.

It can be very helpful if your nutritionist is also an experienced applied kinesiology practitioner. AK can be used, often most effectively depending on the skill of the therapist, to find out precisely what you are short of and exactly how much of it you'll need using on-the-spot muscle-resistance testing. The system can also be used to see whether you have any food intolerances, heavy-metal loads or subclinical infections affecting digestion and nutrient absorption (candida is a common one in those who are very tired, long-term stressed or run down) and be able to suggest appropriate treatment. For AK practitioners in both the UK and the US, try the International College of Applied Kinesiology. For contact details, see in the 'A' section of' Therapies and Therapists' in the Directory.

John Taberman-Pichler suggests the following for men in particular suffering from burnout, since it is the result of long-term chronic stress. All these would also help women, apart from the saw palmetto.

- **Co-enzyme Q** will help the energy powerhouses in each individual cell (the mitochondria) release the maximum amount of energy from the food you eat. You should feel more energetic within a week or two of taking these tablets daily. Often given to recovering ME patients for this very reason. Holland & Barrett do an inexpensive product, Co-Enzyme Q10 High Strength (90 x 10 mg capsules, £6).

- **Vitamin B5** supports the (by now exhausted) adrenal glands. A good source is Quercetin B5 Complex via independent health shops like the Infinity Foods chain in the UK, or a good budget website source is Health Emporium (30 capsules, £6.10).
- **Chromium** will stabilise your blood sugar and help to hold your energy levels steady after you eat. Take up to 200 units twice daily. Try Ultrachrome 200 from Metabolics (60 tablets, £6.02).
- **Vitamin C** is very useful for stress. As it is fast-acting but short-lived, it's best to take a time-release or buffered product at intervals throughout the day. Take 500 mg three times daily or 750mg twice daily. See also Fix 483: Performance Anticipation Stress.
- **Linseed oil** is rich in essential omega-3, -6 and -9 fatty acids, which the brain needs for good cognition and repair. This is also often given to recovering ME patients with good results. Try the top-quality and good-value organic High Barn Oils (100 capsules, £13.50).
- **Saw palmetto** helps stabilise testosterone output, which can go haywire during sustained periods of chronic stress; since testosterone is also a feel-good hormone, this can help your mood to stabilise too if the burnout's been making you feel depressed and unhappy. Take approximately 200 mg once or twice daily. Try Higher Nature's Saw Palmetto and Pygeum Bark Capsules (60 x 120 mg capsules, £14.90).

For all contact details, see under 'Shopping' in the Directory.

453. Retreat and Rethink

Retreats are places where you can have peace, quiet (usually in the countryside, but there are some in major cities), generally with some relaxation techniques, meditation and – only if required and requested – some first-aid spiritual support.

They are excellent places for anyone with burnout to go for a few days, a few weeks or whatever they feel is best – somewhere to stop the world and breathe easier while you take stock. From converted farmhouses to castles, hotels to country houses, monasteries and nunneries to spas, they operate all over the world.

Check out *The Good Retreat Guide* by Stafford Whiteaker, which looks at those in the UK, Ireland, France and Greece, or try www.retreats.org.uk. Or, as this site is informative but can be a bit erratic, see www.retreatsonline.com.

See also General: Stress and Strain on page 95 and Work and Office: Stress on page 530.

Colleagues

454. Bullying

We all hoped that we'd have left bullying behind when we quit school, but this doesn't necessarily happen. Because where have many of them now gone? To work, that's where. Just like us.

Childline figures suggest 80 per cent of children are bullied at school at some point, but TUC survey figures suggest that half the work population is also bullied at some stage, either subtly (e.g. repeated nit-picking, criticisms of work or constant snide jokes at your expense) or overtly (shouting, upbraiding or belittling you in front of colleagues).

You may now be far better able to handle bullies than when you were at school, but it can still make life anything from more difficult than necessary to sheer hell.

Action

1. Log on to www.bullyonline.org for advice and support.
2. Tell your senior manager what's going on.
3. Furnish them in writing with instances, dates, any witnesses and relevant emails.

If the problem *is* your manager – and TUC figures show half of all those bullying workers are their line managers or immediate superiors – go to your company's human resources department, if there is one. If the firm's too small to have one of these, go right to the top (MD or CEO). As at school, workplace bullies rely on their target's ability to sit there and take it. So, like they say in the US, 'grass their a*s'. They're the ones with the problem, not you.

Companies are getting tougher on workplace bullies. Apart from anything else, they are well aware that if someone's being got at, it cuts down their productivity by more than 50 per cent so it is very much in their corporate interests to tackle it.

Essence power

Essences can be powerful emotional tools and effective catalysts for positive change. They are not going to turn a painfully shy person into Ruby Wax, but they will subtly help you find the resources to deal with your situation effectively and enable you to access your reserves of courage and implacability.

Great essences for beating the bullies – at any age – include:

- **Lion** – its maker, spiritual psychologist, abuse-survival counsellor and ex-wilderness guide Daniel Mapel, says, 'This is for those who are fearful and who wish to become fearless.' Go roar! It is made by Wild Earth Animal Essences and is available in the UK from IFER (30 ml, approximately £6.99) and from Healthlines (£8.95); in the US, it can be bought direct ($8.99).
- **Inner Fire** – this is an especially good essence for women. It's the one you use when you need to say, in such a way as to be heard and respected, 'Enough. The line in the sand is *there*.' Great focus remedy for when you need help *now*. Do not take it for more than five days at a time, however: you may find you get a bit strident. You can buy it direct from the maker, Light Heart Essences (10 ml, £5.15).

For all contact details, see under 'Shopping' in the Directory.

455. Angry or Upset Colleague

Stay calm, let them talk themselves out without interruption – all the while seeing in your mind's eye a soothing pale-green light around them.

Pale green has a significant psychological impact: it is the shade used by colour therapists to both soothe fury and alleviate emotional distress (though long term, such as living in a room painted all green, it can be a depressant). And as any meditation teacher, healer or colour therapist can tell you, it can actually be as effective to strongly imagine a colour as it is to physically see it.

Interestingly, when London's Blackfriars Bridge was painted pale green, the number of people jumping off it to commit suicide reduced by 34 per cent.

456. Tiring Colleagues

Do you find that one or two particular work colleagues – or, if you are in the front line and deal with the public in person, many people – leave you feeling drained after they've been talking to you? If so, you need to strengthen your emotional and spiritual boundaries so they can't tire you out.

There are many ways to do this, including meditation, visualisation, prayer or invocation. But a quick (and in the case of the spray below, instant if temporary) way is to use certain protective essences. They may be gentle, but they can be remarkably powerful.

Boundary-strengthening strategies

- the excellent **Guardian gem,** environment and plant essence combination
- the highly effective DIY mix of **Fringed Violet** and **Angelsword bush flower essences**
- the **Bulletproof Screen mind trick** (see Fix 79: Back *Off!*): instant, and it works.

Guardian can be bought from Healthlines (spray, 60 ml, £11.95; stock bottle, 7.5 ml, £7.95); in the US and Canada, buy it direct from Alaskan Essences (spray, 2 fl oz, $11; stock bottle, ¼ fl oz, $7.45). Fringed Violet, made by Australian Bush Flower Essences, is available direct or via Healthlines in the UK (15 ml, £8.95). Angelsword is from the same range and can also be purchased from Healthlines (15 ml, £8.95). For contact details, see under 'Shopping' in the Directory.

Using protective essences to maximum effect

- **Need help now situations** : maybe you've got a meeting coming up with someone who habitually stresses or tires you, or a situation that you know always leaves you feeling washed out? Spray **Guardian** around your head and body before going into battle, preferably in a swift, light, clockwise spiral, working from your feet to just above your head in one continuous movement.
- **Daily stuff**: if you have to sit near someone you don't much like, spray that Guardian around your workstation and desk too first thing each morning. If anyone asks, just tell them it's natural air-freshener: it does smell a bit like one, only far more subtle.
- **Building up your own natural defences** so people can't tire you out (either by taking some of your energy – or even dumping some of their own negativity on *you*) so easily. Essences can work a treat, but in order to do this, they need to be taken more long term as opposed to on a 'need help now' basis. A mix of **Angelsword** and **Fringed Violet** is a terrific combination for this. The *Angelsword* helps protect against taking on other people's dross – it's also great for getting rid of any that you might have collected during the day. And the *Fringed Violet* strengthens the natural energy field everyone has around their body, which usually acts, amongst other things, like a sort of esoteric immune system keeping anything that might literally 'bug' you at bay.

   Take 7 drops of the Angel and Violet mix under your tongue on rising and going to bed for 4-6 weeks and see how you go. People usually notice improvements, i.e. that they are feeling less vulnerable, less tired, or that situations which might usually stress or tire them do not seem to have such an effect any more, after 10-14 days.
- You can also take Guardian internally to build up your own natural protection if you don't want to buy any other essences: see below.

Making up a treatment bottle and taking it: **The Amazing Violet Angel Cocktail**
   Take a clean 30ml dropper bottle (available from Healthlines and other essence retailers), fill it two thirds with natural still spring water,

add 7 drops of Angelsword, then 7 drops of Fringed Violet, top up the last third of the bottle with brandy as a preservative and shake gently. Take 7 drops under your tongue morning and evening.

Shopping note: both the above are from the Australian Bush Flower Essences range: they cost £8.95 each, but Healthlines can also make up customised bottle for you for around £7 which saves you buying the two straight off.

Your Personal Guardian in a bottle

Making up your own treatment bottle of Guardian is easy too. Get a clean 30 ml dropper bottle (chemists sometimes sell them, or you can get them from IFER and Healthlines by mail order for around £1 each). Fill it three-quarters full with pure spring water, add two drops from the Guardian stock bottle, then top up the last quarter with brandy, cognac or, if allergic to alcohol, cider vinegar as a preservative, shake gently to mix and that's it.

Remembering to take it: it helps to do so at specific times – e.g. when cleaning your teeth on a morning and evening and with your lunch and dinner.

Help!

If you feel bad after being with a particular person at work (perhaps you have had an argument, they tried to put you down, patronise, bully or shout at you, or maybe it just feels like they've drained much of your energy), this one's a very powerful 'get rid of the dross – and any continued connection to the person – immediately' trick. And it takes only seconds.

1. Put seven to ten drops of Angelsword on to the palms of your hands and rub them together.
2. Run them lightly over your head, then in two strong, slow, decisive movements down the centre of your body (front and back) as far as your lower back.
3. Now briskly shake your hands away from yourself – as if shaking water off them and saying firmly in your mind, 'Off!'.

Many professional healers do this after they have been with a particularly troubled or negative client, for it works a treat.

Concentration and Performance

457. Endurance Push
If you need an energy boost to stay up and finish an important presentation (or you want to boost your sports performance or sexual stamina) and it's immediate results you need, try taking **rhodiola extract** an hour before expending your energies and you are likely to be able to keep going for longer without getting tired.[1]

Research begun by Soviet-era scientists, then taken up worldwide, has found rhodiola improves work performance, stabilises mood and reduces both the irritability and tiredness that come after prolonged mental effort. One study involved doctors working regular punishing on-call night shifts and rhodiola helped them keep going for longer; it has also been found to improve students' results in exams. However, because this herb is an adaptogen, save it for special occasions – if taken all the time, it seems to stop working after a month or so.

Rhodiola is packaged by many different companies: try Herbal Actives, made by Nature's Plus, available from First Vitality (60 tablets, £17.55). For contact details, see under 'Shopping' in the Directory.

Note: it has more stimulating effect at *lower* doses and a sedating help-you-relax effect at higher ones.

458. Focus and Energy
Aromatherapy can be a great performance-enhancer. If you need to give yourself a boost of energy, or to really focus *now* on your work, **lemongrass** works fast. And if you're on the go or at work, having it in instant, no fuss, use-anywhere format is ideal, so try a **Naturopatch** – aromatherapy in skin-patch form. You wear the patches on your skin under your clothes on the front of your shoulder for up to 24 hours, and they're a highly effective way of delivering a substance into the body, as HRT patches and pain-relieving medication 'plasters' have shown.

You can buy Naturopatch in the UK from Victoria Health (10 patches, £7.99); in the US and Canada, you can buy them direct from Naturopatch of Vermont (10 patches, $15). The company also makes arnica patches for sore muscles and sports strains, eucalyptus, peppermint and camphor patches for coughs and colds (wear on upper chest area) and several others. For contact details, see under 'Shopping' in the Directory.

Note: take the lemongrass patch off when you go home unless you want to keep on buzzing (perhaps you're off out for the evening) or you may have trouble getting to sleep

Test run

Aromatherapy oils may be gentle, but occasionally some people find that certain ones disagree with them. So to be on the safe side, it's important to check your compatibility if you haven't tried a particular one before. So snip off a small square of patch and put it on the crease of your elbow – check after eight hours to ensure no redness or irritation has developed. Do not use on broken or irritated skin.

459. Get More Done

If you want to get more work done – go home. Or rather, if you can possibly swing it, have at least a day a week working from home to concentrate on the difficult stuff.

Workplace psychology studies find that it takes up to 15 minutes to regain a state of deep concentration after a distraction e.g. answering the phone, replying even very briefly to an email or responding to someone coming up to your desk and talking to you.[2] A dozen of those in your working day can lose you three hours.

If your boss won't let you have a work day a week off-site, the following can all help preserve precious concentration:

- putting in earplugs
- having a large sign on your desk when trying to get something done that reads, *'If it's not life or death, GO AWAY. Finishing urgent job.'*
- making set times of day to open up emails, and sticking to them (e.g. 9.30 a.m., 12.30 p.m., 4 p.m., then maybe just before you leave the office). Otherwise you are continually side-tracked by jokes and chat flying to and fro on everyone's screens, and by demands and queries pouring in from outside. (Many people get more than a hundred emails a day that they actually need to reply to and that's not counting the incoming junk, or cheery soundbytes from friends.)

460. Concentration: dropping

When your concentration starts dropping at work, restore it by drinking a glass of water. And if you have a day of continuous concentration ahead, sip cool water throughout. Research in Liverpool's Merseyside showed that both mental focus levels and exam results improve just with this simple measure – possibly because the brain is 90 per cent water, and water is essential for efficient neurological transmission. For more information, see Fix 280: School Test Results.

461. Mid-Afternoon Slump

Next time you feel it coming, instead of heading for the coffee machine, get your head down on that desk and take a speed-nap.

Cornell University psychologist James Maas advocates a regular shut-eye mini-break of 20 minutes every afternoon. While those who wish to be seen as super-achievers will be plodding on at their desks without pause, the *real* achievers (you know them: the ones that can still think clearly and creatively at 5.30 p.m.) will be taking a refreshing pause before powering ahead.

'Sometimes those 20 minutes give you the energy to carry on for many more hours, rather than faking lucidity for the rest of the day.' *Frank Legis, US business analyst*

Others, including Harvard University, have also researched the power-nap phenomenon, and arguments over whether it should be 60–90 minutes or just ten are still going. The bottom line, however, is, who's got time for an hour and a half's sleep at work? But we've all got time for 10–20 minutes, a mini-chunk of downtime whose benefits are confirmed by several studies, including one with Japanese workers in 1999.

So speed-naps may be going in and out of fashion with bosses, but if it works for you, do it. Even if it's in a loo cubicle or parked car. As Darrell Drobnich of the Sleep Institute says, 'Be productive. Take a nap.'

Professional Tips for Speed-Nap Success
- Drink a glass of fresh water first (to rehydrate the brain).
- Time your speed-nap for approximately eight hours after you woke that morning to ensure the kip doesn't interrupt the natural biorhythms of your sleep-wake cycle.
- Set your watch beeper to wake you in 15–20 minutes. That way, you won't spoil your rest by worrying about oversleeping.
- Make this part of your daily routine. It works best if you don't wait until you're exhausted to do it.

462. Working Late

It's 5 p.m., you have been looking forward to going home on time (it's been a tough day and you're tired), but suddenly you get landed with some urgent last-minute work. Terrific – you'll be stuck here for at least a couple more hours (possibly more) and you can't refuse it since this isn't the sort of job where everyone arrives at 9 a.m. and leaves at 5 p.m. every day.

Energy action

Try and stay off the sugar-laced vanilla lattes if you possibly, possibly can – they'll just pick you up for an hour, then drop you down the well of exhaustion again. Instead, drink as much pure water as you are able to face (to rehydrate your brain and help it perform better), then take some of the Brazilian rainforest stimulant herb **guarana** instead – great for short-term pushes and used by busy (tired, multi-tasking) mothers, athletes, performers and executives alike.

Try taking two – or, if you are really wasted, three. Guarana capsules are available from many chemists, most health food shops, including Holland & Barrett, or via Rio Health (20 x 500 mg vegicapsules, £6.99).

Hot shots

The liquid phials of guarana are even more effective, work quickly (within 20 minutes or so) and are invaluable to keep in your desk drawer (by Rio Health, 10 x 125 ml phials, £15.99, or from high-street Holland & Barrett outlets). And handing some out to co-workers who are in the same situation as you will win you many friends.

Partying power

Guarana can also be immensely helpful if you have to go out straight from work but are rather tired, as the effects last three to four hours. But try not to take it too often. It'll get you through, won't give you a sudden rushing high (just steady energy) and won't clash with alcohol, but it does encourage you to use energy you don't actually have, so it's really important to catch up on some rest as soon as you can.

For all contact details, see under 'Shopping' in the Directory.

Day From Hell?

463. How to Clear It

If you get home from a difficult day at work feeling drained or bad, especially if you have had to deal with someone pretty negative or exhausting, **angel power** can clear it in minutes for you. All you'll need is five minutes peace, a bottle of **Angelsword essence, a hot bath** and **a small candle** (a little nightlight or tealight is fine)

> #### Angelic help
>
> It doesn't much matter whether you really believe in these powerful benign energies or not (though it helps). Just try asking for a bit of help like you mean it and see what happens.

All you need to do is:

1. Run a bath the exact temperature you like, turn the lights off and light a candle, dedicating it to Michael, Archangel of Courage, Protection and Strength.
2. Add seven to ten drops of Angelsword to the bath. Swirl it round.
3. Get in and soak. Now, ask very firmly, either out loud or in your head:

> **Dear Archangel Michael – please can you help me?**
> **I ask you to remove all negative energies and sever all negative thought connections sent to me by others, both at their end and my own – ensuring I am totally, and utterly, free of them.**
>
> **Please also ensure that anything and everything that is of a negative nature – whether within me or upon me – is hereby removed, and transmuted to 100 per cent positive vibration by the silver violet flame of transmutation and grace . . .**
> **Please – do this – NOW.**

On the word 'now', take a deep in-breath and imagine a great, shining, silvery wave of light washing over you, taking away every single scrap of unpleasantness.

As you breathe out again, do so strongly and deeply, imagining that you are blowing it all away from you for ever.

It is important to ask that any negative energy is 'transmuted to 100 per cent positive vibration', otherwise it may let go of you all right, but could remain in the room, potentially rejoining you – or even someone else – later on.

Basic version
If you are not comfortable with the idea of talking to angels – simply do the Angelsword in the bath bit. It works pretty well on its own. Just lie back for ten minutes, eyes closed, feeling the unpleasantness of the day simply dissolve, and perhaps imagining you're bathing not in water but silver light (which adds a bit of easy visualisation to strengthen the effect)

See also Work and Office: Burnout on page 488.

Note: you buy Angelsword (one from the Australian Bush Flower Essences range) via IFER or Healthlines (15 ml, £9.95), from selected health shops, or direct. For contact details, see under 'Shopping' in the Directory.

Desks and Workstations

464. The Desktop Health-Booster
What improves concentration levels, reduces stress and cuts headaches in half just by sitting on your desk? A flashy ioniser? A pricey anti-glare computer screen? No, it's a house plant.

Not just any old house plant either. According to research by Washington State University, workers who've got a plant on their desks do not get as tired and stressed as their colleagues and it's **peace lilies** and **fine-leafed figs** that are the most effective. Oslo University also found these plants reduced the amounts of pollutants emitted by man-made materials in the office, such as paints and carpets, led to better concentration levels and even reduced headaches by 45 per cent.

465. Desk-Sitter's Shoulders
This is an effective but quick and easy stretch for those who spend a lot of time at a desk or working on a computer, says Canadian chiropractor Trevor Mains. This technique:

- stretches the anterior shoulder muscles and chest muscles. (Can you feel your chest caving inwards a bit after hours at a keyboard?)
- counteracts rounding shoulders
- improves posture: for better breathing, fewer headaches and a more comfortable back.

Do the corner stretch

1. Stand facing a corner of the office, or in an open doorway.
2. Raise your arms into the T-position, elbows at shoulder height.
3. Put one foot ahead of the other.
4. Breathe out and lean your upper body forwards, *keeping your back straight*. Feel that easing stretch in your arms and across your chest?

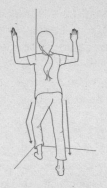

5. Keep your chest and head up, and hold for 20–30 seconds.
6. Repeat three to five times.

481. Position – where to sit for success

FS lore suggests the following for good luck in your business and career, if you work in an office:

- Never sit with your back to a door. It could encourage colleagues to 'stab you in the back'.
- Never sit with your back directly to a window or, symbolically, you will be lacking in support.
- Keep some good luck Chinese coins tied together with a red thread or tassel hanging by your desk or chair. Feng shui practitioners reckon this attracts wealth and good fortune in business and career – perhaps in the form of a promotion, wage rise, more substantial commissions or unexpected bonuses.

466. Computer Emissions

Office workers are reporting fewer health problems – notably less headaches, itchy eyes, skin problems and fatigue – if they work on flat-screen LCD monitors. This is probably because these do not emit any electromagnetic radiation, whereas the older sort give out eight types, from X-rays and ultraviolet to infrared, radio frequencies and both pulsed and static electromagnetic (EM) fields.

But have you got one, or are you stuck with some old round-bellied dinosaur of a monitor screen?

If you think you're working on an old-style one, a fast low-tech way to check if it's sending out harmful EM emissions is to put a small vase of flowers (nothing fancy – a couple of blooms in a jam jar will do) next to it and another a metre away. Watch which wilts first. If it's the one by the screen that's dead next day, call your boss, trade-union rep or human resources department and flatly insist on a modern flat screen.

Prickle power

Another tip if stuck with an old-style VDU: cactuses will mop up some of its harmful energy emissions. According to Switzerland's Institute de Recherches en Geobiologie, which has checked out the ability of many different plants to mop up radiation, a cactus called *Cereus peruvianus* comes out top.

Crystal calm

An **amethyst crystal** – from 8 cm across is big enough – placed below the screen is also said to help absorb static.

467. Keyboard Hands

Wrists and the first joint on the thumb are key areas for soreness and stiffness (actual repetitive strain injury is a different kettle of fish – see General: Repetitive Strain Injury (RSI) on page 79. However, a couple of minutes a day for a DIY hand aroma-massage helps keep inflammation and pain away.

According to former pathologist and medical aromatherapist Dr Vivian Lunny (she is also ex-head of the Aromatherapy Organisations Council's scientific research division) both **lavender** and **chamomile Roman essential oils** have painkilling and anti-inflammatory properties, so they are great ones to use. Try Baldwin's Chamomile Roman (5 ml, £7.85) and Lavender (10 ml, £4.09). For contact details, see under 'Shopping' in the Directory

For an even faster fuss-free fix, spray on some Microvita Pain Spray (also available as a cream) and rub it in to the affected areas: the stuff's so good it is used in 16 different state hospital pain clinics and units around Australia, and is becoming a favourite with sports injury clinics in Europe. (Available direct from Living Essences in Australia or in the UK via The Essence Shop; also from Victoria Health as Body Soothe cream: see 'Shopping' in Directory.

Hands-on recipe

Pour 50 ml almond or apricot-kernel oil (though ordinary kitchen sunflower will do at a pinch) into a screw-top or atomiser-spray glass bottle. Add 10–15 drops of lavender, ten of chamomile Roman and shake well to mix.

To use, drop a 10p-sized puddle of the scented oil into one palm and apply in firm, relaxing, circular motions all over your hands and wrists with the other. Then change hands. If a work colleague asks what you are doing, suggest a reciprocal end-of-day hand rub (if you like them, that is).

Email

468. Accentuate the Positive

It is possible to encourage only good things like co-operation from co-workers and contacts, positive messages, great jokes, helpful offers and good news to come to you via your email, for providing you've already got a rock-solid firewall to keep out spam, there is something very simple you can do which attracts only the good stuff.

Saying thank you

Every single time you open up your inbox – before the messages have even begun to display – take a few seconds to say a friendly, heartfelt thank you to your email system *for only ever bringing you good things*. Something along the lines of 'Thank you for always bringing me that which is positive and good – all the news that I want or need to hear, and the things that help me – and for never, ever bringing me anything negative.'

It is also good to add (if you don't feel awkward doing so), 'I send you love, and I bless you for this,' as this considerably strengthens the positive energy you are directing towards it.

Every single time you do that, you put another small charge of positivity on to your email system. Over the days, weeks and months this builds up so your email coordinates become very positively charged indeed, which acts as an increasingly powerful attractant to other good things.

Why this works

It is based on one of the major laws of the universe, Like Attracts Like, and also upon the spiritual idea that giving (genuine and enthusiastic) thanks produces more abundance. Abundance is the esoteric term for anything that enriches you in any way, whether it's generous help from a friend when you most need it, a valuable new business contact or a large cheque with your name on it arriving out of the blue.

Internationally acclaimed spiritual health teacher Louise Hay recommends the 'Thank-you method' for increasing positive traffic of phone calls (do the same to the handset and connection point) or good things to come to you via the post (thank and bless the letterbox every morning, or each time post comes through it). Since I started using it on my email, it's worked a treat: may it do the same for yours.

Note: if anything negative does arrive, barely give it the time of day. Remain calm and unimpressed, either deleting it right away or, if it needs sorting, dealing with it swiftly and without emotion before you either obliterate it entirely, or (if you need to keep a record of it) relegate it smartly to another folder, out of sight.

Eyes

469. Dry Office Eyes

Central heating, air-conditioning and computers dry out the eye's natural viscous layer. The following all help and work way better than ordinary eye drops from the local chemist – those 'eye-moisturising' ones can create smeary vision; many others that are touted as eye-fresheners just shrink the blood vessels near the eye surface to make them look whiter without actually *feeling* much better.

A recent survey of 500 UK workplaces by Leeds Metropolitan University found one in eight was 'as dry as the Saharan Desert', thanks to air-conditioning and central heating.

Smart ways to moisturise eyes

- Put a **bowl of water** on your desk, or if you are near a radiator, put two on that. It evaporates and helps humidify Death Valley-style office air. Change daily.

- Try **Tulsee Eye Drops** from Victoria Health (approximately 8 ml, £4.99). These contain 17 different Ayurvedic herbal extracts to help alleviate dry eyes and computer vision syndrome (see Fix 471: Sight Going Due to Computer Work?). Many people swear by these; however, a few find they sting their eyes a bit. If this is so for you, try . . .
- Use **White Tea Eye Gel**. Cooling and soothing, tea is often used for sore eyes (remember the old 'resting with cold teabags on them' trick? It even works with PG Tips). However, white tea seems to work especially well, probably because it has a high polyphenol content. Polyphenols are substances found in certain plants that protect against free-radical damage as well as being an ace soother of inflammation. White Tea Eye Gel is from Neal's Yard (10 ml, £18).

Some people find white-tea gel itself a bit sticky; if you do, make it up into an eyelid spray with distilled water for tired, itchy office eyes: immensely soothing and invigorating. Alternatively, you can do your own white-tea infusion: steep loose white tea leaves in freshly boiled water for ten minutes, then use the tea when it's cooled. You could try the white peony strain, which is available in the UK from the Tea House (75 g, £6).

For all contact details, see under 'Shopping' in the Directory.

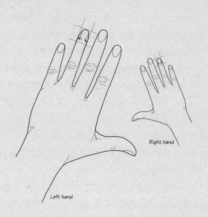

Right hand

Left hand

470. Eye Strain

Try this fast-format acupressure tip suggested by Phil Beech, a top London naturopath, osteopath, acupuncturist and senior lecturer at the British School of Osteopathy.

1. Hold up the fourth finger of either hand. Mentally draw a square grid to enclose the nailbed and nail-base (see diagram on the previous page).
2. See the point in each of the lower corners of the box you've sketched? These are important finger medial and lateral nail points in acupressure.
3. Stimulate them gently for a minute or two at a time with the nail edge of one of your fingers of your other hand to produce a painkilling effect for aching eyes.

471. Sight Going Due to Computer Work?

Around nine out of every ten people whose work involves extended and regular computer use suffer from what the American Optometrist Association calls computer vision syndrome (CVS), according to the National Institute for Occupational Safety and Health. Anti-glare screens and glasses can help, as can regular computer breaks: the rule's 20 seconds every 20 minutes, though if you're on a roll with a piece of work you're doing, this can be irritating and hard to implement.

However, if you don't want your eyesight to deteriorate because of your job, further weapons in your armoury are:

- eye exercises like the **Bates method**
- eye exercises plus eye-relaxation techniques, like the **Schneider method**
- a good **pro-eye nutrition programme** containing antioxidants, like vitamins A, C and E, with substances such as bilberry extract, which helps increase blood supply to the retina.

Schneider method

Meir Schneider, who was declared legally blind at the age of seven after five unsuccessful cataract operations, developed a system that restored his own sight. His method stresses good nutrition, yoga techniques and ways of relaxing the eyes as well as exercising the muscles that control the lens and help us to see near and far at need.

Schneider's method involves techniques such as 'sunning' (exposing closed eyes to sunshine, said to stimulate the rods and cones); 'palming' (holding palms over closed eyes and 'looking' into the velvety dark you've created); strengthening peripheral vision by trying to see with your sight obscured by increasingly large bits of paper stuck to your forehead (looks a bit daft, but devotees of the method say it works); and 'swinging' (leaning from side to side, looking at the same spot opposite by moving your head, not your eyes).

For further information, see the School for Self-Healing website (www.self-healing.org) or, if you are in the US, contact them direct. You can also try the audio CD *Meir Schneider's Miracle Eyesight Method: the Natural Way to Heal and Improve Your Vision*, available via Amazon (£15.38/$24.95).

There are a number of holistic vision therapists worldwide who are trained in his methods. For contact details, see under 'Training Courses' in the Directory.

The Bates method

The Bates exercises for better eyesight, which is where Schneider got his sunning, palming, swinging and many other techniques from, were developed in the 1920s. Though there are no clinical trials on this method, the encouraging level of anecdotal evidence to support it means these exercises are still recommended by some forward-thinking optometrists and opticians.[3]

Bates was the first to suggest that short-sight and long-sight problems were due to a weakening of the muscles that controlled the eye lens and could therefore be corrected by exercising. However, as with all exercise regimes, users need to stick to the system, practise as often as it says you have to and perhaps expect improvements rather than miracles.

To find a practitioner trained in the Bates method, see the website of the Bates Association for Vision Education (www.seeing.org), which has a worldwide directory.

Recommended reading: see *The Bates Method for Better Eyesight Without Glasses*, or Thomas R. Quackenbush's *Re-Learning to See*.

Food

472. Brain-Booster Breakfasts

If you want to arrive in the office primed for the day and firing on all cylinders, eat (a healthy) breakfast first. Studies with schoolchildren show what a difference this makes to their ability to both concentrate and problem-solve accurately – see Fix 348: Peak Performance : Mental. It does the same for adults.

For maximum effect choose:

• something with complex carbohydrates (e.g. muesli or porridge with a little honey and fruit chopped in)
  or
• something protein-rich (e.g. low-fat grilled bacon with wholemeal toast and tomato, or a boiled egg).

Snack attack

If you're someone who feels nauseous at the very thought of eating before 11 a.m. or are in a tearing hurry most mornings, just take a small banana and a good-quality health bar to work then eat them as soon as you can face them. Ensure the health bar is:

• **seed- or nut-packed** as well as containing dried fruit or cereal, so you get some protein and essential fatty acids in your breakfast – essential for brain function both in work and outside it
• **low in refined sugars**, so its effects last longer – i.e. not a processed breakfast cereal bar like a Frosties or Ricicles one. Many so-called health bars contain high levels of refined sugar. Check the labels for weasel wording like 'glucose syrup' appearing second or third on the list of ingredients. The higher up the list something is, the more of it the bar contains.

Browse Holland & Barrett or your local health store for any that catch your eye. Some good ones to try which are additive-free, low in refined sugars and *actually taste good* –an important consideration when some resolutely healthy low-sugar, additive-free bars taste like guinea-pig food – include:

• Flax 9 from the **9 Bar** range (3 for £1.79)
• Organic **Shepherd Boy** Fruit and Nut With Sunflower Seeds (approximately 35p each). You may need two: they're not that big.

- **Eat Natural** (80p each). There are several varieties, and having tried the lot, I can confirm they are all tasty, especially the Yoghurt-Coated Almond and Apricot, the Macadamia and Fruit or the Organic Fruit and Nut bars.

All of the above are available in health shops and good supermarkets.

473. Lunch Smart

Got a free 19 minutes and 42 seconds? Great! Let's do lunch . . . because that's how long the average British worker now gets, according to a 2006 survey by Post-It Notes. What's more, three-quarters of workers eat at their desks as it is. But taking a proper break at lunch to eat a light, nutritious meal boosts brain power, efficiency and concentration.

One of the smartest lunch choices is an omelette, suggest researchers at Boston University, as eggs are rich in choline, which the body uses to make the neurotransmitter acetylcholine, a good supply of which is vital for fast thought processes and deductive thinking.

Goal Achievement

474. Try Tree-Power

Formulating goals for work or your career path is one thing; making them happen can be quite another, as it is so easy to slide off track or be deflected by others.

There is, however, a powerful holistic way of helping ensure your goals turn into solid achievements, recommended by Joe H. Sale, professor of psychology at Athens State University, which he teaches to his own students. It is goal affirmation using a living tree as an anchor. Sale calls it **Tree-Power Infusion**. And before you think, 'No, no, not *tree-hugging*,' here's what it did for a group of the college's underachieving students.

The first time he tried it was with a group who had come in for a remediation programme in the summer holidays because they hadn't managed to get the grades they needed to qualify for a full college programme the following autumn. It was part of an initiative called

'Summer Start', which also involved tuition in the students' weaker subjects and counselling. At the end of it, all 30 originally underachieving students got into the college's proper four-year degree programmes, and all completed the demanding international baccalaureate degree, a third doing so with honours.

Here's how you work with a tree to ensure you reach your goals:

1. First, pick a tree you like the look of (perhaps it's especially beautiful, strong-looking, ancient or has a 'friendly' feel). Ensure it's growing somewhere you could put your hands on it for a few minutes without being stared at by passers-by.
2. Formulate your goal or goals in your head – e.g. 'I wish to redesign that accountancy computing package', 'I will devise a creative campaign by the end of this month', 'I will find a satisfying new job in my chosen area within three months' or 'I will study for and pass these professional qualification exams.'
3. With your hands resting on your chosen tree, ask it in your own words, either out loud or in your head, to be your partner in helping you achieve this goal.
4. Gently stroke the trunk. Begin to feel your connection with the tree and its response. Let that energy flow through you and out through your feet into the ground, spreading out like roots of your own.
5. With your hands still on the trunk, imagine your tree as a powerful antenna that connects you to the energy of the universe itself. Again, state your goal or goals and thank the tree for agreeing to help you achieve them.
6. Finish the exercise with an affirmation. This is the one Professor Sale teaches his students, but you can make up your own, whatever feels right for you: 'All the energies of my being are now balanced and attuned. I have limitless growth potential. And I am fully empowered, mentally, physically and spiritually, to reach my highest goals.'

Do this every day if you can; if not, as often as you can.

Interviews

What Works, What Doesn't

Most of us reckon (unless we have had special training) that it's what you say during the interview that matters and that the easy bits are 'hello' and 'goodbye'.

In fact, psychologically speaking, *the first minute and the last are the most sensitive times of all.* 'Like take-off and landing for a plane, the start and the finish of an interview can be the most dangerous times,' says body-language expert and best selling author Judi James, whose training courses for major corporates have been in high demand for the last 15 years. James recommends:

Beginning well

1. **Make a good entrance:** hold your head up, smile, come in at a smart pace but without rushing and carry any bags in your left hand so you can shake the interviewer's hand without bumbling.
2. **Sit in the chair offered,** but know you can move it a little. This still shows respect for the interviewer's territory, but a small shift in position suggests initiative and may also make you feel more comfortable.
3. **Try to limit your own movements at first,** such as hand gestures and crossing and uncrossing your legs.

Note: If you can feel your hands just longing to fidget or grasp each other anxiously, just fold them quietly on your lap for now until it's time to make a few (a few) illustrative gestures – psychologists and NLP practitioners say people take in far more of what's said if the speaker also 'talks' a bit with their hands, but they may need to get used to looking at you first.

> **Key dos and don'ts**
> ✓ Sit forward a bit in the seat to show enthusiasm and interest in what the interviewer is saying.

✓ Keep eye contact constant, but vary it so you aren't eyeballing the interviewer unblinkingly throughout.

✓ Nod a little while listening. But make sure you don't overdo it – it's easy to appear ingratiating.

✗ Never, ever interrupt the interviewer. Even by a twitch of your hand.

Ending well

The 'Do you have any final questions?' bit can be awkward. Do not shrug, or simply shake your head. Instead, breathe in then either ask the interviewer something relevant or interesting – or say nicely that they seem to have covered everything, and smile.

- Don't get up first – it looks like you can't wait to get out of there. Wait for the interviewer to stand up and mirror them by rising gracefully to your feet.
- Follow if they shepherd you out. If they don't start to actually show you out but use one of those 'You may leave now' hand gestures, or half rise, that's OK. Just thank them, then smile and go.

Hands off?

Keep a lookout for a goodbye handshake, but if it doesn't seem to be forthcoming, don't initiate one. It will look clumsy and a bit pushy, as if you're asking for more politeness or personal contact than they want to give you.

For more information, see *Body Talk at Work,* by Judi James. Details of her seminars are available on www.judijames.com

Lighting

Fluorescent lighting flickers at a rate that saps energy and promotes headaches and eye strain. It has also been implicated in behavioural problems, which office workers feel might explain a lot about certain of their colleagues . . .

However, if you know where to look, you *can* get more health-friendly, ergonomic lighting (at least over your own workstation) quickly and easily. As to getting it for the entire office – not so easy: employers will usually baulk at the idea of spending their profits changing the firm's entire lighting sytem to, say, full-spectrum units when they feel there is a 'perfectly good' (flickering, over-bright, nasty) fluorescent system in place already even if the former has been shown, which it has, to cut headaches, eyestrain and absenteeism and improve productivity.

For making your own desk a headache-and-eyestrain-free zone, try the following:

- Ask that the fluorescent light strip nearest you be turned off if your nearby co-workers agree. Explain to your GP that you are experiencing work-related headaches because of the lighting system there and feel it would be helpful to try a broad- or full-spectrum lamp on your desk and to switch off any existing office lighting directly over your head. Ask him to write a note to your employer to this effect, and also to say that if your employer will not provide this, you would need to do so yourself, since you fear your productivity as well as your health are suffering.
- Put an inexpensive natural-daylight, broad-spectrum, non-flicker lamp on your desk to illuminate your work. It mimics natural daylight, is much less stressful to use, and eyes can see print better using it. Decent products to try for broad-spectrum desk lamps in the UK include the Happy Eyes Reading Lamp from Just Natural Stuff (£49.95); in the US, try Full Spectrum Solutions' Solartech lamp ($49.98). For contact details, see under 'Shopping' in the Directory.

For more products and information, see Fix 298: Light Therapy.

Money

475. Want to Make More?

If you'd like too make more, according to esoteric law, start by giving some away.

Not to charity, or even to help a friend (though do this too whenever you feel it's best!), but scrupulously and whole-heartedly gift a tenth of your income as soon as every bit comes in, each time it comes in, to anyone or anything that has given you spiritual inspiration recently. It can be all given to one person or divided up among several, depending on who's impressed you.

Remember, spiritual doesn't have to mean 'church-style religious', but literally anything that lifts your soul. This can be an inspirational book you've read, a remarkable dance class you've been to, a healing or health worker you've heard of who's doing great stuff, an extraordinary new essence you've found that develops the intuition, a free sacred celebration you went to, a community singing session, a great meditation class or a local 'Working With Angels' day . . . anything that really did it for you.

The practice is very old and respected, and it is called **spiritual tithing**. Some report that the amount of abundance (i.e. not *just* money) coming back to them greatly increased when they began to do this; others report more modest gains, but all to whom I've spoken say it's worth it. I've been doing it too – I'm not sure whether it's a coincidence, but my book-advance payments have been rising (when the publishing-payment trend is static) and unexpected extra opportunities have been coming in, too many to take up all at once.

Many people send a letter (not signed with their full name or bearing any contact details) explaining why this money is arriving out of the blue so the recipients understand that their work is really appreciated and acknowledged by someone; others just pop a cheque in the post. Why not try it for six months and see? You'll be spreading joy and appreciation among your tithe-recipients – they may not usually get much and you could get back more than you ever hoped for yourself.

476. Prosperity Enhancement

If you'd like to earn more money, the compact oriental **coin ball**, traditionally used for prosperity enhancement in China for many hundreds of years, is very practical for using in an office. It's constructed as a square (representing the earth) inside a sphere (which represents the heavens) and the threads that bind it and its hanging tassels are red, the most auspicious (lucky) colour in Chinese lore. Widely available from Chinese supermarkets and artefact shops, Chinatown areas of the city or via the School of Natural Health and Wellbeing website (£5.99).

The best places to hang it are by your phone point or computer. Or, for greater precision, use the bagua grid to determine the 'fortunate blessings (wealth) corner' of your workspace (and, yes, it is possible to feng-shui a desk: the area size is unimportant) – you take the front door as the direction from which you approach your desk to sit down. For how to do this, see Fix 423: Bagua Your Space (No. 4).

For a useful little hardback pocket-sized book on the basics of attracting wealth using traditional FS techniques, see *Feng Shui for Wealth* by international FS master Lillian Too, available from the School of Natural Health and Wellbeing website or via Lillian Too's website.

For all contact details, see under 'Shopping' in the Directory.

Networking

477. Beat the Fear: Become a Networking God(dess)

Want to overcome shyness and get seriously good at networking? Use a mixture of:

- emotional-intelligence manoeuvres
- NLP techniques
- body-language tips.

Carole Stone, the networking queen, holds salons half of London wants to be invited to, has the ear of Downing Street, 24,000 names in her address book and quite literally seems to know everybody worth knowing. Part of her secret is that she deeply interested in other people and seems genuinely – visibly – delighted every time she makes a new contact. The other part is focus and good organisation. The following advice comes from both Stone and top body-language expert Judi James, taken from their excellent seminar on professional networking for the Guild of Health Writers in 2005.

Preparing, walking in and entering conversations

Follow all the advice given in Fix 78: *Parties – How To Walk in and Be Accepted Immediately*, as this really does the business. Crucially for professional networking though – remember to do your homework by getting some background information on the event's organisers, hosts and speakers. You'll be able to slip the odd nice bit in if you are talking to a relevant person, without seeming to overdo it – 'You're XS Theatre Management's PR? Didn't your company sponsor that comedy marathon for Children in Need this year?' This makes you look both informed and positive – very desirable qualities in a new contact.

Joining a new group effortlessly

Pick one you sort of like the look of – any one. Go up to them, wait, and listen to whoever's talking, and look interested. When you've worked out who the dominant speaker is here, pick up on the next thing *they* say and take it further: 'You mentioned you'd had Boris Johnson as an after-dinner speaker at your last company conference. Did you catch him taking on Paul Merton in *Have I Got News For You?* last night?' Before you know it, you are one of the gang and chatting away nineteen to the dozen.

If, by any small chance, it doesn't work out (perhaps they prove to be boring, or are bitching about the rest of the room?) smile briefly, say 'Excuse me' quietly and slide away. Then try another group.

Overcoming panic

If you have just arrived and are hovering on the edge of the room thinking, 'Oh my God: they all look like they know each other, they'll never want to meet *me*,' don't panic. They *will* want to meet you. In fact, they are going to love you. And you needn't take my word for it: because you are about to find this out for yourself if you follow Stone's advice (which, like all good things that really work, is simplicity itself) right now, immediately. She suggests doing two things. Just two:

1. Setting yourself a goal. (It can be a small one.)
2. Giving yourself a time limit. (It needn't be very long.)

The goal can be something like 'I will talk to three people *now* and find just *one* contact who may be of help in the future.'

The time limit can be short: 'I'm only staying for the next 20 minutes.'

Tell yourself that after doing both, you are free to go.

Stone's suggestions work. Why? Because psychologically, the idea of only having to do a little bit and then being off the hook takes away the stress. Then you will usually find you end up staying far longer because by the time you've taken the plunge with those three new people, you're in the swing of it and well away talking to several more, some of whom will indeed prove useful contacts.

And if you don't want to stay on, you can at least leave knowing that you have achieved your goals and feeling proud that you didn't take the easy way out (going home right away). This in itself builds up confidence for the next time.

Follow up

- **Follow up arrangements,** offers of possible future cooperation, work or invitations to other events by email within 24 hours (no later). If it's work, you may want to send a short CV 'just as background, in case you might like to have it on file', but send it as an attachment, not in the main email. This shows you are both professional and reliable but not pushy.
- **Pass on contacts** that will help other people ('Good to meet you yesterday. That training organisation I mentioned? The number is . . .'). This builds you a reputation for having useful contacts and remembering relevant details.
- **Compliment people** on good work, if appropriate ('I enjoyed your book on X. It was really well researched'), particularly if they are high-profile. If you think they made an interesting speech or presentation, this is your chance to tell them you liked it. Everyone is pleased to be complimented on their work, as positive feedback never palls.

- **Put forward your views** on a bit that rang a bell with you ('I think you made a really interesting point about Y, by the way, but what about such and such . . . ?') and see if they take you up on it. Do this by email if they are very eminent and you feel a bit shy of saying, 'Great speech,' face to face (the Net has totally democratised communication) or if they're in the middle of being inundated with congratulations from others and you fear yours may get lost in the social scrum.

Read up
Recommended reading: *Networking: the Art of Making More Friends* by Carole Stone, *Nonstop Networking: How to Improve Your Life, Luck and Career* by Andrea R. Nierenberg and *Bodytalk at Work* by Judi James.

New Jobs

478. How to Be Ethical Yet Properly Paid

> 'Choose a job that you love – and you will never have to work a day in your life.' *Confucius*

Stuck working for a global polluter when you have the heart of an eco-warrior? Sick of greedy corporates when you long to be an ethical entrepreneur? If your spirit and emotions are not aligned with your work, this is one of the prime causes of chronic, hard-to-treat health problems, including anxiety, fatigue, depression and burnout. You need a new job.

Options
You've got lots of ethical job options so long as you don't want a fairly glamorous career and decent money: absolutely anything from setting up an organic vegetable-delivery business or health food shop to working for a local-government sustainable-transport campaign. But what if you're an ambitious medium- to high-flyer who wants to stay in the better-paid finance side of things rather than work in the charitable or grass-roots sectors – could you settle for (often much) lower wages?

If not, the following tips from the inside track come from team-leader Emma Hunt who works for Mercer, one of the UK's top ethical investment consultancies. She has advised everyone from the United Nations to the Carbon Trust and offers the following suggestions for ethical-finance career-hunters. This information is invaluable because you are unlikely to find these hip, increasingly sought-after and satisfying jobs via recruitment agencies.

Where to find them

Reading up? Check out the following magazines (and their job ads).

- *Ethical Performance* (good-quality jobs for middle managers) – www.ethicalperformance.com/recruitment
- *Ethical Consumer* – www.ethicalconsumer.org
- *Green Futures* – www.greenfutures.org.uk
- the *Guardian* – www.jobs.guardian.co.uk/browse/environment

Hot Networking Tip

'CSR' stands for ethical buzz-phrase 'corporate social responsibility'. CSR Chicks (www.groups.yahoo.com/group/csr-chicks) is a well-established email network for CSR news, views and, especially, job opportunities. Emma Hunt calls this one a 'fabulous phenomenon. It started in London and now has international coverage and is really a great source of jobs to plug into.'

Note: there is also a CSR Blokes site (www.finance.groups. yahoo.com/group/csrblokes), though this is not as extensive as Chicks. However, men are welcome on Chicks.

'Hard-core' companies that operate to strong CSR principles include:

- Co-Operative Insurance Services (CIS)
- the Co-Operative Bank
- Novo Nordisk – a Danish pharmaceuticals company
- Unilever

- Interface Corporation – an international carpet manufacturer, which may not sound exciting, but it has been a renowned trailblazer worldwide
- Nike.

Nike? Nike of the child-labour scandals back in the 1990s? 'It's a spectacular company to look at now,' says Hunt. 'It has started to completely transform the way it does business and is now seen as the gold standard in ethical performance.'

479. Starting a New Job

There's reams of advice written on this one, but there are a couple of good measures no one ever mentions that are simplicity itself.

For more confidence

For three days before you start, morning and evening, take **Confid** essence – known as the *You can do it* remedy. Take seven drops under the tongue. Continue taking every day for a couple of weeks, longer if you feel you need the support. In the UK, it is available from Healthlines and Neal's Yard (30 ml, £8.50).

Also try **Lion,** by Wild Earth Animal Essences, available via IFER (30 ml, approximately £6.99) and Healthlines (£8.95); in the US, it can be bought direct ($8.99). It's courage in a bottle.

For all contact details, see under 'Shopping' in the Directory.

> **Tip**
> You can also surreptitiously take some more each time you have to do something new and possibly alarming at work, whether it's a welcome lunch with the boss or talking to your sales team for the first time.

For moving on more easily

Walnut essence can help dissolve the ties binding you to your last job (both actual place of work and the people there) if you feel them tugging on you regretfully, or catch yourself thinking, 'It was better there,' before you've given your new place a real chance. Try a Bach-style one, available via health shops, major chemist outlets or through Healing Herbs (10 ml, £3.20). Ideally, take it for a week before moving and three weeks afterwards, then see how you feel.

If it's a first job and marks going from being a student at college or school to being a paid worker with all that involves, **Bottlebrush** from the Australian Bush Flower range can be very helpful, as this is the one that eases transition between two major new phases of life and helps open the mind up to new opportunities and new ways of doing things. In the UK, contact Healthlines (15 ml, £8.95).

For all contact details, see under 'Shopping' in the Directory.

Promotion: getting it

480. Laughter Lines

If you can make your boss and subordinates laugh (with, not at you), American research shows you will be rated better at your job and have a considerably higher chance of promotion.

Laughter is a side-effect-free, proven health-enhancer that packs such a powerful feel-good factor that it's increasingly used to treat conditions as diverse as depression, anxiety, pain, chronic stress, cancer and burnout. Remember laughter-medicine pioneer Dr Patch Adams and his remarkable Gesundheit Institute (commemorated in the film *Patch Adams* with Robin Williams in the lead)?

In the UK, managers at the BBC, BT, Sony and the Body Shop have been sent on laughter workshops to good effect. Major US companies currently using humour as a management tool include Paramount Pictures, Columbia Pacific, Home Savings of America, 20th Century Fox, Universal Studios and Californian International Technology.

Hewlett-Packard awards its managers positive points if they can make their employees smile. Having found a boss with a sense of humour reduces work tension, absenteeism and boredom and improves productivity, the McGrath's restaurant chain gives its managers a 20 per cent bonus and more likely to promote them if employees rate them as funny.

If you'd like to improve your promotion prospects this way and are in the UK, have a look at Jack Milner's courses. A successful stand-up comedian himself, his corporate clients include Channel 4, Lloyds of London, CSE-Demos and the Greater London Authority. In the US, try Laughing At and Understanding Humor Seminars (LAUGHS), established by Dorothea Keely, adjunct clinical associate of the College of Nursing at Boston's Northeastern University. For contact details, see under 'Training Courses' in the Directory.

Sick Office Syndrome (SOS)

Sick Building Syndrome may be old news but it's still happening everywhere. It causes sick office syndrome, or SOS, also known as the Office Bug Cycle (OBC: *One gets it, we all get it*) whereby coughs, colds and other bugs go round office workers like a bushfire, especially in winters when the central heating's up and the windows won't open. In fact if you are really unlucky, you may be constantly either going down with something, fighting something off, or recovering (while still having to come into work every day) from November to March and your immune system will be in tatters. Sounds familiar? Read on for what helps protect you.

481. (Office) Coughs, Colds and Flu

A cold-killing combination and a half is **echinacea** and **goldenseal**, with **Citricidal** added in for good measure.

Echinacea is one of the most extensively researched herbs on the commercial market; goldenseal works so well (especially taken with echinacea, as the two seem to complement each other) that it has equal status with echinacea in the US; and Citricidal is a proven fungi- and viral-hammer.

Try Nature's Best Echinacea and Goldenseal (60 tablets, £12.95). Take one tablet daily for preventative protection throughout winter. Citricidal is available in the UK from Higher Nature (45 ml, £6.90; 100 tablets, £10.50); in the US, it is called just grapefruit-seed extract and is available from NutriTeam (2 fl oz, $6.45). For contact details, see under 'Shopping' in the Directory.

The combination of echinacea and goldenseal can be taken continuously in one daily tablet as maintenance. At the first sign of a cold or bug, go up to two or three tablets daily spaced throughout the day.

See also General: Colds and Flu on page 36; Sinusitis page 89, and Immune system booster on page 60.

Sleep

482. Work-Related Insomnia

Before you ask your GP for sleeping tablets (which, depending on the medication, can be addictive and may give you a 'hangover' the morning after), consider **Valerian and Ashwagandha Formula** from Pukka Herbs. Valerian is a useful traditional sleep-encouraging relaxant and has been used as such for many hundreds of years. Ashwagandha is a good general tonic and energy-regenerator for the exhausted. The Ayurvedic practitioner who formulated them, Sebastian Pole, says the formula helps with:

* getting to sleep
* night-waking
* inability to go back to sleep after waking
* restless leg syndrome – see also General: Restless Leg Syndrome (RLS) on page 81.

The dosage is two capsules two to three times throughout the evening during periods of stress. Or use for 6–12 months if you have chronic insomnia. Valerian and Ashwagandha Formula can be purchased from Victoria Health (90 capsules, £13.95).

See also General: Sleep on page 92 and Work and Office: Burnout on page 488.

Stress

483. Performance Anticipation Stress

If you're getting stressed – maybe you've got a major presentation or perform-ance approaching, there's a huge row with your partner coming up tonight (you just *know* it) or a house move looming – try good old **vitamin C.**

Possibly the least expensive, simplest, most widely researched and frequently used nutritional supplement in the world, it's great to take when you are up against it, either in the long term or, as it is very fast-acting, short term.

One German study put 120 volunteers through a sure-fire stressful day: making a public speech and then having to solve a lot of maths problems with insufficient time. One half were given 1 g vitamin C, the other nothing. The C group's levels of cortisol (the hormone that is produced when someone's anxious or frightened) and blood pressure were significantly lower than the group who weren't given vitamin C, and they said they felt calmer too.

Use time-release vitamin C – the majority of ordinary C taken in large quantities (i.e. above 500 mg in one go) is merely peed out. Try Nature's Best Time-Release Vitamin C (60 x 1,500 mg tablets, £7.50). For contact details, see under 'Shopping' in the Directory.

484. The Stress-Busting Breath

This one is highly recommended by the remarkable Dr Andrew Weil, 'America's favourite family doctor' and director of the ground-breaking Program in Integrative Medicine at the University of Arizona, which now teaches a fifth of all the graduate doctors in the US about integrated healthcare.

Called the **Relaxing Breath**, the method is a quick and simple yoga technique and has an immediate calming effect. If you practise it every day, it progressively reduces anxiety levels, enabling you to take office and career stresses more in your stride.

'This is the most effective – and time-efficient – relaxation method I have ever found,' says Dr Weil. Effective *and* time-efficient? What more could you ask of a workplace technique?

Here's how you do it:

1. Touch the tip of your tongue to the inner surface of your upper front teeth.
2. Still on the inner surface, slide your tongue just above your teeth now until it rests on the soft tissue between your teeth and the roof of your mouth (called the alveolar ridge). Keep it right there during this exercise.
3. Exhale fully through your mouth, making an audible 'phooosh' sound.
4. Now close your mouth and inhale quietly through your nose, counting to four in your head.
5. Hold your breath for a silent count of seven.
6. Finally, exhale audibly through your mouth for a count of eight.
7. Repeat this cycle four times, then breathe normally again.

It doesn't matter how fast or slowly you do this. It's that ratio of *four, seven and eight for inhaling, holding and exhaling* that does the trick. Practise as often as you can – once in the morning and once in the evening will help raise your calmness levels all day.

Long term, says Dr Weil, this exercise aids calm because it increases the ratio of parasympathetic to sympathetic nervous-system activity, reducing anxiety that you'd otherwise keep inside and enabling the digestive and circulatory systems to work more harmoniously, which is why it is used successfully in a clinical context to treat high blood pressure, IBS and anxiety and panic disorders.

Recommended reading: for further information, see Dr Weil's book (he is also one of the top-selling authors in the US) *8 Weeks to Optimum Health*.

Stuck or Stymied

Feeling stuck or trapped in your job, bogged down by life, frustrated with your lot, or fearing you may be becoming set in your ways but unable to summon the mental energy (or perhaps the confidence) to break free? These may all be familiar sensations to anyone who has ever had a long-term job whose attractions were wearing thin.

Springing the Trap

If you feel discontented at work but lethargic about it, or perhaps secretly fear change or what it might bring – which is entirely reasonable, human and universal – and would like a fresh perspective, now's the time to try a terrific motivation essence called, appropriately enough, **Stuck in a Rut**. Subtle but persistent, it works powerfully on an emotional level, helping you feel '*I can do this. Let's go . . .*'

Made from several of the tough but beautiful plants growing wild on the Yorkshire Moors, this can be a very good one for anyone who feels insecure about accepting their own (often very great) potential to develop, perhaps in new directions, or receiving the recognition for their work that they've not yet had. It takes on average between two to seven days for you to start feeling a difference, after which you may find that you are beginning to think along new lines and considering different options that had not previously occurred to you. However, you may need to keep taking it for between two and six weeks, depending on how long you've been 'stuck' for.

It's also a very good one to use before seeing a headhunter, a job agency, or whilst working with a good life coach or therapist to talk about how you feel and what you really want to do next with your life, for *Stuck in a Rut* helps someone to to be open to the many new possibilities and fresh options that will probably come up during their professional guidance discussions, or counselling sessions.

This essence is available from Bailey Flower Essences (10 ml, £5.15). For contact details, see under 'Shopping' in the Directory.

See also Fix 478: How to Be Ethical Yet Properly Paid, and Burnout, Fix No 488

Travel

485. Commuting

Commuting can be horrible. In fact, commuters may experience greater stress levels than a fighter pilot going into battle or a policeman facing a rioting crowd, according to research carried out in 2004 by psychologist David Lewis for Hewlett-Packard. The worst aspects were found to be:

- the cattle-truck factor
- feeling helpless and not in control of the situation (say, your train's broken down, cancelled, or delayed). Though policemen and fighter-plane aces may be in danger, at least they can get proactive about it.

The Blue-Shield Breath

According to a recent RAC survey, London workers spend, on average, three hours a day commuting. That's nearly two whole working days a week. If there's no room to work on a laptop, kick back and relax or even read, commuting is wasted time. It also uses up a lot of your energy on anxiety and the stress of coping with too many people crowding into what used to be your personal space, or worrying about delays over which you have no control but which are making you late.

However, you can make this time work for you by using it to 'rest' – or at least ensure it is less stressful – with the **Blue-Shield Breath**.

You can do it as you stand or sit, whether on a Tube, train or bus. It is very easy, and takes all of two minutes.

1. Close your eyes. If it's summer, put on sunglasses. They act as an additional barrier. Also, no one can tell you've shut your eyes.
2. Take a deep breath. As you let it out, send it down through your feet, imagining it going deep into the earth.
3. Repeat three times.
4. When you send out the next deep breath, imagine it starting to form a sapphire-blue oval round you. This blue is the shade esoteric therapists use when they want strong protection or concealment.
5. Do the same with your next breath. And the next. See that deep-blue oval barrier getting stronger and stronger. Imagine it pushing away the energies of all those around you to create a clear space around yourself.
6. When you reckon it's strong enough and you are feeling less crowded, rest in the space you have made for yourself.

7. *Reinforcement*: keep seeing the blue sphere around you, clear and strong, at intervals. Whenever you begin to feel impinged upon again, do a couple more blue-shield breaths to keep strengthening your protection.

8. When you are ready, if you need to, open your eyes again.

Note: if you have an MP3 player or an iPod, it also helps to play some calm music.

See also For Travel Rage on page 433.

486. Travel for Business: how to feel at home in a hotel

If you travel a lot as part of your job, there's a lovely way to help ensure you get a better night's sleep and feel more settled, even when you are staying in (yet another) faceless Holiday Inn a long way from home.

It's a way of taking your own bedroom with you wherever you go. The Balinese have traditionally done this for many centuries, which may explain why they have a reputation for being able to sleep anywhere perfectly happily. Here's how you do it:

1. Before you leave your home, sit on your bed and place both hands where you usually sleep.
2. Stroke the bed a little and then still them, mentally absorbing the peaceful *'Mmm, my bed'* energy up into your hands.
3. Put your hands to your heart and hold them there for a few moments. Imagine you are sending the energy you just picked up through your hands into your heart so you can take it with you.
4. Repeat three times.
5. When you get to your hotel room, do the same in reverse. Imagine you are sending the energy you brought from your own bed and carried in your heart into this bed.
6. Repeat three times.

487. Uneasy and oppressive atmospheres

When you get to the hotel, if your room doesn't have a very nice atmosphere (there may be a good reason for this, since all sorts of stuff happens in hotel rooms) and you can't change to another, this can give you a bad night's sleep – leaving you tired the next day when you need to be on the ball for back-to-back business meetings. Try the following:

1. Open the windows and do a quick blast of the **Silver-Violet Flame** technique. For how to do this, see Fix 310: Their Room – a Fetid Teenage Pit? Send it through the mattress, under the bed, into the corners of the room and especially into and above the cupboards, flamethrower-style.

2. If you happen to have some, spray a mixture of Purification and Guardian (the former essence is dross-removing, the latter protective) about the room, especially around your bed. It's useful to carry a little pre-prepared spray with you in your case for this reason. If you haven't got any, don't worry – just do the Silver-Violet Flame three times instead.

Purification is made by Alaskan Essences. In the UK, buy it via Healthlines (spray, 60 ml, £11.95). Guardian is also made by Alaskan Essences and is available from Healthlines (spray, 60 ml, £11.95; stock bottle, 7.5 ml, £7.95); in the US and Canada, you can buy both products direct (spray, 2 fl oz, $11; stock bottle, ¼ fl oz, $7.45). For contact details, see under 'Shopping' in the Directory.

Appendix 1: Cleansing and Programming Crystals and Gems

Cleansing

Gems and crystals – whether they are those little pieces of coloured polished stone from the gift shop ('tumbled' gems, the ones displayed any old how in piles, trays or baskets) or majestic great chunks of raw crystal quartz – usually need a bit of a clean-up before you use them.

Why?

They pick up all sorts of energy very easily, which is why programmed quartz, for instance, is used to keep time in watches. Gems' sensitivity ensures they can be positively charged and used effectively for enhancing well-being. But these lovely stones can also acquire and store other stuff – not only general dross, but actual negative energy – hence the historical stories of unlucky jewels.

If we bought an exquisite 18th-century sideboard, most of us would clean out all its drawers and give it a good polish before using it. If we found a stunning 1930s silk dress in an antiquarian market, we'd gently hand-wash it or get it dry-cleaned before wearing it out to dinner. What do we do this for? To get rid of any dirt or mustiness, to eradicate all traces of former owners, to freshen the article up, to make it ours – and it's the same with gems or crystals.

So it's vital to always cleanse a stone before you work with it. And if it's been used for a while, cleanse it at intervals in the same way you would wash a beautiful piece of clothing you've worn several times.

If you buy a gem or crystal, say a piece of rose quartz to place on a child's bedhead for encouraging peaceful sleep, chances are that, like a 50p coin, it will have been held and handled by a wide variety of people before you came along. You wouldn't let a toddler chew a 50p coin for that very reason (*'Take that out of your mouth, George – you don't know where it's been'*), so would you use a grubby – from an energetic point of view – item to help promote well-being?

The cleansing bit

There are several slightly differing methods for cleansing a gem or crystal's energy. This one works well and is both easy and quick.

1. Take a glass bowl, fill it up with pure spring water and add a handful of rock salt. Swish the salt round until it dissolves.
2. Gently place the gem or crystal in the bowl, then take it into the garden or backyard and place it in a clear space (i.e. not near the rubbish bin or a tangle of garden implements) on a white towel in a patch of sun. Alternatively, put it on a windowsill indoors in sunlight.
3. Let it stay there for, say, ten minutes. Remove, run under cool water and pat dry with the white towel.
4. Fold the towel into as small a square as is practical, place the gem or crystal on it and put it back in the patch of sun.
5. Let it bask and absorb the sun's energy for as long as feels right – say, an hour or so. Don't leave it in the sun for too long, though, as these stones are created over millions of years in the dark of the earth and don't like to be overexposed to bright sunlight.

Programming

Before you start programming a crystal or gem for a particular purpose, you first need to clear yourself and get rid of any bits of negativity you have, whether they be irritation, worry, tiredness or anxiety. If you don't, you'll be passing some of that into the stone or crystal.

The instant self-cleanse

1. Close your eyes.
2. Take six slow, deep, calming breaths, breathing in for six, holding for six, then out for six.
3. Next, imagine a golden light settling all around you, warm and comforting.
4. Feel this light gently dissolving all negativity (tiredness, irritation and worries) that you may have. Sense it melting away for now.
5. Open your eyes and stretch.

That's it.

The programming bit

1. Pick up your newly cleansed stone. It should be sparkling with sun energy if it's a crystal – or if it's a tumbled, polished gem, it may be looking sleeker or somehow a bit more brightly coloured than before. Hold it in your cupped hands.
2. Access your chosen source of positive power to energise the gem – i.e. decide whose help you would like for programming your stone with energy. Some people call upon the Universal Source of Love and Light, others upon their God, some upon Mother Nature, a particular Angel or Archangel. There is no 'right' or 'best' way. Just do whatever feels right for you. If you would like to work with the energy of one of the powerful archangels, see 'Which archangel helps with what?' on page 540 for a very brief guide. You can use a formal prayer or make a respectful but heartfelt request.
3. Now, take slow, easy breaths, close your eyes and speak either out loud or in your head, something along the lines of:

'Dear . . . [say the name of the source of help you have chosen]: **First of all, I thank you from the bottom of my heart for all that you have done for me and for mankind up until this point, and send you blessings of my own.**

Please help me, as I should like this crystal/stone to be filled with the energies of . . . [say what you need – e.g. love, healing or protection]. **I ask that you should send this energy through me to it and that it should work thereafter for the highest possible good. Please – do this – NOW.'**

4. Upon the word 'now', see in your mind's eye a waterfall of golden light pouring down upon you. Feel it warming, calming and protecting you.
5. Let it wash all the way through you. As it reaches your hands, begin to send it from your palms into the stone. You may experience this as warmth coming from your hands or a slight prickling. However, it doesn't matter if you can't feel anything in particular: trust that it'll be happening anyway. Let this golden warmth pour in until you feel 'that's enough'. Then say:

'Dear . . . [say the name of the source of help you have chosen], **I thank you for this energy, and I now have enough for my needs. Please could you cease sending it.** [Imagine the golden waterfall slowing, then stopping.] **Let me be closed down now, and fully grounded.'**

This last sentence is important, since if you're not closed down or grounded, you may remain receptive ('open') so could end up feeling spacey and drained.

6. Stretch and stamp your feet on the ground. If you do feel a bit vague, go and have a drink or even a small snack.
7. Now place the crystal where you need it to be. And know that it will do its work.

Which Archangel helps with what?

- If you would like your stone or crystal to be filled with get-better, **healing** energy (perhaps someone is unwell and you want to use it to help them), call upon *Archangel Raphael.* Raphael is also in charge of helping **children** of all ages.
- If you would like it to be charged with the energies of **love** and **calm** (perhaps for using in a child's bedroom at night), call upon Archangel *Chamuel,* archangel of unconditional love.
- If you want to use it for **getting rid of negative energy**, the best way to do this is to request that the stuff be transmuted (changed) into positive energy. This follows one of the first laws of the universe – and also the first law of physics – which is that *energy can neither be created nor destroyed, merely changed from one form into another.* For this, call upon *Zadkiel,* Archangel of, among other things, **transmutation** and **grace**.
- If you want the crystal or gem to be used for **protection**, call upon *Archangel Michael,* most powerful of them all, who gives courage, protection and strength to all those who ask.
- If you need to enhance your **understanding, intuition** or **ability to see the truth** (maybe there are a lot of people all giving you different advice about what to do at the moment), ask that *Archangel Gabriel,* who oversees birth, death and shows humans the blueprint of their true life's purpose, to send energy into the crystal or stone.
- If it is to help a **woman** or **girl**, especially if she is a **mother**, call upon *Mary, Queen of Heaven* (also known by many other names, such as Isis and Hathor, 'Mistress of the Sanctuary of Women'), who represents the mighty female principle of the Universe.

Recommended reading: for fuller information, see also *A Little Light on Angels* by Diana Cooper, which is straightforward, immensely practical and lovely.

Appendix 2:
The Forgiveness Process

When someone makes a conscious, deliberate and considered choice to award forgiveness freely (no strings attached), it is one of the most powerful forces there is. It's also the one that can finally set you free. Free of whoever has upset or wronged you, no matter how bad it was. Free to get your own energy back – since much of it may have been taken up by keeping in and carrying around feelings of distress, resentment, anger, loathing or hurt for months, if not years (emotional baggage – we've all got it by the bucket-load). Free, in fact, *to get on with the life that you want* and to be who you want. At last.

> Being unhappy or angry long term is physically, emotionally and spiritually exhausting, because it hijacks energy we would usually be putting into other, far nicer things. That is why people who are clinically depressed feel so washed out, why those who are angry much of the time feel tired, why those who are bereaved or broken-hearted say they have no energy left.

Breaking the ties that bind
Resenting someone with all your heart, feeling long-term furious with them (whether justifiably so or not) and pining for them – perhaps after

a break-up – also ties you to them. You can never get away properly, even if you very much want to move on. Yet when it's freely given, forgiveness can sever those ties at a single stroke, no matter how long they've been there nor how strong they seem.

Forgiveness doesn't mean 'letting the person off', nor saying that what they did to you doesn't matter (it may do a great deal). What it means is making a conscious choice to let it go, to stop resenting that person, and to move forward – without them.

> 'There is only one activity which sets you above the laws of cause and effect, and that is forgiveness.'
> *St Germain*

The dictionary defines forgiveness as **'to cease to bear resentment against; to give up the desire to punish; to stop being angry with; to pardon or to overlook'**.

If someone wants to truly forgive another so they can be free of them, doing so in a structured way will make the process especially powerful and effective.

The technique below was taught to me by the National Federation of Spiritual Healers as part of their advanced practitioner training. It was also given in a slightly different form by healer and essence-developer Ian White, who makes the Australian Bush Flower Essences range (some of which are mentioned in this book) in one of his practitioner-teaching programmes.

I have merged the two and changed them slightly. You may well want to alter it a bit too, so it fits what you would like to say better; but try and keep to the basic format, for this is what works.

> It is particularly important to observe the 'three times' rule, since one of the major laws of the universe is that if you ask for something to be done three times – providing it is for the best, and harms no one – it will be.

The beginning

Find a place that's safe, comfortable and where you won't be disturbed for a while. Ensure it is also somewhere you will not be overheard if you talk out loud.

The Forgiveness Process can be quite a long one if there are several people towards whom you feel resentment and from whom you would like to free yourself. It can all be done at one sitting, but you may find that after the first two or three people you feel a bit tired and it is enough for the moment. Many people spread it over more than one session, doing as much as they can comfortably manage each time.

It can be helpful to space those sessions, say, two to seven days apart, to give each one the opportunity to settle. This process, though it's simple and straightforward, deals with big issues, and any changes may take a little time to digest.

It may help to take some **Angelsword** essence (usually seven drops under your tongue, though three to five may be enough if you are very sensitive) both as protection and also to help you 'see' clearly and accurately what is happening during the Forgiveness Process. You can buy Angelsword via IFER or Healthlines (15 ml, £8.95). For contact details, see under 'Shopping' in the Directory.

If you are comfortable with the idea, also ask your guardian angel to draw close and help you.

The middle

1. Get comfortable. Some people like to sit in a straight-backed chair; others lie on a bed or on the floor with a pillow under their head.
2. Take several deep, easy breaths – breathe in for six, hold for six, out for six. Let this become a comfortable rhythm. Feel yourself relaxing. Allow yourself to become receptive.
3. Ask to be shown, visually, the main person whom you hold resentment against without actually naming who you think it is – you may be surprised. You will either get a picture of them in your mind's eye or you may simply just know who it is. Only one person will present

themselves at a time. The first person to appear for you is usually one of your parents, the next is often the other parent – whether or not they are alive.

4. When you see that person or feel you know who it is, see in your mind's eye a cord coming from their navel and connecting with another separate cord coming from your own. This is a visual representation of the tie that is binding you to each other.

5. Say out loud, or very firmly in your head, 'X [say their name], I hold the following resentments against you . . . [list these clearly one by one].'

6. When you've completed that list, say, 'X [say their name], all the resentments I hold against you *I now release*. I love you – and I forgive you.' As you say the words 'I forgive you', physically make a pair of scissors with your fingers and cut right through the imaginary cord connecting you both.

7. Repeat this process twice more.

8. Now it's their turn – since there are two sides to everything (no matter how flimsy theirs may seem). See those two cords connect you both once again. Having imagined cutting them, many people tend to see the two ends being tied back together, rather than seamlessly rejoining.

9. Say out loud, or in your head, 'X [say their name], you hold resentment against me for . . . [list these clearly one by one].'

10. When you have finished, say, 'X [say their name], for all these things for which you hold resentment against me, I now forgive you. I love you and *I now release you*.'

11. Then, making those scissors with your fingers again, once more cut the cord.

12. Repeat this process twice more.

13. If you feel you would like to keep going, let this one fade away and ask to be presented with person number two.

The end

Continue until no one remains or until you feel you have done enough for now. Take a deep breath open your eyes and stretch.

Appendix 3:
Meeting your
Guardian Angel

It is said that we all have our own special guardian angel who chooses to be assigned to us at or just before our birth, and whose job it is to help and protect us for our 'highest possible good', in any and every way they can, throughout our entire lives. *Highest good* is a phrase that often crops up these days in spiritual writing and training: it just means ' *the best possible Big Picture outcome'* – and carries the added proviso that this shall never be something that might harm anyone else.

Some people talk to their guardian angel perfectly normally, as if they are having a conversation with a special friend in their head. Others do so in the form of a short, respectful prayer, explaining what they need help with and why. Many formalise it slightly, as follows. There is no official 'best' way: the best way is whatever feels right to you personally, done with love and respect.

How to connect with your guardian angel

1. Sit down somewhere quiet where you won't be distracted or disturbed.
2. Light a small white candle and place a beautiful flower, or flowers, in water next to it.
3. Take nine deep, peaceful, easy breaths and imagine you are breathing *in* love – and breathing *out* peace each time.
4. Ask in your head 'in the name of Light' that you should first be grounded and protected – and then that your own special guardian angel draw close to you.
   Do this three times.
5. Now just wait a little. You do not need to strain to sense anything in particular – simply be still.
6. You may soon sense warmth or a feeling of quiet peace; some people report an emotional sensation such as a gentle rush of affection or love being showered on them ('like a soft hug' as one woman put it); many people sense light – often golden or silvery gold – near or around them. Some people sense nothing much at all, and that's fine too.
7. First, it is usual to say a (genuine) thank-you for all your guardian angel's past help and protection. Someone's far more likely to give you their full cooperation next time you ask if you were appreciative before, and angels are no exception. Know they have been giving this to you whenever they could, even if you weren't aware of it at the time.
8. Next, send them some of *your* love as well, as a gift.
9. If you just wanted to meet them for the first time, this is all you need to do. Now just sit peacefully, enjoying their company, love and protection for as long as it feels right to do so. Then, when you are ready, thank them for being with you, and move on to No. 11.

However, if you would like some help with something in particular:

10. Politely ask for what you need keeping it clear and simple.
11. Explain that you would like this to be done now – or you could end

up getting that help sometime in the future when the moment's passed somewhat. Add that you'd like this help to be for your 'highest possible good'.

. . . then finally . . .

12. Thank them. And know the help you asked for will come.
13. To end, ask that you may de-attune from your Angel for now, and that they help you close down. *This is important, or you may stay 'open' i.e. receptive, which can, amongst other things, make you feel tired and spacey if you walk about like that all the time.*
14. Open your eyes, yawn, stretch, stamp your feet on the floor a bit – then get up whenever you feel ready.

Leave the candle to burn down of its own accord. If you find you're feeling a bit vague, stretch and stamp a bit more, then go have a small snack or something to drink.

When you have met your angel in this way a few times, you will have established a good line of communication with them. This means that you will be able to access their help quickly when you are out and about if necessary, by just 'asking' them (silently, in your head) to come and help you – without having to sit down in privacy, light a candle etc.

Different feelings

If, when you are trying to connect with your guardian angel, you happen to sense anything that makes you even the slightest bit uncomfortable, that won't be your angel. So just tell it, firmly and calmly, to go away: it is not whom you invited, and therefore has no business here. Open your eyes, stretch, blow out the candle, and go off to do something else for a bit. Then try again later.

Notes

Fix 15: Anti-Arthritis Jewellery

In hospital trials, including the highly publicised one in 1997 by the Baylor Institute for Rehabilitation Research in Houston, which showed magnets could alleviate post-polio pain, the magnets tend to be placed on the person's body for a limited period of time each day, rather than worn all the time as jewellery.

Serious research continues, and while conclusions are mixed, a study in the *British Medical Journal* in 2005 pointed out that any poor results were invariably linked with the use of weaker magnets and that stronger ones (over 47 mtesla) did far better.

Encouragingly, America's National Institute of Health Office of Alternative Medicine also reckons there's sufficient mileage in the idea to have recently given a multi-million-dollar grant to the University of Virginia's School of Nursing to study use of magnets as pain relief for many different types of patients, including those with chronic fibromyalgia.

Fix 19: The Buteyko Method and Fix 235: Buteyko Breathing

There are no good studies recording resounding clinically trialled successes for Buteyko breathing and asthma – just some smaller or rather equivocal ones such as in the *British Medical Journal*[1] and the *Medical Journal of Australia.*[2]

However, we've included Buteyko because of the sheer volume of enthusiastic anecdotal evidence. Check it out, gather as much information as you can from websites, users and respiratory specialists, maybe try it out and see what you think.

Fix 72: Bright Light, Fix 96: Treatments for SAD and Fix 298: Light Therapy
Full spectrum or broad spectrum: what's the difference?
Full-spectrum light bulbs are made to try to imitate natural sunlight, and like sunlight, they also produce UV rays. Typically, full-spectrum bulbs have a colour rendering index (CRI) of 90 or above (100 is actual outdoor light). Full-spectrum light is described as having a purple or bluish cast. Most lightbox companies using full-spectrum light bulbs now block these UV rays through their diffuser screen, though it's good to check to be sure.

Broad-spectrum light bulbs are described as being a pure white light. Broad-spectrum lightboxes are described as being as close to natural full spectrum as you can get without the UV rays. Typically, they have a CRI of around 82. Most lightbox companies use a broad-spectrum light bulb so that there is no danger of UV rays.

Directory

Please note that unless otherwise stated all contacts are in the UK.

Shopping

AAAMagnetic (US)
800 499 3936
www.aaamagnetic.com

Academy Health (worldwide)
0845 370 3203
www.academyhealth.com

Active Herb (US)
858 324 1782
www.activeherb.com

Ainsworths
01883 340 332
www.ainsworths.com

Alaskan Essences (US and Canada)
800 545 9309 (orders), 406 642 3670 (customer service)
www.alaskanessences.com

Alaska Northern Lights (US and Canada)
800 880 6953
www.alaskanorthernlights.com

Allergy Matters
0208 339 0029
www.allergymatters.com

The Allergy Shop (US and Canada)
613 737 5183
www.theallergyshop.ca

All Star Health (US and Canada)
800 875 0448
www.allstarhealth.com

Alternative Medicines
0800 138 0864
www.alternativemedicines.co.uk

American Lifestyle (worldwide)
585 586 1878
www.aragonproducts.com

Amphora
www.amphora-retail.com

Apitherapy Health
01263 761 525
www.apitherapy.biz

Araretama Rainforest Essences (worldwide)
5 11 5531 9068
www.araretama.com.br

Arthro Vite
0800 018 1282
www.arthrovite.com

AuraVita
08700 84 11 14
www.auravita.com

Auro (worldwide)
01452 772 020
www.auro.co.uk

Auroma (US)
800 327 2025
www.auroma.com

Australian Bush Flower Essences (worldwide)
61 29 450 1388 (international)
www.ausflowers.com.au

Bach Flower Essences
(00) 1877 455 8859 (US)
www.essencesonline.com

Bailey Flower Essences
01943 432 012
www.baileyessences.com

Baldwin's
0207 703 5550
www.baldwins.co.uk

Barefoot Botanicals
0870 220 2273
www.barefoot-botanicals.com

Barlean's (US)
800 445 3529
www.barleans.com

Bay House
01273 601 109
www.bay-house.co.uk

Bee Health
0800 695 5295
www.naturalwayhealth.co.uk

Beehive Botanicals (US)
800-BEEHIVE
www.beehivebotanicals.com

Bergen e-Books
PO Box 295
River Edge
New Jersey 07661
USA

Betty Hoops (US)
303 746 4388
www.bettyhoops.com

BioCare
0121 433 3727
www.biocare.co.uk

Bioforce
01294 277 344
www.bioforce.co.uk

Bio Skin Care (UK and US)
866 647 0655
www.naturalbioskincare.com

Biovea
0800 612 9600
www.biovea.net

Black Seed Europe
01323 504 904
www.black-seed-europe.com

Bloesem Remedies (worldwide)
31 77 398 7826
www.bloesem-remedies.com

Body Kind
0800 043 5566
www.bodykind.com

The Body Shop (UK and US)
www.thebodyshop.com

Born to Love (US)
www.borntolove.com

Britannia Health
01732 742 345
www.britannia-health.co.uk

Brunel Healthcare
0117 959 7040
www.bruhealth.co.uk

By the Planet (US)
888 543 9294
www.bytheplanet.com

Canada Drug Superstore (US and Canada)
604 714 0832
www.canadadrugsuperstore.com

Cedar Health
0161 483 1235
www.cedarhealth.co.uk

Centre for Alternative Technology (CAT)
01654 705 980 (product orderline)
01654 705 959 (leaflets)
www.cat.org.uk

CEVA Animal Health
01494 781 510
www.dap-pheromone.com

Children's Lacteeze (US and Canada)
gelda@golbalserve.net (email)

Cisca
0191 373 4425
www.thesaltpipe.co.uk

Colief
www.colief.com

Crest Whitestrips
www.crestwhitestrips.co.uk

Crown Pet Foods
01935 410 600

Cygnus Books
www.cygnus-books.co.uk.
UK order line 0845 456 1577, order line for overseas customers
(including US, Australia and Europe) + 44 1550 777 701.

Dealtime
www.dealtime.co.uk

Dermal Laboratories
01462 458 866

Diamond Organics (US)
www.diamondorganics.com

Dri-Pak
0115 932 5165
www.dripak.co.uk

Early Learning Centre
08705 352 352
www.elc.co.uk

Earth Friendly (UK and US)
01892 616 871 (UK)
847 446 441 Ext. 13 (US)
www.ecos.com

Earth Spirits Herbal Apothecary (US)
(00) 1 508 347 1180
www.earthspiritsherbals.com

Eat Natural
www.eatnatural.co.uk

Ecos Organic Paints
01524 852 371
www.ecos.me.uk

Education and Resources for Improving Childhood Continence (ERIC)
www.ericshop.org.uk

Elixir Health Foods
01208 814 500
www.elixirhealth.co.uk

Equazen
0870 241 5621
www.equazen.com

The Essence Shop
01264 850 176
The Essential Oil Company (US)
800 729 5912
www.essentialoil.com

Express Chemist
0800 542 1203
www.expresschemist.co.uk

Findhorn Flower Essences
01309 690 129
www.findhornessences.com

First Vitality
0800 881 8022
www.1stvitality.com

Florihana Distillerie
00 33 493 09 06 09
www.florihana.com

Flower Essence Services (US)
www.fesflowers.com

Flower Sense
01494 671 775
www.flowersense.co.uk

Flower Vision Research (worldwide)
973 746 5798 (US)

001 973 746 5798 (international)
www.flowervr.com

Food and Vitamins (US)
310 373 2955
www.foodandvitamins.com

Fresh & Wild
www.freshandwild.com

Full Spectrum Solutions (US)
888 574 7014
www.fullspectrumsolutions.com

Gaiam Direct
www.gaiamdirect.co.uk

The Garden Pharmacy
0207 836 1007
www.garden.co.uk

Genesis (US and Canada)
253 226 1263

GloryBee (US and Canada)
800 456 7923
www.glorybee.com

Goodness Direct
0871 871 6611
www.goodnessdirect.co.uk

Graminex (US)
877 472 6469
www.graminex.com

Greatest Herbs on Earth (US)
775 996 1327
www.greatestherbsonearth.com

Green People
01403 740 350
www.greenpeople.co.uk

Green's
0207 976 0649

The Green Shop
01452 770 629
www.greenshop.co.uk

Green Tea Lovers (US)
516 374 6538
www.greentealovers.com

Grey's Teas
01926 419 180
www.greysteas.co.uk

Growing Lifestyle
www.growinglifestyle.co.uk

Hair Formula 37 (US)
888 849 8686

Healing Herbs
01873 890 218
www.healingherbs.co.uk

Healing Waters (US)
1 877 455 8859
www.essencesonline.com

Health and Yoga (US, Japan and India)
www.healthandyoga.com

Health Emporium
01462 436 881
www.health-emporium.co.uk

Healthlines
01539 568 761
0845 223 5436
www.healthlines.co.uk

Healthspan
0800 731 2377
www.healthspan.co.uk

Healthy Direct
0800 107 5757 (24 hours)
www.healthydirect.co.uk

Healthy4You (US)
www.healthy4youonline.com

Helios
01892 537 254
www.helios.co.uk

Herbal Remedies (US)
866 467 6444
www.herbalremedies.com

High Barn Oils
01403 730 326
www.highbarnoils.co.uk

Higher Nature (UK and US)
0800 458 4747 (orders)
01435 884 572 (queries)
01435 884 668 (East Sussex shop)
01435 882 880 (US customers)
www.highernature.co.uk

Hippy Chick
www.hippychick.co.uk

Holland & Barrett
www.hollandbarrett.com

Home Herbs
01942 670 911
www.homeherbs.com

Homeopathic Educational Services
800 359 9051
www.homeopathic.com

Igennus
0845 130 0424
www.igennus.com

Immunocorp (worldwide)
1582 W. Deere Avenue
Suite C
Dept 12IU
Irvine
CA 92606
USA
800 446 3063
www.immuderm.com

Indigo Essences (worldwide)
353 1 201 8029
www.indigoessences.com

International Flower Essence Repertoire (IFER)
01583 505 385
www.ifer.co.uk

The Irlen Institute
www.irlen.com
Island Spice
01524 271 655
www.islandspice.co.uk

Jembush
01403 823 924
www.jembush.co.uk

Just Buy Online
0870 740 8835

Kittykins
www.kittykins.co.uk

Lamberts
www.supportme.co.uk/lamberts.htm

Leppin Health
0121 779 6619
sales@leppin-health.com (email)

Lichtwer Healthcare
0800 652 7150
www.lichtwer.co.uk

Life Plus Vitamins (US)
www.lifeplusvitamins.com

LifeSource
01623 490 141
www.lifesource.co.uk

LifeTime Vitamins (UK and US)
800 333 6168
www.lifetimevitamins.com

Light Heart Essences
01986 789 168
www.lightheartessences.co.uk

The Litlington Crystal Store
01323 871 226

Livespan Nutrition (US)
800 247 5731
www.lifespannutrition.com

Living Essences of Australia (worldwide)
61 894 435 600 (international)
www.livingessences.com.au

Living Tree Orchid Essences
See IFER on page 562.

Lollypop Publishing
0121 600 0150

Love Lula (worldwide)
0870 242 6995
www.lovelula.com

The Maca Company
www.maca.co.uk

Magna Therapy/Magna Jewellery
0208 421 8848
www.magna-health.com

Manuka Honey
01252 330 850
www.manukahoney.co.uk

Maplin Electronics
0870 429 6000
www.maplin.co.uk

Massive Member (US)
www.massivemember.com

Materia Aromatica
0208 392 9868
www.materiaaromatica.com

MEDesign
01704 542 373
www.medesign.co.uk

Medshop
www.medshop.co.uk

The Men's Health Centre
Suite 20
Harmont House
20 Harley Street
London W1G 9PH
0207 636 8283

Metabolics
01380 812 799
www.metabolics.co.uk
You will need your nutritionist's prescription to buy items.

Milkaid
www.milkaid.com

Mother Nature (US)
800 439 5506
www.mothernature.com

Napiers
0131 343 6683
www.napiers.net

The National Supplement Center (US)
800 369 1039
www.nationalsupplementcenter.com

Natremed
01422 371 139
www.theraflex.co.uk

The Natural Approach
01577 830 649

Natural Collection
0870 331 3333

Natural Dentistry (US)
727 446 6747

The Natural Healing Centre
01482 222 089

Naturally Does It
01525 860 535
www.naturallydoesit.co.uk

Natural Salt Pipes (US)
312 224 2710
www.natural-salt-lamps.com

Nature's Answer (US)
800 439 2324
www.naturesanswer.com

Nature's Best
01892 552 117 (order line)
01892 552 118 (general queries)
01892 552 175 (nutrition advice line)
www.naturesbest.co.uk

Nature's Gift (US)
615 612 4270
www.naturesgift.com

Nature's Menu
0800 018 3770
www.naturesmenu.co.uk

Nature's Way (US)
801 489 1500
www.naturesway.com

Naturopatch of Vermont (US and Canada)
800 340 9083
www.naturopatch.com

N B Nutrition
www.nbnutrition.com

Neal's Yard Remedies (UK and US)
0845 262 3145 (mail order)
01747 834 634 (customer advice line)
www.nealsyardremedies.com (UK)
www.nealsyard.hostcentric.com (US)

Nelsons
0207 629 3118
www.nelsonspharmacy.com

New Forest Soaps
www.newforestsoaps.co.uk

No-Jet-Lag (worldwide)
www.nojetlag.com

Nutrica (US)
800 278 8002
www.nutrica.com

The Nutri Centre
0207 436 5122
www.nutricentre.com

NutriTeam (US)
800 785 9791
www.nutriteam.com

Nutrivea USA (US)
561 912 0912
www.nutrivea-usa.com

NZ Health
0208 850 4539

Omlet (Eglu)
www.omlet.co.uk

1001 Herbs (US)
866 340 3404 (orders)
800 223 8225 (queries)
www.1001herbs.com

Only Hair Loss (worldwide)
888 849 8686
www.onlyhairloss.com

The Organic Gardening Catalogue
0845 130 1304
www.organicgardening.com

Original Organics
01884 841 515
www.originalorganics.co.uk

OttLight Systems (US)
800 234 3724

Outside In
01954 780 500
www.lumie.com

Pacific Essences (US and Canada)
250 384 5560
www.pacificessences.com

Parentsmart (US)
714 99 8617
www.parentsmart.com

Perfect Poultry
01276 453 777
www.perfectpoultry.co.uk

Petite Fleur Essences (US)
817 293 5410
www.aromahealthtexas.com

Pet Planet
0845 345 0723
www.petplanet.co.uk

Physician Formulas (US)
877 225 2466
www.physicianformulas.com

Planta
0208 761 3114
www.planta.co.uk

Postal Pet Products
01531 633 985
www.postalpetproducts.co.uk

Powerwatch
www.powerwatch.org.uk

Pretty Rock (US)
704 641 9107
www.prettyrock.com

Proof (worldwide)
0870 444 9886 (UK)
212 563 0132 (US)
www.proof.co.uk (UK)
www.proofmagazine.com (US)

ProSolution (UK and US)
800 370 5054
www.prosolutionpills.com

Provillus (worldwide)
0207 669 4750 (UK)
800 238 1413 (US)
www.provillus.com

Pukka Herbs
0845 375 1744
www.pukkaherbs.com

Regency Poultry
01246 854 647
www.regencypoultry.com

Relax Kids
0870 350 5035
www.relaxkids.com

Rentokil
0800 917 1989
www.uk.rentokil.com

Revital
0800 252 875
www.revital.co.uk

Rio Health Trading Co
01273 570 987
www.riohealth.co.uk

Safe 2 Use (US)
800 931 9916
www.safe2use.com

Salt Pipe
See Cisca on page 556.

Sarakan
01420 544 424
www.sarakan.com

School of Natural Health and Wellbeing
01276 367 978
www.come-alive.co.uk

Sea-Band (worldwide)
01455 639 750 (UK)
401 841 5900 (US)
www.sea-band.com
usa@sea-band.com (US email)

Simplers Botanical Company
800 652 7646
www.simplers.com

The Sivananda Yoga Centre
0208 780 0160
www.sivananda.co.uk

Skin Energizer (US)
888 909 1658 Ext. 2
www.skinenergizer.com

Slendertone
0845 070 7777
www.slendertone.com

SMARTbomb (US)
800 425 3115
www.smartbomb.com

Solgar (worldwide)
01442 890 355 (UK)
800 645 2246 (US)
www.solgar-vitamins.co.uk (UK)
www.solgar.com (US)

So Organic
0800 169 2579
www.soorganic.com

South African Essences (worldwide)
27 21 794 6762
www.safloweressences.co.za

Space NK
0208 740 2085
www.SpaceNK.co.uk

Special Gifts (US)
330 733 4283
www.specialgifts.com

Star Child (worldwide)
01458 834 663
www.starchild-international.com
Supersmile (US)
800 784 7645
www.supersmile.com

Takara (US)
866 448 1789
www.takarapatch.com

The Tea House
07880 550 751
www.theteahouse.co.uk

Terra Firma Botanicals (US)
800 837 3476
www.terrafirmabotanicals.com

Think Natural
0845 601 1948
www.thinknatural.com

This Works
0845 652 9591
www.thisworks.com

Tisserand Aromatherapy (UK and US)
01273 325666
707 769 5120 (US)
www.tisserand.com

Tower Health
08450 066 077
www.tower-health.co.uk

Tranquil Living
01264 850 176
www.tranquil-living-online.com

United Field (US)
610 310 2490
www.theunifiedfield.com

USA Homeopathic Pharmacies (US)
www.homeopathyhome.com

Vet UK
www.vetuk.co.uk

Victoria Health
0800 389 8195
www.victoriahealth.com

Victoria's Health and Beauty
0117 957 5080
www.victoriasbeauty.co.uk

VitaDigest (US)
626 965 8308
www.vitadigest.com

Vitamin Express (US)
800 500 0733
www.vitaminexpress.com

Washington Homeopathic Products (US)
1 800 336 1695
www.homeopathyworks.com

Web Vitamins (US)
800 919 9122
www.webvitamins.com

Wellbeing UK
0121 444 6585
www.wellbeing-uk.com

Weleda
0115 944 8200
www.weleda.co.uk

What Doctors Don't Tell You (UK and US)
0870 444 9886
www.wddty.co.uk

Wild Earth Animal Essences (US)
800 871 5647 (US)
540 363 4615 (international)
www.animalessences.com

Wilderness Family Naturals (US)
866 936 6457
www.wildernessfamilynaturals.com

Worldwide Shopping Mall (UK and US)
0808 144 0842
www.worldwideshoppingmall.co.uk

Zipvit
0800 028 2875
www.zipvit.co.uk

Zooscape (US)
800 760 8783
www.zooscape.com

Therapies and Therapists

Animal Behavioural Therapists
The Association of Pet Behaviour Counsellors
01386 751 151
www.apbc.org.uk

Applied Kinesiologists
The International College of Applied Kinesiology UK
01403 734 321
www.icak.co.uk

Kinesiology Connections
0208 856 7717
www.kinesiologyconnections.com

US
The International College of Applied Kinesiology US
913 384 5336
www.icakusa.com

The Touch for Health Kinesiology Association of North America
31 0313 5580
www.touch4health.com

Aromatherapists
The Aromatherapy Council
0870 774 3477

Brain Reprogramming
See 'Dyslexia, Dyspraxia and ADHD' on page 593.

Chiropractors
The British Chiropractic Association
0118 950 5950
www.chiropractic-uk.co.uk

US
The American Chiropractic Association
703 276 8800
www.amerchiro.org

Colour Therapists
Worldwide
The International Association of Colour (IAC)
0208 349 3299
www.iac-colour.co.uk

Cosmetic Surgeons
The British Association of Aesthetic Plastic Surgery (BAAPS)
0207 405 2234 (advice line)
www.baaps.org.uk

Counsellors
The British Association for Counselling and Psychotherapy (BCAP)
0870 443 5252
www.bacp.co.uk

US
The American Counseling Association
800 347 6647
www.counseling.org

Cranial Osteopaths
UK and US
The Sutherland Society
www.cranial.org.uk

(Holistic) Dentists
The British Homeopathic Dental Association (BHDA)
0167 548 1535
www.bhda.co.uk

The British Society for Mercury-Free Dentistry
0207 370 0055
www.mercuryfree.co.uk

Patients Against Mercury Amalgams
0207 256 2993

US
The International Society of Mercury-Free Dentists
800 504 4977
www.mercuryfreenow.com

The Foundation for Toxic-Free Dentistry
800 331 2303

Canada
Canadians for Mercury Relief
www.talkinternational.com

Doulas
Doula UK
0871 433 3103
www.doula.org.uk

US
Doulas of North America/Dona International
206 324 5440
www.dona.org

Feng Shui Practitioners
The Feng Shui Society
0705 028 9200
www.fengshuisociety.org

UK and US
Karen Kingston
01373 461 280 (UK)
877 917 7223 (US)
www.spaceclearing.com

Lillian Too
www.lillian-too.com
US
The American Feng Shui Institute
626 571 2757
www.amfengshui.com

Floatation-Tank Therapy
The Floatation Tank Association
0207 627 4962
www.floatationtankassociation.net

Floatopia
0208 994 0708
www.floatopia.co.uk

Healers
The National Federation of Spiritual Healers
01932 783 164
www.nfsh.org.uk

US
The American Association of Healers
www.americanassociationofhealers.com

See also 'Reiki Practitioners' on page 583.

Herbalists
The National Institute of Medical Herbalists
01392 426 022
www.nimh.org.uk

Homeopaths
The British Homeopathic Association
0870 444 3950
www.trusthomeopathy.org

The Society of Homeopaths (SOH)
0845 450 6611
www.homeopathy-soh.org

US
The National Center for Homeopathy
www.homeopathic.org
877 624 0613

For homeopathic vets, see 'Vets' on page 584.

Hypnotherapists
The British Society for Medical and Dental Hypnosis (BSMDH)
01132 619 292
www.bsmdh.com

US
The American Psychotherapy and Medical Hypnosis Association
(APMHA)
509 662 5131
www.apmha.com
See also 'Self-Hypnosis' on page 589.

Naturopaths
The British Naturopathic Association
0870 745 6984
www.naturopaths.org.uk

Neuro-Linguistic Programming Therapists
The Association of NLP Practitioners
020 8275 1175
www.anlp.org

US
NLP-Practioners.com
www.nlp-practitioners.com

Nutritionists
The British Association of Nutritional Therapists (BANT)
0870 606 1284
www.bant.org.uk

The British Dietetic Association
0121 200 8080
www.bda.uk.com

The British Society for Ecological Medicine
(incorporating the British Society for Allergy and Environmental Medicine)
01547 550 378
www.ecomed.org.uk

Food and Behaviour Research
0870 756 5960
www.fabresearch.org

The Institute of Optimum Nutrition
020 8614 7800
www.ion.ac.uk

The Natural Health Advisory Service
(incorporating the Women's Nutritional Advisory Service)
01273 609 699
www.naturalhealthas.com

US
The American Academy of Environmental Medicine (AAEM)
316 684 5500
www.aaem.com

The American Dietetic Association
800 877 1600
www.eatright.org

The Institute for Functional Medicine
800 228 0622
www.functionalmedicine.org

Australia
The Australasian College of Nutritional and Environmental Medicine
61 3 9589 6088
www.acnem.org

See also 'Naturopaths' on page 581, as naturopaths also use nutrition as a major part of their treatment.

Osteopathy
The General Osteopathic Council
0207 357 6655
www.osteopathy.org.uk

US
Osteohome
www.osteohome.com

See also 'Cranial Osteopaths' on page 578.

Physiotherapy
The Sports Injury Clinic
www.sportsinjuryclinic.net

Canada
Sport Physiotherapy Canada
613 748 5794
www.sportphysio.ca

Reiki Practitioners
The Reiki Association
0770 427 0727
www.reikiassociation.org.uk

Worldwide
The International Association of Reiki Professionals (IARP)
603 881 8838 (based in US)
www.iarp.org

See also 'Healers' on page 579.

Spirit Release Practitioners
The Spirit Release Foundation
01684 560 725
www.spiritrelease.com

Therapeutic Touch (TT) Practitioners
British Association of Therapeutic Touch
01267 232 715
www.sacredspace.org.uk

US
Healing Touch International
303 989 7982
www.healingtouchinternational.org

Timeline Therapy
See 'Neuro-Linguistic Programming Therapists' on page 581.

(Holistic) Vets
The British Association of Homeopathic Veterinary Surgeons
For a list countrywide, send a stamped, addressed envelope to:
The Alternative Veterinary Medicine Centre
Chinham House
Stanford in the Vale
Oxon SN7 8NQ
01367 710 324

The British Holistic Veterinary Medicine Association
01273 725 951
www.spvs.org.uk

US
The American Holistic Veterinary Medical Association (AHVMA)
410 569 0795
www.ahvma.org

Training Courses

Animal Communication and Animal Whispering
Animal Communication Training (ACT)
0845 419 49 51 (enquiries)
01428 685 944 (consultations)
www.reikicare.co.uk

UK and US
Amelia Kinkade
www.ameliakinkade.com

US
Carol Gurney
818 597 104
www.animalcommunicator.net

Animal Shiatsu and Massage
Jacqueline Cook
01547 530 871
www.shiatsu-for-horses.com
(for dogs and horses)

The Institute of Complementary Animal Therapies (ICAT)
01626 852 485
www.theicat.co.uk

US

The Bancroft School of Massage
508 757 7923
www.bancroftsmt.com

The Northwest School of Animal Massage
425 222 3703
www.nwsam.com

Autogenic Training (AT)

The British Association for Autogenic Training and Therapy (BAFATT)
For information and classes on AT, send a stamped, addressed
envelope to:
BAFATT
c/o the Royal Homeopathic Hospital
Great Ormond Street
London WC1N 3HR

The British Autogenic Society
0207 391 8908
www.autogenic-therapy.org.uk

The Centre for Autogenic Training (CAT)
01803 312 098

Bates Method

The Bates Association for Vision Education (BAVE)
www.seeing.org

Biodynamic Gardening

The Biodynamic Agricultural Association (BDAA)
www.biodynamic.org.uk

Emerson College
01342 822 238
www.emerson.org.uk

US
The Biodynamic Farming and Gardening Association
541 998 0105
www.biodynamics.com
The Pfeiffer Center
845 352 5020
www.pfeiffercenter.org

Buteyko Method
The Buteyko Breathing Centre
01789 298 290
www.buteyko.co.uk

Worldwide
The Buteyko Institute of Breathing and Health (BIBH)
61 3 9419 4211 (based in Australia)
www.buteyko.info

US
Buteyko International
353 91 756 229
www.buteykointernational.com

Eco-Friendly Building and Design
The Centre for Alternative Technology (CAT)
01654 705 981 (courses)
www.cat.org.uk/courses

Healing
The National Federation of Spiritual Healers
0845 123 2767
www.nfsh.org.uk

The Reiki Association
0770 427 0727
www.reikiassociation.org.uk

Worldwide
The International Association of Reiki Professionals (IARP)
603 881 8838 (based in the US)
www.iarp.org

Hooping
Sharna Rose
01622 814 670

Laughter Therapy
Jack Milner
01494 772 908
www.jackmilner.com

US
LAUGHS (Laughing At and Understanding Humor Seminars)
508 588 2382
www.laughsrus.com

Linden Method
The Linden Centre
0870 119 0298
www.thelindenmethod.co.uk

Meditation
Transcendental Meditation Independent UK
0191 2132 179 (North)
01843 841 010 (South)
www.tm-meditation.co.uk

Rites of Passage
Circle of Life
01273 470 793
www.circleoflifediscovery.com

The Dolphin Connection
Amanda Stafford
01273 882 778
www.dolphinconnectionexperience.com

Kate Shela (The Maiden's Voyage)
01273 736 598
kate.shela@virgin.net (email)

US
Soul Awakening
800 707 4566
www.soulawakening.org

Youth Vision Quest
707 537 1927
www.ritesofpassagevisionquest.org

Safety Courses
Kidscape
www.kidscape.org.uk
0207 730 3300

StreetWise Safety Centre
01202 591 330
www.streetwise.org.uk

US
Kidspower
(also runs courses called Teenpower and Fullpower)
800 467 6997
www.kidspower.org

US
The School for Self-Healing
415 665 9574
www.self-healing.org

Self-Hypnosis
The National Register of Hypnotherapists and Psychotherapists (NRHP)
01282 716 839
www.nrhp.co.uk

UK and US
Marisa Peer
www.marisapeer.com

US
Riquette Hofstein
800 747 8388
www.riquette.com

See also 'Hypnotherapists' on page 580.

Tellington Touch
Mark Simmons
01959 561 774
www.animal-problems.co.uk

Yoga
British Wheel of Yoga
01529 306 851
www.bwy.org.uk

Useful Helplines, Websites and Contacts

Alcohol
Alcohol Concern
0800 917 8282 (helpline)
www.alcoholconcern.org.uk

ParentLine Plus
0808 800 2222 (helpline)
www.parentlineplus.org.uk

US
The National Drugs and Alcohol Treatment Referral Routing Service
800 662 4357
www.niaaa.nih.gov

Andropause
The Andropause Centre
0207 636 8283

US
The Men's Health Center
250 979 0300

Anorexia and Bulimia
The Eating Disorders Association
0845 634 1414 (helpline)
0845 634 7650 (youthline)
help@b-eat.co.uk
www.eatingdisorders.org.cuk

Anti-Aging Facial Exercises
Eva Fraser
0207 937 6616
www.evafraser.com

UK and US
Carole Maggio (Facercise)
800 597 3555
www.facercise.com

Anxiety
AnxietyPanic.com
www.anxietypanic.com

National Panic and Anxiety Disorder News
www.npadnews.com

Asthma
The National Asthma Campaign
08457 01 02 03
www.asthma.org.uk

US
The Asthma and Allergy Foundation of America
800 727 8462 (hotline)
www.aafa.org

Bed-Wetting (Enuresis)
Education and Resources for Improving Childhood Continence (ERIC)
0845 370 8008 (helpline)
www.enuresis.org.uk

US
The National Enuresis Society
800 697 8080

Body Language
Judi James
www.judijames.com

Cellulite and Body-Brushing
Leslie Kenton
www.lesliekenton.com

Disabilities
Canine Partners
08456 580 480
www.caninepartners.co.uk

Ducks and Hens
The British Waterfowl Association
www.waterfowl.org.uk

The Indian Runner Duck Association
01558 650 532
www.runnerduck.net

Dyslexia, Dyspraxia and ADHD
Dyslexia, Dyspraxia and Attention Disorder Treatment (DDAT)
01926 514 033 (UK)
877 855 3673 (US)
www.dore.co.uk (UK)
www.doreusa.com (US)

Dyspraxia Connexion
0115 963 2220
www.dyspraxiaconnexion.org.uk

The Dyspraxia Foundation
01462 454 986 (helpline)
www.dyspraxiafoundation.org.uk

The Hyperactive Children's Support Group
01243 539 966
www.hacsg.org.uk

The Irlen Institute
www.irlen.com

Matt's Hideout
www.matts.hideout.co.uk

Millennium Volunteers
www.millenniumvolunteers.gov.uk

US
Adders
www.adders.org.usa

Eco-Friendly Building and Design
The Centre for Alternative Technology (CAT)
01654 705 991 (consultancy services)

Eco-Friendly Cleaning
Low-Impact Living Initiative
01296 714 184
www.lowimpact.org

Electomagnetic Pollution
The Mobile Manufacturers Forum
www.mmfai.org

Powerwatch
01353 778 814
www.powerwatch.org.uk

Ethical Jobs
CSR Blokes
http://finance.groups.yahoo.com/group/csrblokes

CSR Chicks
http://.groups.yahoo.com/group/csr-chicks

Ethical Consumer
www.ethicalconsumer.org
0161 226 2929

Ethical Performance
www.ethicalperformance.com/recruitment

Green Futures
0207 324 3660
www.greenfutures.org.uk

Guardian
www.jobs.guardian.co.uk/browse/environment

Fertility and Preconceptual Care
Baby Hopes
www.babyhopes.com

The Endometriosis and Fertility Clinic
www.endometriosis.co.uk

The Healthvibes Clinic
0845 671 0160
www.healthvibes.co.uk

Infertility Network UK
www.issue.co.uk

More to Life
www.moretolife.co.uk

UK and US
Foresight
178 Hawthorne Road
West Bognor
West Sussex PO1 2UY
01243 868 001
www.foresight-preconception.org.uk

US
The Center for Occupational and Environmental Medicine (COEM)
843 572 1600
www.coem.com

Green Gyms
UK Nappy Helpline
01983 401 959

Pests
Pest Control Direct
01323 846 854
www.pestcontroldirect.co.uk

The Pesticide Action Network
www.pan-uk.org

Rentokil
0800 917 1989
www.uk.rentokil.com

Premature Babies
Bliss
0500 618 140 (helpline)
www.bliss.org.uk

Prematurity.com
www.prematurity.com

US
The Pregnancy and Newborn Health and Education Center
914 997 4488
www.marchofdimes.com

Seasonal Affective Disorder (SAD)
Outside In (Lumie)
01954 780 500
www.lumie.com

Self-Harm
The Bristol Crisis Centre
0117 925 1119 (helpline)

Palace.net
www.palace.net

Self-Injury and Related Issues (SIARI)
www.siari.co.uk

US
Self-Abuse Finally Ends (SAFE)
800 366 8288 (hotline)
www.selfinjury.com

Smoking
Giving Up Smoking
www.gosmokefree.co.uk

Quit
0800 00 22 00
www.quit.org.uk

Volunteering
Do It
0207 250 5700
www.do-it.org

Time Banks
01452 541 439
www.timebanks.co.uk

Walking Buses

The Walking Bus Guide
0121 602 0150
www.thewalkingbus.co.uk

Safe Kids Walking
01536 454 994
www.safekidswalking.org.uk

School Run
08700 780 225
www.school-run.org

Recommended Reading

Please note that all titles are published in the UK unless US prices are given. Almost all are, however, available internationally via Internet sites, such as Amazon.

Adams, Zoe, *The Colloidal Silver Report*, Another Country Verlag, Berlin (£2.50).

Allatt, Tracy, and Marshall, Sarah, *The Walking Bus Guide*, Lollypop Publishing, 2005 (£25).

Anthony, Diana, *Creative Sustainable Gardening*, CAT Publications, 2000 (£12.99).

Ashton, Chris and Mike, *The Domestic Duck*, Crowood Press, 2001 (£19.95).

Bates, William, *The Bates Method for Better Eyesight Without Glasses*, Harper-Collins, 2000 (£9.95)/Owl Books, 1981 ($13).

Billinghurst, Ian, *The Barf Diet for Cats and Dogs,* Ian Billinghurst Publications, 2001 (£11.50).

Billinghurst, Ian, *Give Your Dog a Bone*, Ian Billinghurst Publications, 1993 (£20.30).

Bradford, Nikki, and Chamberlain, Professor Geoffrey, *Childbirth Doesn't Have to Hurt*, Vega, 2002 (£8.99).

Bradford, Nikki, *Heal Yourself With Flowers and Other Essences*, Quadrille, 2006 (£7.99).

Bradford, Nikki, *Men's Health Matters: the Complete A–Z of Male Health*, Vermilion, 1995 (£9.99).

Bradford, Nikki, and Chamberlain, Dr David, *The Miraculous World of Your Unborn Baby*, Chrysalis, 2002 (£12.99).

Bradford, Nikki, *Natural Fertility*, Hamlyn, 2003 (£14.99).

Bradford, Nikki, *Your Premature Baby 0–5 Years*, Frances Lincoln (UK edition with Tommy's Campaign, US and Canadian editions with the Toronto Hospital for Sick Children and the Duchess of York), 2000 (£9.99/$15).

Brewer, Sarah, *Increase Your Sex Drive*, HarperCollins, 1999 (£7.99).

Carruthers, Malcolm, *The Testosterone Revolution: Re-Discover Your Energy and Overcome Symptoms of the Male Menopause*, Thorsons, 2001 (£10 including worldwide postage and packaging via the Men's Health Centre, London).

Cooper, Diana, *Angel Inspiration*, Hodder & Stoughton, 2001 (£12.99).

Cooper, Diana, *A Little Light on Angels,* Findhorn Press, 2000 (£9.99/$11.95).

Cooper, Diana, *Living With Angels*, Piatkus, 2003 (£9.99).

Etcoff, Dr Nancy, *Survival of the Prettiest*, Abacus, 2000 (£9.99)/Anchor, 2000 ($14.95).

Ewing, Dawn, *Let the Tooth Be Known*, Holistic Health Alternatives, reprint 2002.

Feltwell, Ray, *Small-Scale Poultry-Keeping*, Faber & Faber, 1992 (£8.99).

Franzen, Suzanne, *The Healing Touch*, Southwater, 2001 (£7.95/$12.25).

Fraser, Eva, *Eva Fraser's Facial Workout*, Penguin, 1992 (£7.99).

Gallop, Rick and Dr Ruth, *The Family GI Diet*, Virgin, 2006 (£10.99).

Gimbel, Theo, *Healing With Colour*, Gaia, 2005 (£9.99/$14.95).

Gurney, Carol, *The Language of Animals*, Bantam Dell, 2001 ($15).

Hall, Christine, *Rites of Passage*, Capall Bann Publishing, 2000 (£9.95).

Hannay, Pamela, *Shiatsu for Dogs*, Allen Photographic Guides, 1998 (£4.95).

Hannay, Pamela, *Touching Horses: Communication, Health and Healing Through Shiatsu*, J. A. Allen & Co., 1995.

Harland, Edward, *Eco Renovation*, Resurgence Books, CAT, 1999 (£9.99).

Holick, Michael, MD, *The UV Advantage*, ibooks, 2005 (£6.99/$7.99).

Huggins, Dr Hal A., *It's All in Your Head*, Avery, Penguin, 1993 ($13.95).

Ingraham, Caroline, *Aromatherapy for Animals*, Orphans Press, 2002 (£24.50).

Irving, Dr Andrew, *How to Cure a Hangover*, Little Books, 2005 (£9.99).

James, Judi, *Bodytalk at Work*, Piatkus, 2001.

James, Judi, *Sex Signals: Decode Them and Send Them*, Piatkus, 2003 (£7.99).

Johnson, Pam, *Twisted Whiskers: Solving Your Cat's Behaviour Problems*, Crossing Press, 1994 (£12.95/$12.99).

Kingston, Karen, *Creating Sacred Space With Feng Shui*, Piatkus, 1996 (£8.99).

Kinkade, Amelia, *The Language of Miracles*, New World Library, 2006 (£11.99/$15.95).

Kinkade, *Straight From the Horse's Mouth*, New World Library, 2005 (£9.99/$15.95).

Kirby, Dr Amanda, *Dyspraxia, the Hidden Handicap*, Souvenir Press, 2002 (£12.99/$24.95).

Kollerstrom, Nick, *Gardening and Planting by the Moon*, Quantum, 2006 (£8.99).

Lansky, Vicki, *Baking Soda: Over 500 Fabulous, Fun and Frugal Uses You Probably Never Thought Of*, Book Peddlers, 2004 (£4.70).

Linn, Denise, *Sacred Space*, Random House, 1995 (£8.99).

Lockie, Dr Andrew, *The Family Guide to Homeopathy*, Hamish Hamilton, 1998 (£16.99).

Ludington-Hoe, Susan, *Kangaroo Care: the Best You Can Do to Help Your Preterm Infant*, Bantam, 1993 ($15).

Luttmann, Rick and Gail, *Chickens in Your Backyard*, Rodale Press, 1976 ($12.95).

MacDonald, Carina Beth, *Raw Dog Food: Making It Work for You and Your Dog*, Dogwise Publishing, 2003 ($12.95).

Mack, Allison, *Dry All Night*, Little, Brown, 1990 ($5.95).

Maizels, Max, MD, Rosenbaum, Diane, and Keating, Barbara, *Getting to Dry: How to Help Your Child Overcome Bedwetting*, Harvard Common Press, 1999 ($28).

Mercer, Renée, *Seven Steps to Night-Time Dryness*, Brookeville Media, 2004 ($14.95).

Nierenberg, Andrea R., *Nonstop Networking: How to Improve Your Life, Luck and Career*, Capital Books, 2002 ($19.95).

Orbach, Dr Susie, *Fat Is a Feminist Issue*, Arrow, 1996 (£7.99).

Ott, Dr John, *Health and Light: the Effect of Natural and Artificial Light on Man and Other Living Things*, Ariel Press, reprint 2000 ($7.99).

Ott, Dr John, *Light, Radiation and You: How to Stay healthy*, Devin-Adair Publishing, reprint 1999 ($11.95).

Ott, Dr John, *The UV Advantage*, I Books, 2004 (paperback edition, $7.99).

Pavlovec, Meli, and Vazvary, Dr Ivette, *You Can Influence the Sex of Your Unborn Child*, Bergen e-Books ($29).

Peiffer, Vera, *Regrowing Hair Naturally*, Peiffer Press, 2004 (£14.99).

Philips, Alasdair and Jean, *EMF and Microwave Protection for You and Your Family*, Powerwatch (£8.50).

Puri, Dr Basant, *The Natural Way to Beat Depression*, Puri & Boyd, Hodder Mobius, 2004 (£10.99).

Quackenbush, Thomas R., *Re-Learning to See*, North Atlantic Books, 2000 ($27.50).

Salomon, Thierry, and Bedel, Stephane, *The Energy-Saving House*, CAT, 2003 (£12).

Scott, Martin, and Mariani, Gael, *Crystal Healing for Animals*, Findhorn Press, 2002 (£7.95).

Sheehy, Gail, *Understanding Men's Passages: Discovering the New Map of Men's Lives*, Random House, 2004 (£7.99)/1998 ($14.95).

Shettles, William, MD, *How to Choose the Sex of Your Baby*, Bantam, reprint 1997 ($13.95).

Stacey, Sarah, and Dooley, Dr Michael, *Your Change, Your Choice*, Hodder Mobius, 2004 (£7.99).

Stone, Carole, *Networking: the Art of Making More Friends*, Random House, 2001 (£7.99).

Tan, Robert S., *The Andropause Mystery: Unraveling the Truths About Male Menopause*, Amred Consulting, 2001 ($11.50).

Too, Lillian, *The Complete Illustrated Guide to Feng Shui*, Element Books, 2002 (£14.99).

Too, *Feng Shui for Wealth*, Konsep Books, 1996 (£2.50).

Walters, Derek, *The Feng Shui Handbook: a Practical Guide to Chinese Geomancy and Environmental Harmony*, Aquarian Press, HarperCollins, 1991.

Weil, Andrew, *8 Weeks to Optimum Health*, Time Warner, 2005 (£7.99).

Whiteaker, Stafford, *The Good Retreat Guide*, Rider & Co., sixth edition, 2004 (£12.99).

Wormwood, Valerie, *The Fragrant Mind*, Bantam, 1991 (£9.99).

Wormwood, *The Fragrant Pharmacy*, Bantam, 1997 (£9.99).

Ziff, Sam and Dr Michael, *Infertility and Birth Defects*, Bio-Probe Inc, Orlando, 1987 ($14.95).

References

General

[1] Cooke, B., and Ernst, E., 'Aromatherapy: a Systematic Review', *British Journal of General Practice*, 2000, 50.

[2] *British Medical Journal*, June 2005.

[3] Vas, A. L.,'Therapeutic Activity of Oral Glucosamine Sulphate in the Management of Osteoarthritis of the Knee in Outpatients', *Current Medical Research and Opinion*, 1982, 3 (3).
  Drovanti A. et al., 'Therapeutic Activity of Oral Glucosamine Sulphate in Osteoarthritis: a Placebo-Controlled, Double-Blind Investigation', *Clinical Therapeutics*, 1980, 4.

[4] *Seminars in Arthritis and Rheumatism*, 2005, 35: 77–94.
  Altman, R., and Gray, R., 'Inflammation in Osteoarthritis', *Clinics in Rheumatic Diseases*, 1985, 11.

[5] *Scandinavian Journal of Rheumatology*, 1983, 12: 85–8.
  British Journal of Rheumatology, 1991, 30: 370–2.
  Leventhal, L. J. et al., 'Treatment of Rheumatoid Arthritis With GLA', *Annals of Internal Medicine*, 1993, 119.

[6] *International Journal of Immunopharmacology*, 2005, 5: 1749–70.

[7] *J. Med. Food*, 2005, 8: 125–32.

[8] Bliddal, H., Rosetsky, A. et al., 'A Randomised Placebo-Controlled Cross-Over Study of Ginger Extract and Ibuprofen in Osteoarthritis', *Osteoarthritis Cartilage*, 2000, 8: 9.

[9] Bingham, R. et al., 'Yucca-Plant Saponin in the Management of Arthritis', *Journal of Applied Nutrition*, 1975, 27.

Fosters, S., and Duke, J. A., *A Field Guide to Medicinal Plants: Eastern and Northern America*, Houghton Mifflin, Boston, 1990.

[10] Gibson, R. G., Gibson, S. L. M. et al., 'Homeopathic Therapy in Rheumatoid Arthritis: Evaluation by Double-Blind Clinical Trial', *British Journal of Clinical Pharmacology*, 1980, 9.

[11] *Annals of the Rheumatic Diseases*, 1997.

[12] Walker, W. R. et al., 'An Investigation Into the Therapeutic Value of the Copper Bracelet: Dermal Assimilation of Copper in Arthritic/Rheumatic Conditions', *Agents Actions*, 1976, 6.

Blake, D. R. et al., 'Copper, Iron, Free Radicals and Arthritis', *British Journal of Rheumatology*, 1985.

Sorensen, J. R. J., 'Copper Boosts Activity of Anti-Inflammatory Drugs', *Progress in Med. Chem.*, 1978, 15.

[13] Harlow, Tim, Greaves, Colin et al., 'Randomised Controlled Trial of Magnetic Bracelets for Relieving Pain in Osteoarthritis of the Hip and Knee', *British Medical Journal*, 28 June 2005.

[14] Hodge, L. et al., 'Increased Consumption of Polyunsaturated Oils May Be the Cause of Increased Prevalence of Childhood Asthma', *Australian and New Zealand Journal of Medicine*, 1994, 24: 727.

Hodge, L. et al., 'Consumption of Oily Fish and Childhood Asthma Risk', *Medical Journal of Australia*, 1996, 164: 137–40.

[15] *Thorax*, 1981, 44: 1.

[16] *Annals of Allergy, Asthma and Immunology*, 1997, 39.

[17] 'Bronchodilator Effects of Caffeine in Coffee: a Dose-Response Study of Asthmatic Subjects', *Chest*, March 1986.

[18] Ledezma, E. et al., 'Efficacy of Ajoene, an Organosulphur Derived From Garlic, in Short-Term Therapy for Tinea Pedis', *Mycoses*, 1996, 39 (9–10): 393–5.

[19] Satchell, A. C. et al., 'Treatment of Inter-Digital Tinea Pedis With 25 Per Cent and 50 Per Cent Tea-Tree-Oil Solution: a Randomised Placebo-Controlled Blinded Study', *Australasian Journal of Dermatology*, 2002, 43 (3): 175–8.

[20] *The Lancet*, 2003, 362.

[21] Collacott, E. A., and Zimmerman, J. T., 'Bipolar Permanent Magnets for the Treatment of Chronic Low-Back Pain', *Journal of the American Medical Association*, 2000, 286: 1322–5.

Brown, C. S., Ling, F. W. et al., 'Efficacy of Static Magnetic Field

Therapy in Chronic Pelvic Pain: a Double-Blind Pilot Study', *American Journal of Obstetrics and Gynaecology*, 2002, 197: 1581–7.

Valbona, Carlos, Hazelwood, Carlton F., and Jurida, Gabor, 'Response of Pain to Static Magnetic Fields in Post-Polio Patients: a Double-Blind Study', *Archives of Physical and Rehabilitation Medicine*, 1997, 78 (11): 1200–3.

[22] Kaplan, B. L. et al., 'Dietary Replacement in Pre-School-Age Hyperactive Boys', *Pediatrics*, 1989, 83.

[23] *Proof*, May 2005.

[24] Bauer, U., 'Six-Month Double-Blind Randomised Controlled Clinical Trial of Ginko Biloba Extract vs Placebo in Two Groups in Patients Suffering From Peripheral Arterial Insufficiency', *Arzeneimittelforschung*, 1984, 34.

[25] *Journal of the American Medical Association*, 267, 1992.

[26] Janatuinen, E. K. et al., 'No Harm From Five-Year Ingestion of Oats in Coeliac Disease', *Gut*, 2002, 50 (3): 323–5.

[27] Bernstein, J. et al., 'Depression of Lymphocyte Transformation Following Oral Glucose Ingestion', *American Journal of Clinical Nutrition*, 1977, 30.

Sanchez, A., 'Role of Sugars in Human Neutrophilic Phagocytosis', *American Journal of Clinical Nutrition*, 1973, 26.

[28] 'Systematic Review: Vitamin C for Respiratory-Tract Infection', *Cochrane Library Database*, 1997.

[29] Barret, B. et al., 'Echinacea for Upper Respiratory Infection', *Journal of Family Practice*, 1999, 48.

Schulten, B. et al., 'Efficacy of Echinacea Purpura in Patients With a Common Cold: a Placebo-Controlled Randomised Double-Blind Clinical Trial', *Arzeneimittelforschung*, 2001, 51.

[30] Scheller et al, 'Biological Properties and Clinical Application of Propolis', *Arzneittelforschung*, 1977, 27: 1395.

[31] *British Homeopathic Journal*, 1970, 59: 42–3.

Ibid., 1971, 60: 97–104.

[32] Rose, J. E., and Behm, F. M., 'Inhalation of Vapour From Black Pepper Extract Reduces Smoking Withdrawal Symptoms', *Drug and Alcohol Dependence*, 1994, 34.

[33] *Behavioral Th.*, 1988, 19.

[34] Avron, J. et al., 'Reduction of Bacteria and Pyuria After Ingestion of Cranberry Juice', *Journal of the American Medical Association*, 1994, 271.

Sobota, A. E., 'Inhibition of Adherence by Cranberry Juice', *Journal of Urology* 1984, 131.

Edwards, B. et al., 'Cranberry Concentrate: UTI prophylaxis', *Journal of Family Practice*, 1997, 45 (2): 185–7.

[35] 'Aromatherapy: a Systematic Review', *British Journal of General Practice*, 50, 493.

[36] Murck et al., *Neuropsyhcopharmacology*, 2004, 7: 1–19.

Su, K. P. et al., 'Omega-3 Fatty Acids in Major Depressive Disorder: a Preliminary Double-Blind Placebo-Controlled Trial', *European Neuropsychopharmacology* 13 (4).

[37] Puri, Dr Basant, *The Natural Way to Beat Depression*, Puri & Boyd, Hodder Mobius, 2004.

[38] Tame, David, *The Secret Power of Music: Transformation of Self and Society Through Musical Energy*, Destiny Books, Vermont, 1984.

[39] *Annals of Behavioral Medicine*, 1997, 19.

[40] Scattner, P., and Randerson, D., 'Tiger Balm as a Treatment of Tension Headaches: a Clinical Trial in General Practice', *Austral. Fam. Psych.*, 1996, 25.

[41] *Neurology*, 28 December 2004.

[42] *What Doctors Don't Tell You*, 16 (10).

[43] Molan, P. C., and Betts, J. A., 'Using Honey as a Wound Dressing: Some Practical Considerations', *Nursing Times*, 2000.

Lusby, P. E. et al., 'Honey: a Potent Agent in Wound Healing?' *Journal of Wound, Ostomy and Continence Nursing*, 2002, 29 (6).

Molan, P. C., 'Reintroducing Honey in the Management of Wounds and Ulcers: Theory and Practice', *Ostomy and Wound Management*, 2002, 48 (11).

Allen, K. L., and Hutchinsoin, G., 'The Potential for Using Honey to Treat Wounds Infected With MRSA and VRE', paper presented at the First World Wound Healing Congress, September 2000, Melbourne, Australia.

[44] 'A Comparative Multi-Centre Study of the Efficacy of Propolis, Acyclovir and Placebo in the Treatment of Genital Herpes', *Phytomedicine*, 2000, 7, 1: 6.

[45] Petrie, K., Dawson, A. G. et al., 'A Double-Blind Trial of Melatonin as a Treatment for Jet Lag in International Cabin Crew', *Biol. Psych.*, 1993, 1: 33.

Suhner, A., Schlagenhauf et al., 'Comparative Study to Determine the Optimum Melatonin Dosage From for the Alleviation of Jet Lag', *Chronobiology International*, 1998, 15: 655–66.

[46] Daan S., and Lewy, A. J., 'Scheduled Exposure to Daylight: a Potential Strategy to Reduce Jet Lag Following Transmeridian Flight', *Psychopharmacol. Bull.*, 1984, 20: 566.

Wever, R. A., 'Light Effects on Human Circadian Rhythms: a Review of Andechs Studies', *Journal of Biological Rhythms*, 1989, 4: 161.

[47] Kumar, Prof. K. and Criglington, A. J., 'Effect of Homeopathic Remedy No-Jet-Lag on Passengers During Long-Haul Flights', unpublished, College of Pharmacy, Western University of Health Sciences, Pomona, California, USA, and Research Department, Miers Laboratories, Wellington, New Zealand.

[48] Hambleton-Jones, Nicky, *10 Years Younger*, Transworld, 2005.

[49] Boublik, J. H., 'Coffee Contains Potent Opiate-Receptor-Binding Activity', *Nature*, 1983, 301.

[50] *Canadian Medical Assocation Journal*, 1976, 15: 217–22.

Folic Acid in Neurology, Psychiatry and Internal Medicine, Botez & Reynolds, Raven Press, New York.

[51] *Journal of the Florida Medical Association*, 1973, 60: 29–31.

[52] *J. Clin. Psych.*, September 1978.

[53] *Acta Med. Scan.*, 1953, 145.

Neurology, 1960, 10: 868–73.

[54] Ebner, F. et al., 'Topical Use of Dexpanthenol in Skin Disorders', *American Journal of Clincial Dermatology*, 2002, 3 (6).

[55] Fink, M., 'Treatment of Herpes Simplex by Alphatocopherol (Vitamin E)', *British Dental Journal*, 1980, 148: 246, letter.

Nead, D. E., 'Effective Vitamin-E Treatment for Ulcerative Herpetic Lesions', *Dent Survey*, 1976, 52 (7).

[56] Wheatley, D., 'Hypericum in Seasonal Affective Disorder (SAD)', *Current Medical Research and Opinion*, 1999, 1 (5): 33–37.

Kasper, S.; 'Treatment of Seasonal Affective Disorder (SAD) With Hypericum Extract', *Pharmacopschiatry*, 1997, 30: 89093.

Martinez, preliminary trials of 20 SAD patients comparing efficacy of broad-spectrum light treatment with hypericum extract, 1994.

[57] Martindale, *The Extra Pharmacoepia*, Pharmaceutical Press, 26th edition, 1972.

'The Effects of Aloe Vera on Cutaneous Erythema and Blood-Flowing Following Ultraviolet B (UVB) Exposure', *Clinical Research*, 1987, 35.

Strickland, F., Pelley, R. P. et al., 'Prevention of Ultra-Violet-Induced Radiation Suppression of Contact and Delayed Hypersensitivity by Aloe Barbadenesis Gel Extract', *Journal of Investigative Dermatology*, 1994.

58 Stahl, W., Heinrich U. et al., 'Dietary Tomato Paste Protects Against UV-Produced Erythema in Humans', *Journal of Nutrition*, 2001, 121: 1149–51.

59 John, T. J. et al., 'Viruses Inhibited by Tea, Caffeine and Tannic Acid', *Indian Journal of Medical Research*, April 1979.

60 Freidman, M. et al., 'Fluoride Concentrations in Tea', *Clinical Preventive Dentistry*, January–February 1984.

61 'American Study on Green Tea and Weight Loss', *American Journal of Clinical Nutrition*, 1999, 70: 1040–5.

62 'Japanese Study on Green Tea and Weight Loss', *American Journal of Clinical Nutrition*, 2005, 81: 122–9.

63 *International Journal of Obesity*, 1997, 21, suppl. 2, S61.

Diabetes and Obesity Metabolism, 2004, 6: 171–80.

J. Nut. S. Vitaminol., Tokyo, 2002, 48: 128–33.

64 *Am. Journal Bariatr. Med.*, 1993, summer 17–19.

65 *What Doctors Don't Tell You*, 16 (10).

66 Colditz, G. A. et al., 'Diet and Lung Cancer: a Review of the Epidemiologic Evidence in Humans', *Arch. Int. Med.*, January 1987.

Menkes, M. S. et al., 'Serum Beta Carotene, Vitamins A and E, Selenium and the Risks of Lung Cancer', *New England Journal of Medicine*, 13 November 1986.

Women

1 Cheek, Dr David, 'Are Telepathy, Clairvoyance and Hearing Possible In Utero? Suggestive Evidence as Revealed in Hypnotic Age-Regression Studies of Prenatal Memory', *International Journal of Pre- and Perinatal Psychology and Medicine*, winter 1992, 7 (2): 125–37.

'Maternal Emotionality During Pregnancy and Reproductive

Outcome: a Review of the Literature', *Int. J. of Behav. Dev.*, 2: 343–76.

[2] Rossi, N. et al., 'Maternal Stress and Fetal Motor Behaviour: a Preliminary Report', *International Journal of Pre- and Perinatal Psychology and Medicine*, 1989, 3 (4): 311–18.

Verny, T., *The Secret Life of the Unborn Child*, Warner Books, 1991: 57–9.

Van den Bergh, B. R. H., 'The Influence of Maternal Emotions During Pregnancy on Fetal and Neonatal Behaviour', *International Journal of Pre- and Perinatal Psychology and Medicine*, winter 1990.

[3] Abraham, M. et al., 'Inhibiting Effect of Jasmine Flowers on Lactation', *Indian Journal of Medical Research*, 1979, 69: 88–92.

Shrivastav, P. et al., 'Suppression of Purpureal Lactation Using Jasmine Flowers (*Jasminum Sambac*)', *Austral. New Zeal. J. Obs. Gyn.*, 1988, 28: 68–71.

[4] *Journal of Nutrition and Environmental Medicine*, 1995, 5: 205–8.

[5] *Journal of the American Medical Association*.

New England Journal of Medicine.

[6] Johnson, R. L. et al., 'Foetal Acoustic Stimulation as an Adjunct to External Cephalic Version', *Journal of Reproductive Medicine*, 1995, 40.

[7] Royal College of Obstetricians and Gynaecologists professional Guidelines for Episiotomy, June 2004.

[8] *British Journal of Obstetrics and Gynaecology*, 1 January 2004.

[9] Barrington, J. W. et al., 'Selenium Deficiency and Miscarriage: a Possible Link?', *British Journal of Obstetrics and Gynaecology*, 1996, 103 (2): 130–2.

[10] George, L. et al., 'Plasma Folate Levels and the Risk of Spontaneous Abortion', *Journal of the American Association*, 2002, 288 (15): 1867–73.

[11] Nelen, W. L. et al., ' Hyperhomocysteinemia and Recurrent Early Pregnancy Loss: a Meta-Analysis', *Fertility and Sterility*, 2000, 74 (6): 1196–9.

Nelen W. L. et al., 'Homocysteine and Folate Levels as Risk Factors for Recurrent Early Pregnancy Loss', *British Journal of Obstetrics and Gynaecology*, 2000, 95 (4): 519–24.

[12] Cnattingius, S. et al., 'Caffeine Intake and the Risk of First-Trimester Spontaneous Abortion', *New England Journal of Medicine*, 2000, 343 (25): 1839–45.

Wisborg, K. et al., 'Maternal Consumption of Coffee During Pregnancy and Stillbirth and Infant Death in First Year of Life: a Prospective Study', *British Medical Journal*, 2002, 22 (326): 420.

13 Li, D. K. et al., 'Exposure to Non-Steroidal Anti-Inflammatory Drugs During Pregnancy and Risk of Miscarriage: Population-Based Cohort Study', *British Medical Journal*, 2003, 327 (7411): 368.

14 'Biochemical Profile of Osteoporotic Patients on Essential Fatty Acid Supplementation', *Nutrition Research*, 15 (3): 325–34.

15 *J. Agric. Food Chem.*, 2005, 5 (53): 191–6.

16 *J. Psychosomatic Res.*, 1993, 37: 127–33.
    Brit. J. Clin. Psych., 1995, 34: 447–60.

17 *Journal of Reproductive Medicine*, 1991, 36: 131–6.

18 *J. Clin. Endocrin. Metab.*, 1987, 64: 1246–50.
    American Journal of Clinical Nutrition, 1989, 49: 1179–83.
    Physiol. Behav., 1987, 40: 483–7.

19 *Am. J. Epid.*, 1999, 149: 550–7.
    'Caffeine Worsens PMS', *American Journal of Public Health*, 1989, 79 (67).
    Ibid., 1990, 80: 1106–10.

20 *J. Women's Health Gender-Based Med.*, 2000, 9: 315–20.
    British Medical Journal, 2001: 134–7.
    Brown, D., 'Herbal Research Review, *Vitex Agnus Castus*: a Clinical Monograph', *A Quartlery Review of Natural Medicine*, German surveys of 1,542 women, summer 1994.

21 *Controlled Clinical Trials*, 1996, 17: 60–8.
    Journal of Reproductive Medicine, 1985, 30: 149–53.
    Rec. Adv. Clin. Nut., 1986, 2: 404–5.

22 *British Journal of Clinical Practice*, 1992, 46: 161–4.

23 *British Journal of Obstetrics and Gynaecology*, 1990, 97: 847–52.
    British Medical Journal, 1999, 318: 1375–81.

24 *American Journal of Clinical Nutrition*, 1981, 34: 2364–6.
    Annals of Clin. Biochem., 1986, 23: 667–70.
    Journal of Women's Health, 1998, 7: 1157–65.

25 *J. Orthomolecular Med.*, 1998, 13: 215–22.

26 *American Journal of Obstetrics and Gynaecology*, 1993, 168.
    Ibid., 1998, 179: 444–52.

27 Anderson, 'Professional Care of Mother and Child', 1994, 4: 13–15.

[28] Vutyananich, T. et al., 'Pyridoxine for Vomiting and Nausea of Pregnancy: a Randomised Double-Blind Placebo-Controlled Trial', *American Journal of Obstetrics and Gynaecology*, 1995, 173.

[29] Vutyananich, T. et al., 'Ginger for Nausea and Vomiting in Pregnancy: a Randomised Double-Blind Placebo-Controlled Trial', *British Journal of Obstetrics and Gynaecology*, 2001.

[30] International Congress on Ethnobiology, 1990.

[31] *Archives of Dermatology*, 1988, 134: 1356–60.

Men

[1] Lassus, A. et al., 'A Comparative Study of a New Food Supplement Viviscal, With Fish Extract, for the Treatment of Hereditary Androgenic Alopecia in Young Males', Department of Dermatological Research, ARS-Medicina, Helsinki, Finland, *Journal of International Medical Research*, 1992, 20: 445–53.

Lassus, A. et al., 'Treatment of Hereditary Androgenic Alopecia in Middle-Aged Males by Combined Oral and Topical Administration of Special Marine Extract-Compound (Viviscal)', Helsinki Research Centre and the Dermatological Clinic, Leverkusen, Germany, *Les Nouvelles Dermatologies*, 1994, 13: 254–55.

[2] *British Journal of Urology*, May 2000.

[3] *Public Health Nutrition*, December 2002.

[4] Masson, M., 'Bromelain in Blunt Injuries of the Locomotor System: a Study of Observed Applications in General Practice', *Fortschritte der Medizin*, 1995, 113: 303–6.

Taussig, S. J., and Batkin S., 'Bromelain: the Enzyme Complex of Pinapple (*Ananas comosus*) and Its Application', *Journal of Ethnopharmacology*, 1998, 22: 191–203.

Uhlig, G., 'The Effect of Proteolytic Enzymes (Traumanase) on Post-Traumatic Edema', *Fortschritte der Medizin*, 1981, 99: 554–6.

[5] International Planned Parenthood Federation.

[6] International Congress on Ethnobiology, 1990.

[7] *Journal of Ethnopharmacology*, 2004.

[8] *Journal of Impotence Research*, 1997, 9, suppl. 1.

Young Children

[1] 'Caffeine Affects Cardiovascular and Endocrine Activation at Work and

Home', *Psychosomatic Medicine*, 2002, 64: 595–603.

2 'Effects of Caffeine on Mood and Performance', *Psychopharmacology*, 2002, 164 (2): 188–92.

3 Asthma Audit by the National Asthma Campaign, 2001.

4 *J. Paed.*, 2002, 1451: 71–5.

5 *Journal of Clinical Psychology*, 1998, 59, suppl. 7.

6 *Paed. Neur.*, 2001, 24: 99–102.

7 *Can. J. Psych.*, 1999, 44: 811–3.

8 *Encephale*, 2000, 26: 45–7.

9 *Journal of the American Academy of Child and Adolescent Psychiatry*, 2000, 39, 517.

10 *The Lancet*, 1985, 7: 540.

11 *Biological Psychiatry*, 2002 (6) :233–9.

Stevens, L. et al., 'Essential Fatty Acid Metabolism in Boys With Attention Deficit Hyperactivity Disorder', *American Journal of Clinical Nutrition*, 1995, 62: 761–8.

Stevens, L. et al., 'Omega-3 Fatty Acids in Boys with Behaviour, Learning and Health Problems', *Physiology and Behaviour*, 1996, 59: 915–20.

12 *Biological Psychiatry*, 1979, 14, 741.

13 *Ann. Acad. Med. Stet.*, 1998, 44: 297–314.

14 'Influence of Fluorescent Lights on Hyperactivity and Learning Disabilities', *Journal of Learning Disabilities*, 1976; 9: 417–22.

'Canadian Study on Children, Stress Levels, Behaviour and Full-Spectrum Light Use', *Int. J. Biosc. Res.*, 1982: 10–38.

Hathaway, W. E., Hargreaves, J. A. et al., 'A Study Into the Effects of Light on Children of Elementary-School Age: a Case of Daylight Robbery', Alberta Education Authority, Edmonton, 1992.

15 *Journal of the American Academy of Child and Adolescent Psychiatry*, 1994, 33: 558–66.

16 Banerjee, S. et al., 'Hypnotherapy in the Treatment of Nocturnal Enuresis: a Comparative Study With Imipramine', *Clinical Pediatrics*, 1975, 14: 273–5.

Olness, K. et al., 'Use of Self-Hypnosis in the Treatment of Child Nocturnal Enuresis: a Report on 40 Patients', *Clinical Pediatrics*, 1975, 14: 273.

Banerjee S. et al., 'Hypnosis as a Treatment for Enuresis', *Journal* of *Child Psychiatry and Psychology*, 1985, 26: 169.

[17] Daoud, A. S. et al., 'Effectiveness of Iron Therapy on Breath-Holding Spells', *Journal of Pediatrics*, 1997, 130: 547–50.

[18] *Ann. Clin. Nut.*, 1973, 26: 1180.

[19] *Paed. Adolesc. Med.*, 158.

[20] Anderson, T. W. et al., 'Vitamin C and the Common Cold: a Double-Blind Trial', *Canadian Medical Association Journal*, 1972, 207.

[21] Kanabar, D., 'Infantile Colic', *Journal of Family Health Care*, 14 (2), suppl. 1, 2004.

    Weizman, Z. et al., 'Efficacy of Herbal-Tea Preparation in Infantile Colic', *Journal of Pediatrics*, 1993, 122: 650–2.

[22] Bouldoukian, Joelle et al., *Opthalmic and Physiological Optics*, January 2002, 22.

    Journal of Research in Reading, February 2001, 24: 41.

[23] O'Hare, A., and Khalid, S., 'Evaluation of Exercise-Based Treatment for Children With Reading Difficulties', *Dyslexia*, 2003, 9 (1): 48–71.

[24] Stevens, L. et al., 'Essential Fatty Acid Metabolism in Boys with Attention Deficit Hyperactivity Disorder', *American Journal of Clinical Nutrition*, 1995 62: 761–8.

    Stevens, L. et al., 'Omega-3 Fatty Acids in Boys With Behaviour, Learning and Health Problems', *Physiology and Behaviour*, 1996, 59: 915–20.

[25] Bradford, Nikki, *Natural Painkillers*, Orion 1999.

[26] *Proof*, 1 (3), digest 26.

[27] *New Generalist*, the magazine for the UK's Royal College of GPs, September 2005.

[28] Carruthers, A., 'Therapeutic Touch: a Force to Promote Bonding and Well-Being', *Professional Nurse*, February 1992.

    Daley, B., 'Therapeutic Touch: Nursing Practice and Contemporary Cutaneous Wound Healing Research', *Journal of Advance Nursing*, 25: 1123–32.

    Olsen et al., 'Stress-Induced Immuno-Suppression and Therapeutic Touch', *Alt. Ther.*, 1997, 3 (2): 68–74.

    Quinn, J. F., 'Transfer of the Relaxation Response', *Journal of Holistic Nursing*, 1988, 6: 1.

    'Therapeutic Touch and Post-Operative Pain: a Rogerian Research Study', *Nursing Science Quarterly*, 6: 2.

[29] Whitelaw, 'Skin-to-Skin Contact for Very Low Birth-Weight Infants and

Mothers: a Randomized Trial of Kangaroo Care', *Archives of Diseases in Childhood*, 1988, 63: 1377–81.

Virgin, C., 'The Kangaroo Method Brings the Child Back to the Mother', *Sygeplejersken*, 1987, 11.

Hosseini, R. B. et al., 'Pre-Term Infants and Fathers: Psychological and Behavioral Effects of Skin-to-Skin Contact', *Ursus Medicus*, 1992, 2: 47–55.

[30] 'Promoting Better Health for Young People Through Physical Activity and Sport', a report for the President from the Secretary for Health and Human Services, 2002.

'Physical Activity and Health', the Surgeon-General of America's report, 1996.

[31] Kirkcaldy, B. D., and Shepard, R. J., 'The Saskatchewan in Motion Project: Relative Benefits of Physical Activity...Amongst Adolescents', *Social Psychology and Epidemiology*, 2002, 37 (11).

[32] Ernst, Prof. Edzard, *The Desktop Guide to Complementary and Alternative Medicine: an Evidence-Based Approach*, University of Exeter, Mosby, 2001:103–6 (summary of EPO trials).

[33] *European Journal of Pediatrics*, 2004, 163: 402–7.

[34] Bradford, Nikki, and Williams, Jean, *What They Don't Tell You About Being a Mother and Having Babies*, HarperCollins, 1997.

[35] *Fluoride*, 1995, 28: 189–92.

Pediatric Dentistry, 2000, 22: 269–77.

Proof, July 2005.

[36] *Journal of Contemporary Dental Practice*, 2002, 3: 27–35.

[37] Focht, D. R. 3rd et al, 'The Efficacy of Duct Tape vs Cryotherapy in the Treatment of Verruca Vulgaris (the Common Wart)', *Arch. Paed. and Adol. Med.*, 2002, 156 (10): 971.

Teenagers

[1] Ernst, E., and Huntley, A., 'Tea-Tree Oil: a Systematic Review of Randomised Clinical Trials', *Koplementarmed Klass Naturjeilkd*, 2000, 7: 17–20.

Bassett, B. et al.,'A Competitive Study of Tea-Tree Oil vs Benzoyleperoxide in the Prevention of Acne', *Medical Journal of Australia*, 1999, 153: 455–8.

[2] *Journal of Alternative and Complementary Medicine*, 2000, 6: 31–5.

[3] Gersch, C. B. et al., 'Influence of Supplementary Vitamins, Minerals and Essential Fatty Acids on the Antisocial Behaviour of Young Adult Prisoners: Randomised Placebo-Controlled Trial', *British Journal of Psychiatry*, 2002, 181: 22–8.

[4] Hippchen, L. J. (ed.), 'The Effects of Light and Radiation on Human Health and Behavior', *Biochemical Approaches to Treatment of Delinquents and Criminals*, Van Nostrand Reinhold, New York, 1978: 105–15.

'The Role of Electromagnetic Energy in Human Health and Behavior', *J. Energy Med.*, 1980; 1: 110–13.

'School Lighting', *Churchill Forum*, 1980, 2: 3.

S. J. Optom., 1979, 21: 8–14.

[5] Mayron, L. W., Mayron, E. L., and Nations, R., 'Light, Radiation and Academic Achievement: Second-Year Data', *Academic Therapy*, 1976; 4: 397–407.

[6] 'Canadian Study on Children, Stress Levels, Behaviour and Full-Spectrum Light Use', *Int. J. Biosc. Res.*, 1982: 10–38.

Hathaway, Hargreaves et al., 'A Study Into the Effects of Light on Children of Elementary-School Age'.

[7] *US Diagnostic and Statistical Manual of Mental Disorders*.

[8] *The Lancet*, 1985: 1041–2.

Journal of Clinical Psychiatry, 1898, 50: 456–9.

Journal of the American College of Nutrition, 1992, 11: 694–700.

[9] *Townsend Letter for Doctors and Patients*, November 1993, 1154.

Saffi-Kutti, S., 'Oral Zinc Supplementation in Anorexia Nervosa', *Acta Psychiatrica Scandinavia*, 1990, 361: 14–17.

'Controlled Trial of Zinc Supplementation in Anorexia Nervosa', *International Journal of Eating Disorders*, 1994, 15: 251–5.

[10] *Arch. Gen. Psychiatric*, 1991 48: 556–62.

[11] Dalvitt-McPhillips, S., 'A Dietary Approach to Bulimia', *Physiology and Behaviour*, 1984, 33: 769075.

[12] 'L-Tryptophan as an Adjunct to Treatment of Bulimia Nervosa', *The Lancet*, 1989, 2: 1162–3.

[13] Bouldoukian, Joelle et al., *Opthalmic and Physiological Optics*, January 2002, 22.

Journal of Research in Reading, February 2001, 24: 41.

[14] Onishenko, *Rossiskya Gazetta*, 1 February 2005.

[15] *Journal of Advanced Nursing*, 2004, 48: 380–7.
[16] Dunn, C. et al., 'Sensing an Improvement: an Experimental Study to Evaluate the Use of Aromatherapy Massage and Periods of Rest in an Intensive-Care Unit', *Journal of Advanced Nursing*, 1995, 21: 31–40.
[17] *New Scientist*, 28 May 2005.
[18] Childline survey, May 2004.

Pets
[1] *British Medical Journal*, 2000.
[2] Cats Protection survey, 2003.
[3] Cats Protection survey, 2004.
[4] *Mutat. Res.*, 2003, 539: 195–201.

Houses and Gardens
[1] Roney-Dougal, S. M., and Solfrin, J., 'Field Study on an Enhancement Effect on Lettuce Seedlings', presented at the 45th Annual Convention of the Parapsychological Association, Paris, 2002.
[2] *Journal of the American Medical Association*, 1992, 268: 625–9.
[3] *The Lancet*, 1993, 342: 1295–6.
[4] Adams, Zoe, *The Colloidal Silver Report*, Another Country Verlag, Berlin.

Work and Office
[1] Loehr, Franklin, *The Power of Prayer on Plants*, Doubleday, New York, 1959, detailing 700 experiments using over 27,000 seedlings and seeds (with photos) at Loehr's Los Angeles Foundation. Out of print, but a must for anyone wanting to research this area.
Secrets of the Soil, Tompkins & Bird, Harper & Row, New York, 1989; Viking, 1991.
[2] Tame, David, 'Brandenburg Concerto Enhancing Growth', *The Secret Power of Music*, Destiny Books, 1984.
[3] *International Journal of Sport, Nutrition and Exercise Metabolism*, 2004, 14: 208–307.

Notes
[1] *New Scientist*, May 2005.
[2] Karatz, May Annexton, 'William Horatio Bates MD and the Bates Method of Eye Exercises', *New York State Journal of Medicine*, 75 (7).

Index